Healing through Trigger Point Therapy

Healing through Trigger Point Therapy

A Guide to Fibromyalgia, Myofascial Pain and Dysfunction

Devin J. Starlanyl & John Sharkey

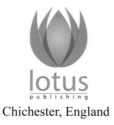

lotus
publishing

Chichester, England

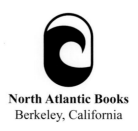

North Atlantic Books
Berkeley, California

First published in 2013 by
Lotus Publishing
Apple Tree Cottage, Inlands Road, Nutbourne, Chichester, PO18 8RJ and
North Atlantic Books
P.O. Box 12327
Berkeley, California 94712

Illustrations Amanda Williams
Text Design Wendy Craig
Cover Design Paula Morrison
Printed and Bound in India by Replika Press Pvt. Ltd.

Acknowledgements
Healing through Trigger Point Therapy: A Guide to Fibromyalgia, Myofascial Pain and Dysfunction is sponsored by the Society for the Study of Native Arts and Sciences, a nonprofit educational corporation whose goals are to develop an educational and cross-cultural perspective linking various scientific, social, and artistic fields; to nurture a holistic view of arts, sciences, humanities, and healing; and to publish and distribute literature on the relationship of mind, body, and nature.

British Library Cataloguing-in-Publication Data
A CIP record for this book is available from the British Library
ISBN 978 1 905367 39 9 (Lotus Publishing)
ISBN 978 1 58394 609 1 (North Atlantic Books)

Library of Congress Cataloguing-in-Publication Data
Starlanyl, Devin.
  Healing through trigger point therapy : a guide to fibromyalgia, myofascial pain and dysfunction / Devin J. Starlanyl and John Sharkey.
    p. ; cm.
  Includes bibliographical references and index.
  Summary: "This guide to trigger points is a comprehensive resource for the diagnostics, care, treatment, and prevention of symptoms related to fibromyalgia, myofascial pain, and other commonly misdiagnosed chronic pain conditions"—Provided by publisher.
  ISBN 978-1-58394-609-1
  I. Sharkey, John, MSc. II. Title.
  [DNLM: 1. Fibromyalgia—therapy. 2. Chronic Pain—therapy. 3. Musculoskeletal Manipulations—methods. 4. Myofascial Pain Syndromes—therapy. 5. Trigger Points—physiology. WE 544]

  616.7'42—dc23
                      2012043017

> *This book is dedicated to pain patients and to the care providers and researchers who seek to understand and relieve their pain.*
> *God bless them all.*
> Devin J. Starlanyl
>
> *To my wife Fidelma, daughters Xsara and Katie.*
> *You bring love, laughter, and joy to my life.*
> John Sharkey

Contents

Foreword

It is my pleasure to write the foreword for the first edition of this work, *Healing through Trigger Point Therapy: A Guide to Fibromyalgia, Myofascial Pain and Dysfunction*, by Devin J. Starlanyl and John Sharkey. This excellent textbook, targeted at patients with musculoskeletal pain, is highly relevant and helpful in these times when chronic pain is one of the epidemics of modern society.

Using a nomenclature that is clear and accessible to patients, the book provides information about myofascial pain and fibromyalgia syndrome. The authors have combined both clinical and scientific experience in order to analyze, integrate, and present useful and clear information and guidelines relevant to their own patients.

The last decade has witnessed increasing interest and advances in the aetiology and diagnosis of trigger points (TrPs). In fact, the referred pain elicited by active TrPs has been associated with several chronic pain syndromes, such as mechanical neck pain, whiplash-associated neck pain, carpal tunnel syndrome, shoulder pain, lateral epicondylalgia, knee pain, low back pain, headaches, and migraine, as well as fibromyalgia syndrome. This book is therefore highly relevant, since it will help patients to gain a better understanding of their symptoms.

The book is divided into three sections. The first covers basic data pertaining to TrPs, muscle pain, fascia, and fibromyalgia, and explains how these conditions can be interconnected. It is interesting to note that the authors have included a chapter about kinetic chains and how the different muscles act in combination with others during a functional task. The second section—the heftiest one in the book—covers the clinical relevance of TrPs in each muscle and how they can affect many activities of daily life. The authors have put a lot of effort into the content by dealing with a wide range of muscles, and the information included for each one is excellent. Finally, the third section suggests future directions for improving our knowledge in the management of TrPs and chronic pain.

The authors, editors, illustrators, and publisher involved in the production of this volume can be justifiably proud of the final product. I hope that patients and readers of the book will find that the important and helpful information which it contains will come in useful in managing pain and improving their own knowledge about the particular syndrome that they may be suffering from.

César Fernández-de-las-Peñas PT, DO, MSc, PhD, DMSc

Department of Physiotherapy, Occupational Therapy, Rehabilitation, and Physical Medicine

Rey Juan Carlos University, Madrid, Spain

and

Center for Sensory-Motor Interaction, Department of Health Science and Technology

Aalborg University, Aalborg, Denmark

Acknowledgments

Thanks go to our publisher contact at Lotus Publishing, Jon Hutchings, who had the foresight to believe in the importance of our work; to our editor, Stephen D. Brierley, who turned our manuscript into a book. Any mistakes in this book occurred after it left his capable hands; to our illustrator, Amanda Williams, who brought our figures to life; to our designer, Wendy Craig; to Cesar Fernandez-de-las-Penas, who has kindly written the foreword and provided great research; and to our mentors, David Simons of blessed memory and Leon Chaitow.

We also thank all those who contributed to this book—especially Rodney Anderson, Ragi Doggweiler, James Earls, Nye Ffarrabas, Lawrence Funt, Yun Hsing Ho, Chris Jarmey, John Jarrell, Justine Jeffrey, Alena Kobesova, Rhonda Kotarinos, Tamara Liller, Thomas Myers, Simeon Niel-Asher, Carol Shifflett, Roland Staud, and David Wise—and the many others who have made this book possible.

Abbreviations

ACh: acetylcholine

ACS: anterior compartment syndrome

ALL: anterior longitudinal ligament

ATP: adenosine triphosphate; basic energy carrier and main cellular energy supplier

AUTOPAP: CPAP with pressure that automatically adjusts as needed

CHD: coronary heart disease

CHF: congestive heart failure

CI: chemical intolerance

CLBP: chronic low back pain

CMP: chronic myofascial pain

CNS: central nervous system

COPD: chronic obstructive pulmonary disease

CPAP: continuous positive airway pressure; machine that provides same

CTS: carpal tunnel syndrome

FM: fibromyalgia

FSM: frequency specific microcurrent

GERD: gastroesophageal reflux

HPA-axis: hypothalamus-pituitary-adrenal axis

IBS: irritable bowel syndrome

IC: interstitial cystitis

IP: interphalangeal

ITB: iliotibial band

LTR: local twitch response

MRI: magnetic resonance imagery

MTrPs: myofascial trigger points

OA: osteoarthritis

OSA: obstructive sleep apnea

OTC: over-the-counter (medications)

PCP: primary care provider

QL: quadratus lumborum

ROM: range of motion

SCM: sternocleidomastoid muscle

STR: soft tissue release

T3: triiodothyronine, the active form of thyroid hormone

T4: inactive form of thyroid hormone

TFL: tensor fasciae latae

TMJ: temporomandibular (jaw) joint

TMJD: temporomandibular joint dysfunction

TOS: thoracic outlet syndrome

TrP: trigger point

TSH: thyroid-stimulating hormone

TSSP: temporal summation of second pain

URI: upper respiratory infection

I

WHAT YOU NEED TO KNOW

Part I contains the latest on what we know about myofascia, how trigger points (TrPs) form, the TrP/fibromyalgia (FM) connection, and what happens when TrPs become chronic. It explains how TrPs interact with each other, and with other conditions. You'll discover how TrPs can cause and/or maintain FM, and why the ability to control TrPs directly affects the control of FM symptoms. Kinetic chains are included here, as is a list of some TrP non-pain symptoms that may surprise you and give you a sense of hope. The key to controlling many symptoms rests with the control of TrPs, and the key to controlling TrPs is identifying and controlling perpetuating factors. This information is contained in this segment as well.

This part is packed with information you will need in order to understand Parts II and III, so strap on your seat belt and let's begin.

1 General Overview

What This Book Is

Healing through Trigger Point Therapy: A Guide to Fibromyalgia, Myofascial Pain and Dysfunction is written primarily for patients with chronic pain and those with other previously unexplained symptoms associated with fibromyalgia (FM), trigger points (TrPs), and chronic myofascial pain (CMP), and for their care providers of *all* varieties. It is designed to facilitate communication among them, and to be used as a tool for FM, TrP and CMP diagnostics, care, treatment, and prevention. TrPs are one of the main factors generating and perpetuating FM pain and other symptoms, no matter what initiated the FM. The FM amplifies the pain and other symptoms. TrPs can cause acute or chronic pain, as well as a surprising diversity of seemingly unrelated symptoms that are often mistakenly linked to FM. The TrPs can mimic many conditions, causing diagnostic confusion. TrPs tend to refer pain in specific referral patterns. This book can help match symptoms to the TrPs generating those symptoms, and will provide the knowledge you need to bring those symptoms under control. It is also a tool that you can use to help explain those symptoms to others. TrPs can cause such diverse symptoms as impotence, loss of voice, pelvic pain, muscle weakness, cardiac arrhythmia, menstrual pain, irritable bowel syndrome (IBS), clumsiness, toothaches, shortness of breath, headaches (even migraines), and incontinence. The good news is that TrPs can be treated, and they can be prevented. Control of TrPs results in control of CMP and FM, and can help with control of coexisting conditions by minimizing symptom burden.

Everyone needs to be familiar with TrPs. They cause symptoms that mimic conditions seen by general practitioners and every type of specialist. Every medical care professional has seen patients with TrPs, although TrPs are often unrecognized as the symptom cause. TrPs can cause a number of altered sensations, including numbness, itching, dizziness, burning, prickling, heat, or cold. The older population needs to know about TrPs, because they are treatable causes of range of motion (ROM) loss, muscle weakness, pain, and other symptoms often blamed on "old age." Osteoarthritis (OA) may be minimized if related TrPs are promptly treated. Prompt control of TrPs can prevent FM from developing, and minimize its impact once it has. Those involved with children need to know too, because "growing pains" are due to TrPs. Athletes need to know this material, because TrPs are one of the most common sources of musculoskeletal pain. Physical therapists need to know, since strengthening exercises worsen the muscle weakness caused by TrPs. Insurance agencies need to know, because prompt diagnosis and treatment may avoid surgery and other major expenses later. Chronic pain patients need to know, because most chronic pain conditions have a treatable TrP component, and treating TrPs can substantially relieve the symptom burden. For example, pain and ROM in an otherwise well-treated case of arthritis may be significantly improved by treating the TrP component.

This book will enable the medical care team to treat more efficiently, and will teach patients what they need to help regain function and gain some control over symptoms. TrPs may seem complicated, and for the most part they are, but they are also very treatable. This book will show you where and how to look for the TrPs for each symptom. You will learn what can perpetuate each TrP. Both patients and care providers will learn how to treat and prevent them.

This book offers empowerment and hope to patients, and direction to care providers. FM and TrP symptoms are real. Although we don't currently have all the answers, a great deal is known, but the practical applications of the latest research are not often in use. This book will help bridge that gap. We believe that there's already too much pain involved in FM and TrPs, and have attempted to make this book as understandable and pleasant to use as possible.

What This Book Is Not

Healing through Trigger Point Therapy: A Guide to Fibromyalgia, Myofascial Pain and Dysfunction is not a substitute for an education in FM, TrP and CMP medicine. Patients with these conditions need a GREAT medical team. This book will help patients find such a team and help care providers to become part of one. In the best of all possible worlds, every health care team and every patient would be one that considers and understands chronic pain management, including TrPs. This world does not exist yet, but this book is part of the effort to transform medical care into a more efficient, user-friendly experience.

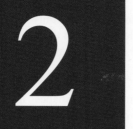

2 Muscles: Your Moving Machine

If you are reading this book, you probably have pain or know somebody who does. You may be a care provider. Unlike other systems of the body, the fascia and muscles have been orphans. Although myofascial texts have been published and documented, and many myofascial research papers are available in the medical literature, tight and rigid minds are more difficult to change than tight and rigid muscles. TrPs are not "controversial"; that term implies scientific evidence on both sides. As you will see, TrPs have been imaged by the National Institutes of Health and the Mayo Clinic. They are very real. Understanding TrPs requires a paradigm shift—it's a different way of looking at something that's been here all along. Myofascial pain is not a "belief system"; it is a medical and scientific reality. As you will later find out, fibromyalgia pain is largely maintained and may be initiated by TrPs. The ability to control TrPs is the ability to control FM. Even many symptoms blamed on "old age" may be at least partially due to TrPs, and those TrPs can be treated. So where and how does TrP pain originate?

Fascia: The Force That Connects

Bones don't hold together by themselves, nor do muscles. You're held together and given shape by connective tissue. Blood vessels, lymph, nerves, and other structures are supported by and meander through fascia (pronounced fass-e-ah or fash-ah). Fascia is connective tissue that forms a three-dimensional network in your body. It's an internal web, providing both structure and a medium through which your body repairs tissue, fights infections, and works its metabolic miracles. The words "fascial" and "facial" look similar, but they're not the same. Your face has fascia, but so does the rest of your body. In the universe of the body, fascia is the force that connects.

When fascia gets stuck to other tissue, your muscles may feel as if they've been tied in knots. In a way, they have. Unraveling stuck, unhealthy fascia is a key to relieving many forms of chronic pain and dysfunction.

Fascia comes in many varieties. Fascia covers the organs and helps support them. The dural tube is a long bag of specialized fascia that contains your spinal cord and the fluid that lubricates it. Specialized fascia forms the linings in your chest and abdominal area, and the bag surrounding your heart. Fascia forms scar tissue and adhesions. Myofascia is fascia surrounding and permeating skeletal muscle. At the molecular level, myofascia has an organic crystalline component that can generate and conduct electrical fields. This piezoelectric (pie-ee-zoh-...) ability is greatly affected by how well your tissues are hydrated. Hydration is dependent not only on adequate water intake, but also on other variables such as the health of your cellular membranes, of your fluid transport system, and of your myofascia itself.

There is important material in myofascia called ground substance. In young, healthy people, ground substance is like soft gelatin, absorbing the traumas of life. Life creates changes, and ground substance reflects those changes. Biochemical and mechanical traumas transform the texture of the ground substance: what was soft and flexible becomes thick and gluey, tightening the myofascia. Your muscles and your cells are wearing a three-dimensional wetsuit that is several sizes too small. It becomes more difficult for nutrients and other biochemicals to move through the myofascial network, and harder for wastes to be removed. The tightening of ground substance is a reversible process, but does not happen on its own.

Muscles: The Inside Story

Anatomical terms are explained in this book because they are specific and useful. Medical appointments can be more efficient when patients arrive, book in hand, saying "I have a typical gluteus minimus pain pattern, just like on this page," rather than a vague "my hip and leg ache." Patients will find it worthwhile to become comfortable with words that describe conditions and anatomical parts. You already use words derived from Greek and Latin every day. For example, the word "muscle" is from Latin for "little mouse," because the biceps brachii muscle looks like a little mouse when it contracts your upper arm. To understand TrPs, you need to know how muscles function in order to learn how they become dysfunctional. Then you can start helping them to heal. We'll start with the muscle types that most of us understand, or think we do:

1. **Skeletal muscle**, the muscle type we will mainly focus on in this book, is under the voluntary control of your nervous system. To move skeletal muscle, your brain—director of the central nervous system (CNS)—communicates with the nerves in the outer areas of your body (peripheral nerves). Once you learn a movement, each time you perform it you will recruit muscles needed to complete the action in the same sequence every time. If you have learned a movement incorrectly the first time, you will perform that movement wrong every time. This can be corrected, but the process requires a lot of patience, commitment, and willpower. The correct movement sequence must be performed many times before it becomes natural. TrPs affect muscle recruitment order.

2. **Cardiac muscle** is heart muscle: it works without being told to do so, which is a very good thing for us! It is therefore involuntary muscle.

3. **Smooth muscle** is also involuntary muscle; it moves things too. This muscle is found in the blood vessels, gut, and stomach, and helps to move blood, digested food, and gases.

Skeletal muscle comes in different shapes. It's formed of muscle fibers and the direction of those fibers helps fingers identify the muscle and the kind of work it does. Each skeletal muscle is infiltrated by myofascia. There's really only one continuous muscle in your entire body; it's just squeezed into 657 individually wrapped fascial envelopes. The belly (or gaster) of the muscle is the central part. Where the muscle fibers end, the sticky myofascia forms ropes called tendons, that attach the muscles to wherever they belong. Tendons have a limited blood supply, so they look pale compared to muscles, and they heal much more slowly.

Tendons link muscles to the lining of the bone by becoming periosteum. The periosteum is the fascia of the skeletal system. It covers all of the bone except for the joint cartilage. Tendons come in assorted sizes and shapes, with a great deal of variation, just as muscles do. Some tendons are big flat sheets that can cover large expanses of your body. These are called aponeuroses, and if there is only one of them, it's an aponeurosis. Tendons can be either thick or thin. There are also areas where the muscle bag blends right in with the tendon. Those tendons are called raphe, from the Greek, meaning a "seam." You can see these tendon types in the figure opposite. Ligaments also come in sheets or bands, and they connect bones to other bones. These are only some of the types of connective tissue in the body. Your body is an ecosystem of its own. Everything is connected to everything else.

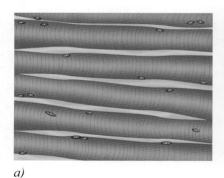
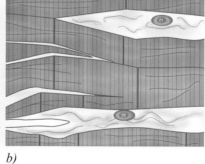
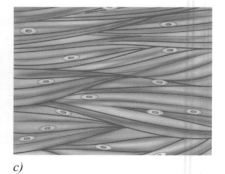

a)   b)   c)

Muscle shapes: a) skeletal muscle, b) cardiac muscle, c) smooth muscle.

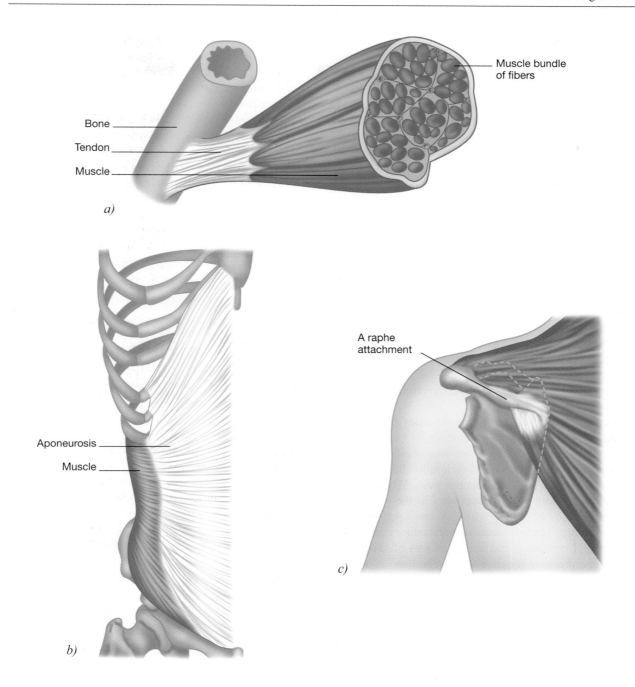

Muscle bundle
of fibers

Bone

Tendon

Muscle

a)

Aponeurosis

Muscle

b)

A raphe
attachment

c)

Muscle attachments by: a) tendon, b) aponeurosis, c) raphe.

Do muscles control movement? The answer is no. Muscles *facilitate* movement. The nervous system orchestrates movement: we cannot have quality movement without first having appropriate information. Special units located throughout the entire body, called "proprioceptors," send this vital information to where it is needed. Proprioceptors tell you where parts of your body are in both time and space, and without this information you'd be forever bumping into things. (When they are dysfunctional from TrPs, you do bump into things.) There are specialized units in your joints, your fasciae, your muscles, and so on, all providing valuable feedback. In response, your nervous system recruits muscles in the most appropriate fashion, creating a tension or force which, in turn, "pulls" on the fascia, resulting in coordinated movement. Amazing! Close your eyes and touch something. Without seeing, you can tell simply by touch if it is wet, moist, soaking, hot, cold, tepid, roasting, cool, freezing, rough, smooth, uneven, metallic—and the list goes on. Wow! If you touched something and it burned your fingers, that information would result in you immediately withdrawing your fingers from the burning surface. This is an example of how the nervous system controls movement.

A muscle doesn't function alone. Muscles function in synergies. A synergy is the interaction of two or more cooperating groups or forces so that their combined effect is greater than the sum of their individual abilities. Muscles can only pull; they cannot push. When one or more muscles lengthen, the opposites of these muscles shorten. These synergies work in conjunction with other systems. Tendons and ligaments move as well, supporting, protecting, and acting as part of the team. Motor coordination requires the integration of a vast number of communications. Messages are continuously traveling throughout the body and mind, allowing the simple acts that we take for granted, such as standing up, walking, and sitting down. These actions require not only the health of the individual components of the systems, but also the coordination of communication among the systems. The brain must be able to talk to the muscles. The sensory receptors in the muscles must be able to integrate those messages with other sensory input, and then provide feedback to the brain. Muscles have sensory units called muscle spindles that are a key component in this feedback system. Muscle spindles respond to muscle lengthening, sending information including how fast the muscle is lengthening and if the muscle is being held in the lengthened position. TrPs can disrupt this system of synergic action by affecting proprioception.

Muscle cells are long cylindrical fibers wrapped in myofascia. The space between the fibers is the critical fiber distance, and when muscles are injured or dehydrated, that distance is not maintained. This creates opportunities for fibers to stick together. Muscle fibers are formed into bundles called fascicles, also wrapped in myofascia. The long cylindrical muscle cells contain mitochondria, the body's energy factories. Muscle fibers contain contractile units called sarcomeres, which are important in the formation of myofascial TrPs. Pain stimuli from the local areas directly affect the CNS, which is composed of the brain and spinal cord. When the CNS becomes overloaded with pain stimuli from peripheral areas, a state of central sensitization, called FM, can result.

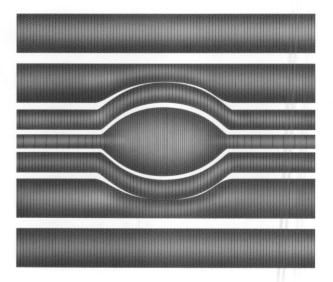

Relationship of trigger point, sarcomeres, and taut band.

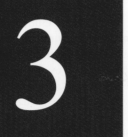

3 Trigger Points: Cause and Effect

Fibromyalgia patients must understand this section, because your pain is directly maintained by peripheral stimuli from pain generators such as TrPs and arthritis. You need to control the peripheral pain generators before you can gain control of the pain amplifier, FM. Nearly everyone has TrPs at one time or another. Have you ever heard stories such as: "I broke an ankle when I was small, and it's been weak ever since"? The bones have healed, so why is the ankle still weak? Most commonly, TrPs were activated at the time of the break or during immobilization after, and the soft tissue damage was never adequately treated. After the TrP treatment, the ankle will no longer be weak. We have successfully treated people who have had such symptoms for decades. Many of these patients had been told they had to "live with" these symptoms. The patients were grateful to receive healing, but some got angry later, grieving for their lost years. Consider the man impotent for 30 years, or the woman with IBS for 25 years. They looked at TrP patterns and recognized themselves. When they learned how long TrP texts had been available, they wondered why former care providers didn't recognize the TrPs causing their symptoms. The universe has many mysteries. This lack of training is one; TrPs are not. Knowledge is power, and this book is about empowerment for patients and care providers alike.

Getting to the (Trigger) Point

Myofascial TrPs are hyperirritable localized spots in taut bands within those muscle sarcomeres you met in the last chapter. You may not always be able to feel those ropy bands, but they're there. Placing the muscle in a lengthened position exaggerates the bands and helps you locate them. Contraction knots—the lumps in the bands—can be small or large, depending on a number of variables, such as how many TrPs make up the contraction knots, the tissue consistencies, and the amount of fluid infiltration involved. When a muscle is burdened with one or more TrPs, it hurts to stretch that muscle out. There is pain at the end of the range of motion (ROM), so you avoid extending the muscle. This is not a sign of mental illness and "pain avoidance behavior": it's logical to avoid doing things that hurt. Some psychologists have trouble with this concept.

TrPs in each muscle cause a recognizable pain and/or dysfunction in a characteristic referral pattern. Sometimes those patterns are in the area of the TrP, but they may cover several muscles. The patterns may not even include the muscle that holds the TrP, because TrPs can *refer* pain elsewhere and can also alter sensations. Imagine having a constant itch you cannot find, or hearing a noise that won't go away—until you find and treat the TrPs causing it. Referred pain is something you already know. Angina and heart attack can refer pain down the arm. (So can TrPs. They can mimic heart attack and other conditions very well, keeping Emergency Department staff busy and frustrated unless they know TrPs.) An irritated gall bladder can refer pain to the top of the right shoulder, abdomen, and upper back. In the body, everything is connected.

The pain patterns in this book do not have "X" to "mark the spot" of the TrP, as in many other books. TrPs can occur *anywhere* in *any* muscle, although they often occur in the muscle belly or where the muscle attaches to other tissue. They can also occur in any *layer* of any muscle, and each muscle layer can have multiple TrPs. You need to know anatomy to find them all. TrPs can also occur in other tissues, including scars, ligaments, tendons, skin, joint capsules, and periosteum, but myofascial TrPs have the most commonly recognizable referral patterns. Fortunately, these patterns have been mapped out, and we have a whole picture gallery of them in this book, and we include anatomical drawings so you can find their source.

Fascia contains protein that contracts it (Schleip et al. 2005). In low back fascia, there can be a thousand times more contractile protein than in surrounding muscles. Myofascia may form contractures slowly, a few sarcomeres at a time, even over the course of years, causing worsening stiffness as we age. Sometimes TrPs twitch. Patients might be able to feel or see that happening, as the muscle seems to jump visibly. Every time a TrP twitches, over 30 irritating biochemicals are released into your body (Shah and Gilliams 2008). These twitches can occur whenever you get successful treatment, and can be visible to the care provider. These biochemicals include nerve toxins, and acidify the surrounding area. When many TrPs twitch, or a few TrPs twitch a lot, patients can feel extremely toxic, with exhaustion, nausea, fatigue, and/or extra achiness. It takes time for these toxins to be processed and eliminated, so they need to be patient patients. Better the toxins are on their way out, rather than being stored within the tissues.

TrPs shorten muscles. Muscle fibers can contract without any input from the nervous system, without adenosine triphosphate (ATP)—the body's main energy biochemical—and even without additional energy. The muscle is in physiological contracture—a tightened state that is different from contraction. A *contracted* muscle is shortened because it has been told by the nerves to tighten. A *contractured* muscle is shortened because the sarcomeres are shortened, without any message from the nerves. This is *physiological. You can't relax a physiologically contractured muscle without outside intervention.* Tissues close to the TrPs develop a serious energy deficit. Because of increased tissue tension, which can itself cause pain, they get less oxygen. This worsens the energy crisis around the TrP, and adds to fatigue.

TrPs can cause dysfunctions of the autonomic nervous system, including itching, burning, redness, goosebumps, or other sensations, often in the typical referred pattern. TrPs can also cause proprioceptor dysfunction. Proprioceptors are sensory units that tell your body parts where they are in relation to the world around them. This includes the positions of other body parts. If your teeth don't know where your cheek or tongue is, they can chomp down on part of *you* rather than on that sandwich you are eating. Your legs don't lift your feet quite high enough when you walk, and you stumble over them. You are forever stubbing your toes or walking into doorjambs.

If this happens, it doesn't mean you're clumsy. You are simply proprioceptively impaired. Not only do some TrPs cause all of the above, but also their little (figurative) myofascial fingers wrap around nerves, blood vessels, lymph vessels, and maybe even ducts. So you can have nerve entrapment, which can feel like you are being hit with jolts of lightning, zapped by tongues of fire, or impaled on a sword of pain. You can experience swelling of the hands and feet if TrPs are entrapping blood vessels in your neck. Your breast may be lumpy from TrP duct entrapment. These localized symptoms are not caused by FM. Diagnosing TrPs is a challenge because they don't show on common tests, and for a long time much of the medical world dismissed them. In 2008, the Mayo Clinic announced it had photographed the taut bands of TrPs (Chen et al 2008). The National Institutes of Health did a study on TrPs using this type of equipment, and verified that TrPs are real (Sikdar et al. 2008). They noted that "as many as 85–93% of chronic pain patients" in pain clinics have TrPs, and "almost 10% of the population of the USA" have them.

The figure here shows the chain reaction of the Integrated TrP Hypothesis as we know it today; it creates and perpetuates TrPs. At first, the flattened end of a local motor nerve, called the motor endplate, is stressed. The motor endplate responds to this stress by releasing excess calcium. The excess calcium prompts the release of excess amounts of the neurotransmitter acetylcholine (ACh). The area becomes more acidic, which inhibits the biochemical that breaks down ACh. These biochemical releases result in tissue tightness, and that tightness restricts the blood supply. This makes it difficult for nutrients and oxygen to get to the muscles and for the

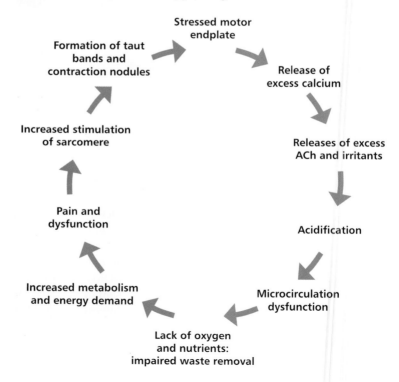

Cycle of misery: trigger point formation hypothesis as we know it today. These individual links in the chain do not always occur in this order.

waste materials of muscle metabolism to be transported away, resulting in a state of energy crisis. The tissues in the area of the motor endplate are starving for oxygen and food, and burdened with excess waste.

The deforming of the sarcomeres creates the characteristic TrP contraction knot. Those knots are the lumps you can feel—or learn to feel—in your muscles. The sarcomeres on either side of the contraction knot lengthen, creating the taut band. Within the dysfunctional endplate area, there is a situation of increased energy demand and lower energy supply that is self-perpetuating. Muscles with TrPs begin the day tired (so do their owners) and become more fatigued more easily and quickly than healthy muscles. These muscles are *physiologically* weak. Repetitious strengthening exercises, like those often found in "work-hardening" clinics, don't help TrPs. These muscles are crying out for more energy, and they are given more work instead, so the energy crisis gets worse. And it can all be amplified by FM.

Active and Latent TrPs

Trigger points can occur directly from an initiating factor (such as repetitive motions) or secondary to another condition, such as arthritis or anything that can induce the energy crisis. They can even result from faulty muscle recruitment patterns. When a person performs an action—any action—many muscles contract to provide the tension and stiffness required to carry out the task without stressing joints. All the muscles don't contract at the same time, but in a specific sequence or order. When "good muscles go wrong," some muscles contract "too early" and others contract "too late," with some muscle fibers not contracting at all! This state is called "dysfunctional muscle inhibition." If the TrPs recur in spite of adequate treatment, look for the *perpetuating factor(s)*. These are mechanical and metabolic factors that keep the TrP(s) active and produce symptoms. The key to controlling TrPs is control of perpetuating factors. TrPs are activated by acute or chronic overload. Your introduction to TrPs may come from a sports injury, inappropriate physical activity, surgery, a fall, an unexpected movement, an auto accident, or a repetitive trauma. Even with acute onset TrPs, there may be delay in TrP formation. Active TrPs can hurt all the time, even at rest. The tendency is to back away from a roaring lion. You restrict your muscle movement and the pain may go away. The TrP does not; it has become latent.

Latent TrPs are like land mines waiting silently under the soil, ready to activate at any provocation. Latent TrPs don't cause spontaneous pain, but they still cause dysfunction: the muscles are still shortened, tight, weak, and in an energy crisis. Younger people tend to have more active, painful TrPs; older people have more latent TrPs, with restricted ROM and muscle weakness, because, in general, they move less. They have decreased their range of motion, because it hurts when they stretch TrP-laden muscles. Then along comes an infection, a fall, or other stressor. *Wham!* Those latent TrPs activate, and there is an unexpected pain overload. This may also occur in sedentary people. Often, one event initiates a TrP and another maintains it. For example, a head cold can cause many symptoms, including headache, stuffy sinuses, and a runny nose. It may also activate TrPs that cause the same symptoms. The TrPs and their symptoms may remain long after the cold is gone. TrPs are dynamic in nature. During the activation process of a TrP, or while it is in the process of becoming latent, spontaneous pain (occurring without outside pressure) may be present in the area of a TrP, without the typical referral pattern. Even with pressure, when the TrP is in this stage, the pain may only be local. For example, a temporalis TrP may cause pain that is restricted to the immediate area around the TrP, without characteristic referral to a tooth, the eyebrow area, or extended areas of the head. These transitional TrPs may be missed and the pain misdiagnosed, because the characteristic referral pattern is absent.

Satellite TrPs

Uneven tightening of muscles caused by TrPs can affect joints. Bones follow muscles, so the bones can be pulled a little bit out of alignment by contractured muscles. This can cause wear and tear on the joints, and result in inflammation known as osteoarthritis (OA). This process includes TrPs that can affect your jaw alignment, causing wear and tear on the temporomandibular joint (TMJ). Others cause gait disturbances that, if untreated, may lead to hip and/or knee replacement. Much of this damage can be prevented, but if TrPs are not properly treated and perpetuating factors are not brought under control, TrPs can spread. This process is not progressive, because it is reversible. Simple TrPs, if diagnosed and treated promptly, can be easy to resolve. If, however, they remain untreated, your body compensates. You limit the way you move to avoid pain at the end of the movement. You set in motion habits that will further perpetuate TrPs, stress other muscles, and take time to unlearn. As muscles weaken from TrPs, other muscles are recruited to take up the work of the weaker ones. These muscles tend to be targets for spasm when others are stressed, including the trapezius, masseter, posterior cervicals, and lumbar paraspinals. Muscles that are in the referral pain pattern of a TrP are also subject to stress. These muscles can develop TrPs too. To find out what happens when one TrP becomes many, we need to explore the world of chronic myofascial pain and fibromyalgia.

Fibromyalgia, Trigger Points, and Chronic Myofascial Pain: A New Understanding

Fibromyalgia: A Hypersensitized Central Nervous System

Fibromyalgia doesn't *cause* aching muscles. It doesn't *cause* numbness and tingling. Yes, patients with FM can have these symptoms and many others, but these symptoms' origins have been terribly misunderstood. So have the patients. We are beginning to understand the process that creates the central sensitization state we know as fibromyalgia. FM is the term given to a family of illnesses that have in common central nervous system (CNS) sensitization and chronic diffuse *systemic* pain. FM is *systemic*, not local. The nervous system is divided into central and peripheral sections, although the dividing line may be fuzzy at times. The CNS is composed of the brain and the spinal cord. The rest of the nervous system is peripheral. These systems blend and meld in places, but the differences are very important to patients with these conditions, and to their care providers, because their treatments are different.

An initiating event or series of events and responses occurs in FM, creating a state of CNS hypersensitization. This affects wind-up, or temporal summation of second pain (TSSP). TSSP is the best indication of FM pain intensity (Staud et al. 2004), and is an important concept for both FM patients and their care providers to understand. If an intense, severe pain or other stressor hits the CNS it is considered "first pain." The brain and spinal cord figuratively cringe and do their best to recover from the assault. If the assault continues, or the pain or other unpleasant stimuli becomes chronic, the next assault is called "second pain." The CNS starts to adapt, changing in an attempt to protect itself. It begins (figuratively again) to tense the shoulders of the brain, clenching the fists of the spinal cord, and causing little nerves to quiver, waiting for the next blow to fall. As you can see in the figure if the stimulation recurs or continues, the base pain level climbs higher, and takes longer to return to its original level. With continuing or recurring stimuli, the pain level may not come all the way down again. The base level may continue to climb as long as assaults continue, and the CNS is further sensitized. In FM patients, CNS sensitization requires less noxious stimuli to spike the pain level, and after-effects are greater and

more prolonged (Staud et al. 2003). TSSP and *central* pain in FM results primarily from *peripheral* stimuli. You *must* gain control of the peripheral stimuli to control the central pain.

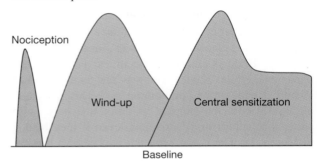

Fibromyalgia pain amplification. Temporal summation of second pain (wind-up). Reproduced with the permission of Roland Staud.

FM is characterized by hyperalgesia (amplified pain) and allodynia (normally non-painful stimuli such as touch, sounds, light, and smells are interpreted as pain by the CNS). Some days, everything can hurt. Even the pounding of rain on the window can seem as if sharp crystals or walls of pressure are whipping at your cells. That's part of the world of FM. Peripheral stimuli, such as TrPs, may initiate noxious sensations such as pain, nausea or dizziness, and FM amplifies them too, and the pain or other sensations can outlast the stimulus. Research verifies that the central sensitization of FM can be initiated and/or maintained by peripheral pain (Staud 2006). The referred pain of TrPs is itself a manifestation of central sensitization (Gerwin 2010). In FM, the filters that protect healthy people from CNS over-stimulation are not working adequately, (Carrillo-de-la-Pena et al. 2006). The FM patient may not be able to pinpoint sources of pain, because his or her brain is totally preoccupied with attempting to handle a deluge of pain and other stimuli. In uncontrolled FM, anything that can shock the CNS—including pain, loud noises, and any other startling stimuli—must be moderated or avoided. Any CNS assault can lead to FM "flare." During flare, old symptoms worsen and new ones may appear as new TrPs activate. Everything is hypersensitive. Since few articles on FM patients account for the coexistence of TrPs, it's not known if the flare response is actually multiple TrP activation. We do know that the CNS may take a long while to calm down, and may never return to its former level of sensitivity (Staud et al. 2004). Relatives may not understand the cost of holiday season demands on an FM patient, and employees with FM may pay heavily for mandated overtime. The lack of external support also adds stress to the patients' lives. Attempts to explain may be met with disbelief or dismissed entirely. Patients pay heavily for the lack of general, medical and legal understanding.

Cognitive dysfunctions may be the most disruptive aspect of FM, although some of those disruptions may be due to the chronic pain itself (Dick et al. 2008). The brain is otherwise employed, processing pain stimuli, and literally can't deal with anything else. It may not be able to recognize a jar of mustard placed on a different shelf, or remember a sequence of numbers—or a sequence of anything. Brain dysfunction specific to FM has been documented (Glass 2008). You may feel as if your head is stuffed with cotton and nothing else. This can cause difficulties with the simplest of tasks, and may cause patients to appear and feel stupid, even if they belong to Mensa. Dr. Glass and her team have shown that for patients with FM, working tasks, executive memory, and semantic memory deficits equal about 20 years of extra aging. Yet you look fine, so people expect you to act accordingly.

Some FM patients have difficulty following a book or television show because they can't remember the characters (Russell and Larson 2009). "The existence of these symptoms has been confirmed by the results of objective tests of metamemory, working memory, semantic memory, everyday attention, task switching, and selective attention. More complex tasks cause greater difficulty, as will distraction. Short-term memory can be especially affected by distraction" (Leavitt and Katz 2006). Cognitive impairments can vary with fatigue and mood. Pain has the greatest effect on perceived language deficits, not concentration or attention, and lack of restorative sleep most affected perceived memory deficits (Williams et al. 2011). FM cognitive deficits can be profound and yet be undetected by conventional cognitive assessment techniques (Leavitt and Katz 2009). Research has "revealed a pattern of impairment in working memory and attention/executive control as well as memory impairment." (Glass 2010). Even when global processing is unimpaired, there is frequently a significant impairment in selective deficits such as specific naming speed skills (Leavitt and Katz 2008). There are new simple tests that may prove useful (Leavitt and Katz 2011). The cognitive deficits of FM are neurological, not psychological. "The present data suggest that associated psychological distress and maladaptive emotional responses that are commonly attributed to the general

FMS population may be largely a distinguishing feature of one subset of patients" (Salgueiro et al. 2011).

Spatial memory may be more impaired in FM patients than verbal memory (Kim et al. 2011). This may be caused by biochemical brain trauma from the sidetracking of tryptophan to the kynurenine pathway. On this metabolic path, instead of needed serotonin, the result is quinolinic acid. This metabolic pathway is utilized in at least a subgroup of FM patients (Schwartz et al. 2003). Quinolinic acid is a neurotoxin that causes spatial memory impairment in rats; they can no longer find their way through their maze. Is quinolinic acid causing the same chemical brain trauma in FM patients? This experiment may be on-going without our knowledge, (perhaps as FM patients attempt to traverse the maze of medical insurance and managed care?) We don't yet know, and certainly haven't given consent. (Neither did the rats.) FM patients can have significant cognitive deficits that tend to increase in times of stress, or if hormones are unbalanced. This is important for care providers to remember, especially as this may make communication difficult in emergency situations, or during stressful office visits or medical procedures. These cognitive deficits could be mistaken for dementia in the elderly. They can worsen dramatically if the FM patient is overexposed exposed to stimuli, such as in a large crowd, with lighting, varying colors and patterns, odors, and noise. This sensory overload can overwhelm the brain, and the patient, quickly. Sensory overload can initiate a panic or shock state. It can also initiate a stress response: fight, flight, startle, or freeze. It's important to remember that this response is neurological, not psychological, and requires decreased stimuli and increased recovery time.

FM is not exclusionary. One may have FM and many other conditions. Impaired balance, falls, dizziness, irritable bowel, sexual dysfunctions, sleep impairment, numbness, dyspnea, burning, etc. often ascribed to FM may be from coexisting conditions such as insulin resistance, TrPs, thyroid resistance or vestibular dysfunction. One of the first steps in managing FM is to discover what condition is causing or contributing to the most significant symptoms. It is important to know that when the CNS is hypersensitized, pain is not the only symptom that is enhanced (Geisser et al. 2008). Fibromyalgia has many invisible symptoms. Along with the pain and cognitive deficits come sleep deprivation and fatigue. Patients may feel anxious or depressed because no one can tell them why they hurt or what they can do about it. They may feel helpless and hopeless. Quality of life can spiral downhill as financial and other resources are depleted. Friends don't know what to do or say, and patients *and* their caregivers may become isolated. So far, we've seen massive denial from the general public and the medical establishment, except, of course, from those pharmaceutical corporations who are now making a tidy sum from FM patients. They have a vested interest in placing all symptoms under the fibromyalgia umbrella.

FM can be divided into subgroups depending on the initiators of the central sensitization state, including (but not limited to) infections, severe or sustained physical trauma or emotional stress, exposure to toxins, severe or persistent pain such as can be caused by TrPs, persistent lack of restorative sleep, and/or existing metabolic imbalances. Many cases of FM have multiple initiating factors. Some cases of FM are initiated by TrPs. We don't know if TrP formation could be an intermediate stage between any initiator such as an infection or trauma and the central sensitization of FM. It takes time for central sensitization to develop after a sudden initiating event. Are TrPs forming during that delay, preparing to set patients up for chronic pain? We don't yet know. Sometimes the FM initiator is slow, such as sustained grief, stress, or overwork, often involving tight muscles and TrPs. Whatever the cause of FM, TrPs help to maintain the central sensitization once FM develops, and are avenues for controlling it. The initiating causes may be helpful guides to FM subsets, offering direction for treatment options.

FM itself affects the energy status of the body in so many ways that FM and TrPs may be the most common interactive conditions. Adaptations to sensory overload may themselves create a variety of biochemical (neurotransmitters, hormones, etc.) cascades that may initiate yet other cascades. These biochemical imbalances vary from patient to patient. As you will discover in the gallery, some TrPs can cause cognitive deficits as well. In FM, there may be a multitude of biochemical imbalances that must be gently brought back into harmony. The good news is that whatever helps FM will indirectly help TrPs, and whatever helps the TrPs will help FM.

Someone can't have FM only in the hands or in the back. The CNS is the brain and spinal cord. It affects the whole body, causing a diffuse pain all over. *FM does not cause localized pain.* If there is localized pain, it's caused by something else, although FM may also be present. Often, but not always, localized pain is caused by one or more TrPs. Many, many symptoms usually blamed on FM are due to other causes, most commonly TrPs. We suspect that all chronic illness may have a myofascial component. For example, people with OA, Parkinson's disease, and other chronic illnesses have a TrP component to their symptoms. This is good news, because the TrP component can be treated and the overall symptom burden can be lightened.

Trigger Points, Fibromyalgia, or Both: Different and Interactive

Since there is much confusion, there are two key facts we must make clear:

1. TrPs and myofascial pain are not part of FM although these conditions often coexist and interact.

2. There is no such thing as a "fibromyalgia trigger point."

FM is neither musculoskeletal nor rheumatic. Once a central sensitization state such as FM exists, minimal pain bombardment from TrPs is enough to maintain it (Staud 2011). To control the FM pain amplification, you must control the pain generators. Far too many have insisted that myofascial TrPs are too complex to understand, and they lump everything under the label "FM," using it as a garbage-pail diagnosis. It should not be so used! It is unjust to the patient, and poor (but currently standard) medical practice. Corporations make money with high-priced "FM" pain medications, and the patients deal with the costs and the side effects. Meanwhile, many treatable TrP symptoms go untreated or mistreated, and many perpetuating factors remain unidentified and out of control, because care providers have not been trained to manage TrPs. Failure to comprehend the combination of TrP pain generation plus the pain amplification of FM leads to undertreatment of the pain itself—yet another perpetuating factor. Care provider and patient alike must understand TrPs as well as FM. You have what you have. Identifying it will not cause harm; not identifying it may do so. That's simple. Every coexisting condition and perpetuating factor identified provides one more way to gain control over symptoms. The FM component—the central sensitization—must be respected. Extra care must be taken not to further sensitize the CNS during treatments or procedures. The nerves have become facilitated, which means that any nerve path that has been stimulated can more easily be stimulated again and again, like any well-worn path. To someone with FM, the person sitting next to them wearing perfume in a closed environment is unknowingly guilty of an assault that may result in increased pain, migraine, or other symptom amplification that may last for days.

Fibromyalgia patients can tolerate slow, gentle strengthening of muscles unless TrPs are in those muscles. You can't strengthen a TrP-laden muscle until those TrPs are resolved. This takes time. Every treatment must be modified when TrPs and FM are both part of the equation. TrPs cause contracture. Contracture from only a few TrPs may be microscopic, but it's there. Usually, the more TrP contraction nodules there are, and the longer they have existed, the more contracture there will be. A lot of contracture is easy to see, but it has to start somewhere, and manual workers must understand this. Repetitious exercises make TrPs worse and muscles with them weaker. Many chronic conditions are interactive (bidirectional) and any treatment plan must take that into consideration. Doctors are now trained in differential diagnoses, but that model doesn't work with multiple chronic illnesses. Chronic pain patients need care providers experienced in *interactive diagnoses*. It takes skill and training to identify FM, CMP and other coexisting illnesses. To do anything else is a disservice to the patient. How can anyone justly accept money to treat a patient if s/he isn't able to diagnose and treat the conditions that the patient has?

Research into the pathophysiology and characteristics of TrPs and FM indicates that "FM pain" is mainly caused by TrPs (Ge 2010). As myofascia twists and sticks to other tissues, it can entrap nerves, blood and lymph vessels, and perhaps even ducts. This can lead to symptoms such as swelling, numbness and tingling, and all sorts of other diagnostic nightmares for care providers and real horror for patients living with them. When multiple TrPs develop satellites and *those* develop satellite TrPs of their own, the whole body may become riddled with interacting TrPs. This is a sign of uncontrolled perpetuating factors, some of which may be coexisting conditions, which also may interact. "Chronic pain syndromes become complex, involving all aspects of the patient's life and, with rare exceptions, include a significant, if not dominant myofascial TrP component … it will require a comprehensive approach to unravel all the intertwining components" (Simons, Travell, and Simons 1999, p. 268). Everyone with chronic pain has a story to tell. It takes time to listen, and patients deserve that courtesy. There are clues in each story that may explain what causes the symptoms and why.

Stage I CMP: How It Is

Helen struggles to her apartment, short of breath. She pulls herself up each step using the handrails, and shuffles slowly down the hall. At her door, she fumbles with her keys, dropping them. When she finally gets the right key into the lock, it hurts to turn the key, and pain shoots through her wrist when she turns the doorknob. At least she made it home in time to reach the bathroom. She always had to urinate. Well, she thought, I'm 65. I have to expect this.

Kerry woke up exhausted every morning, and he always hurt. It was difficult to concentrate in school, because he ached trying to sit still at his desk, and he was sleepy. He'd just gotten new eyeglasses, but his vision was blurry again, and he couldn't see what his teacher wrote on the board. He was clumsy, and kept falling off gym equipment. He tripped over his own feet. His nose ran constantly. Other kids teased him. He didn't fit in. What was he doing wrong?

Mary felt crushing chest pain that radiated down her left arm, coupled with shortness of breath. It felt as if an elephant was on her chest. She was rushed one more time to the Emergency Department, where she was well known as a "frequent flyer." Nobody there took her seriously. It was always something: abdominal pains, chest pains, severe menstrual cramps, sciatica. Every test was negative, and physical therapy made her pain worse. Her family called her a hypochondriac. Her doctor wanted her to see a psychiatrist. She started doubting her own sanity.

These names are not real, but the stories are, and they and many like them are repeated daily across the world. They are the story of chronic myofascial pain (CMP). Anything that can tighten the muscles can cause the first TrPs.

Stage I CMP: What It Is

Although the term "chronic" in medicine is usually taken to mean a condition that has existed for over six months, there are basic problems with a time limit for CMP because CMP covers a wide spectrum. Some patients may have TrPs that are chronic only because they are unrecognized, untreated, or inadequately treated. Some have chronic latent TrPs, and the patients don't even know they are there. Others have chronic TrPs because perpetuating factors have not been adequately controlled; they may only have a few TrPs in one area that have nagged at them for years. CMP is frequently misdiagnosed as fibromyalgia. One of the authors (Starlanyl) saw a patient who came to her because her doctor told her she probably had FM. She didn't, though she had pain in all four quadrants of her body. She had a history of separate traumas over time, and had nine TrPs, but no perpetuating factors and no other conditions. With treatment, her symptoms quickly resolved. Simple chronic TrPs without central sensitization are Stage I CMP.

Stage II CMP with Fibromyalgia

Joe was a healthy jogger who developed chronic pain after promotion from a desk job. The new position meant long hours, frequent travel, and long meetings. He took aspirin. Low back, groin, and hip pain developed over the next four months, followed by neck pain. He couldn't jog. He developed gastric symptoms and jaw pain with bruxism, and his sleep quality declined. He gained weight, mostly around the abdomen. He stumbled frequently, his feet hurt, his right ankle occasionally buckled, and he became impotent. He felt a sensation like water trickling down his outer thighs, and those areas hurt to touch, but Joe didn't tell the company doctor, because his symptoms had already been met with unbelief. He was sent for a psych consult when medical tests failed to reveal anything abnormal except high cholesterol and triglycerides. The psychiatrist denied pain medications, as "there was no demonstrable cause for the pain," and referred him to psychological counseling and a pain clinic.

The psychologist concluded Joe was unhappy with his new job, and this was causing the symptoms. The pain clinic treated Joe with pain language and mannerisms avoidance. Joe was not allowed to mention his pain to anyone, or to grimace, limp, or otherwise indicate that he was in pain. He was put on a work-hardening program; his pain increased exponentially. When he could no longer grip the weights, they were strapped to his wrists; pain became intolerable. When Joe tried to withdraw from the pain clinic, he was called noncompliant and told that his insurance would not pay if he left. His marriage was in trouble. Nobody believed his pain

was real; he knew it was. Joe left the clinic and called a chiropractor, who immediately recognized some TrP patterns and probably coexisting FM. The chiropractor was part of a medical team that included a nutritionist, an MD, a DO, and a myofascial TrP therapist. An exam revealed TrPs in the: trapezius; temporalis; occipitalis; masseter; pterygoid; suboccipital; posterior cervical; digastric; scalene; sternocleidomastoid; longus colli; levator scapulae; supraspinatus; infraspinatus; teres minor; subscapularis; coracobrachialis; deltoid; biceps brachii; brachialis; triceps brachii; supinator; hand and finger flexors and extensors; pollicis muscles; pectoralis major; abdominal obliques; paraspinals; iliopsoas; gluteus minimus, medius, and maximus; piriformis and short lateral rotators; pelvic floor; tensor fasciae latae; R quadratus femoris; R adductors; hamstrings; R tibialis anterior and posterior; R peroneals; R soleus; and R foot muscles and attachments (all TrPs were bilateral unless noted). The exam also uncovered: a number of geloid masses that, because of pain, could not be examined at that time (Starlanyl et al. 2001–2); a rotated pelvis; rotoscoliosis; bilateral Morton's foot; and paradoxical breathing. Testing revealed insulin resistance, possibly developing into metabolic syndrome, and FM.

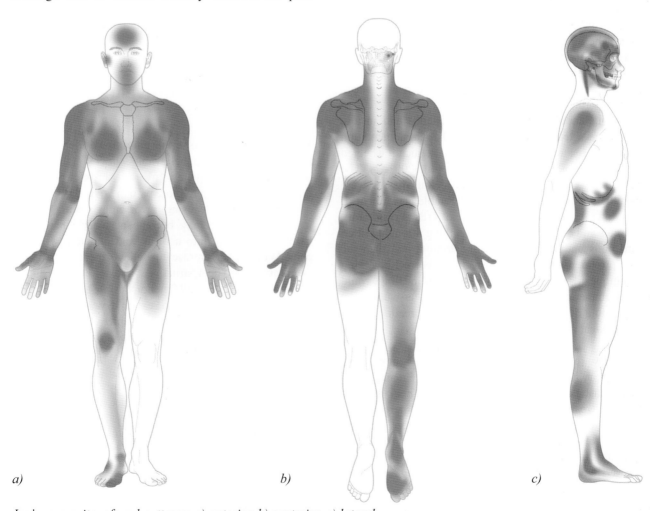

Joe's composite referral patterns: a) anterior, b) posterior, c) lateral.

The most life-impacting symptoms were then listed and contributors identified. Those that could be treated quickly with little negative impact were addressed immediately. This included medicinal and nonmedicinal aggressive control of pain; identification of potential contributing respiratory, abdominal and pelvic floor TrPs; control of perpetuating factors; and gentle, brief sessions of myofascial release, frequency specific microcurrent (FSM), craniosacral therapy, and education in self-treatment. A plan was drawn up for restoration of healthy breathing, and for sleep, diet, and exercise, as well as symptom control. In each category, specific dysfunctions were identified and as many causes and contributors as possible were listed. Sleep deprivation can counteract analgesic medications (Kundermann et al. 2004), as well as adding to pain, cognitive dysfunction, and fatigue. When conditions are interactive, treating one successfully may also relieve others. Jaw clenching and grinding (bruxism) can be caused by micro-arousals and sleep disturbance (Miyawaki et al. 2004). A sleep study can be critical to uncovering sleep dysfunctions (Schneider-Helmert 2003). Joe's sleep study confirmed that he had obstructive sleep apnea (OSA) and GERD. Continuous positive airway pressure (CPAP) treatment helped both OSA and GERD (Tawk et al. 2006), helped balance sympathetic nervous system activity (Smith et al. 1998), and balanced some hormones (Loth et al. 1998), helping the FM. The CPAP was successful for OSA without restoring deep sleep. The use of thyroid-stimulating hormone (TSH) to monitor thyroid function is unreliable in FM, as this test depends on a balanced hypothalamus-pituitary-adrenal axis, and this is often out of balance in FM. Thyroid resistance and insulin resistance often occur together, so T4 supplementation was not indicated. Topical T3 (thyroid) medication helped clear the geloid masses (Starlanyl et al. 2001–2). The TrPs that had been underneath the geloid masses were eventually revealed and became treatable. Treatment of breathing function included release of TrPs in respiratory muscles and education in belly breathing through written directions and a practical demonstration, and then the care provider watched Joe perform the correct breathing technique. There was recognition that healing could begin immediately, but that lifestyle changes would take time and a dogged persistence to retrain breathing from paradoxical respiration.

Joe's new job had required long periods of immobility. The history included examination of pre-accident photos. A whiplash accident had stressed head and neck muscles already weakened by latent TrPs and hyperextended because of a head-forward, round-shouldered posture. History also revealed a poor diet on the road, and difficulty hauling heavy luggage. Many TrPs had been aggravated or initiated by the work-hardening repetitious exercises. Sleep medications and pain alleviation helped relieve some of the fatigue. Suitable bedding was purchased for Joe's needs, and a pillow found to fit his neck curvature, with the understanding that it might change as tissues responded to treatment. The use of an automatically adjusting CPAP (AUTOPAP), *set with the maximum at the highest needed pressure found on the sleep study*, allowed for adjustment of pressures required with the changes of airway flow due to changing amounts of nasopharyngeal congestion and varying levels of TrP contraction. The use of the AUTOPAP also minimized the air going into the gut. This occurrence is common during CPAP therapy and may aggravate gas and bloating symptoms, which add to the misery of both abdominal TrPs and IBS. Joe and his family were given educational materials and counseling on the illnesses involved and control of perpetuating factors, including location of outside resources and support services. Joe started a food diary, and he and his family were given nutritional counseling. His new diet eliminated high-fructose corn syrup, and trans-fats. Also deleted were excitotoxins such as monosodium glutamate and aspartame, which may worsen FM (Smith et al. 2001). Joe lost weight. He was warned that toxic chemicals stored in body fat might be released by weight loss, slowing metabolism and contributing to temporary fatigue (Tremblay et al. 2004). When this occurred, Joe and his family understood it, and this helped them cope.

CMP and FM: Unraveling the Knots

When multiple TrPs cause pain amplified by fibromyalgia, the pain level can be unbelievable *unless* you understand the reasons. Inadequately treated chronic pain may disturb sleep, leading to more pain the next day. Multiple conditions interact, causing a worsening spiral. Without understanding, life may become a steadily narrowing hallway stretching into a bleak and hopeless world of pain. When others refuse to believe the extent of the symptoms, it can be destructive. "Lack of belief in ability to manage pain, cope and function despite persistent pain, is a significant predictor to the extent to which individuals with chronic pain become disabled or depressed" (Arnstein et al. 1999). Patients may go from doctor to doctor, seeking answers until resources are exhausted. Family and companions become skeptical, withdrawing support when it is most needed. Patients feel isolated and can withdraw from society, not just because of symptoms, but also because of neglect, hopelessness, and resulting depression. Diagnosing this combination and coexisting conditions is the first step, but it is a big one.

Knowing individual TrPs is not sufficient. Well-intentioned care providers have again done harm by not understanding this. Any TrP therapy or treatment will be more complex once CMP has developed, especially if FM is involved, and must proceed carefully. Even patient examination may have to be done one area at a time, with extra medication or other support before, during, and after, to ensure that no further central sensitization occurs. No matter how gentle the touch, multiple twitch responses may occur during the exam. They liberate irritating biochemicals from the tissues (Shah et al. 2005), which can result in extra misery after the exam. Patients and care providers need to understand and be prepared, because this can be debilitating. Patients may need extra therapy such as FSM and craniosacral release to calm the CNS after other types of manual therapy or exercise, and extra home help may be required if TrPs are many and FM severe, and/or there are uncontrollable coexisting conditions.

Exercise itself must be prescribed as carefully and individually as any medication. It took time for the fascia to tie itself into knots, and it will take time for fascia to unwind. There may also be tissue changes. Muscles may be fibrotic, and/or areas may be calcified, or there may be geloid masses. Tissues may be so tight care providers can't feel the TrPs. That doesn't mean they aren't there, and a good medical history can indicate where they may be. Many traditional TrP therapies will need to be modified when dealing with the combination of CMP and FM. Sensory overload can result from an overabundance of stimulation and pain during treatment. The brain can handle only so much stimulation. Care providers and patients must monitor comfort levels carefully during an exam and therapy. Be attentive after therapies, and keep communication lines open. Tolerance to therapy can vary considerably: during times of high stress (even good stress such as holidays), therapy tolerance can decrease significantly. With CMP, usual alternatives suggested for individual TrPs may aggravate other TrPs. A telephone headset may prevent stress on arm TrPs but may activate head TrPs. A computer voice-activated system may not work because of throat TrPs or scarred vocal cords due to GERD. A cane to help buckling knees or ankles may not be usable if hand and arm TrPs won't support the cane's use.

How disabling is CMP and/or FM? This depends on many variables, including how many coexisting conditions are present, how severe they are, the possibility of controlling perpetuating factors, the extent of central sensitization, the length of time the patient has been ill, the available support system, the quality of care (including self-care), the ability to modify the environment, patient education and ability to manage conditions, the ability to modify work tasks or job modification, and many other factors. There are always options, but it takes a creative mind to find them. It's easier to think outside the box if you aren't boxed in to begin with.

5 Kinetics: Lines of Power

The word "kinetic" means "relating to movement or motion." The movement of kinetic chains (or lines) is the way the body flows. Kinetic chains are composed of integrated individual links. Any chain is only as strong as its weakest link; in humans, these links are our tissues, and fascia unites them. The body is continually receiving, interpreting, and adapting to numerous everyday stimuli. Events in our lives (physical, emotional, etc.) are stored in our musculoskeletal and fascial systems, imprinting a record of our life experiences—and interpretations of those experiences—through tissue changes, posture, and habit. The body is a reflection of all that we are, physically and mentally, past and present.

If your skeleton were suddenly to disappear, what would happen to the rest of your body? It would fall in a heap on the floor, correct? Now, what would happen to your body if all your soft tissues disappeared? Your skeleton would fall to the floor! Then what is holding us up? The human body holds itself together by a unique relationship between tension and compression. This is called tensegrity. Your bones push out (compression) and your soft tissues pull inward (tension). The end result is lift. With time, we lose our battle with gravity: we round our shoulders, and find it difficult to straighten our knees; our heads poke forward, and our breathing becomes more shallow and rapid. We've set the stage for TrP development. Connective tissue, such as fascia, is predominantly water, which is non-compressible, so physical force (tension, compression) must be distributed throughout the organism. We need to stay hydrated, or our tissues could "dry out" and become sticky. Then they might adhere to other structures, causing restriction, or lack of motion.

In medicine, fascia has long been overlooked, and considered a nuisance to be scraped away to see the muscles. Even today, there's not much attention paid to human fascia and its relation to motion. A recent cadaveric dissection course delivered by one of the authors (Sharkey) at King's College London focused on myotensegrity: the one-muscle hypothesis. This course highlighted the interrelationship of muscles and bones through the fascial oceans, rivers, streams, and pools that flow throughout our bodies and our lives. We hope for more research concentrated in this area. When you view the lovely muscle diagrams in this book or others, please understand that isn't what muscles look like in reality. We often think in a linear fashion; in one-dimension. Two dimensions is possible, but three? It's difficult to portray fascia in a book, yet three-dimensional fascia occurs everywhere in the human body. Our bodies can move in so many ways only with the combined function of all muscles, fascia, and skin. For us to function at our best, tissues must work together in an integrated manner.

Imagine that, while barefoot, you walk on a thumbtack. Would you raise your foot, or your entire leg? Would you hold your breath for an instant, affecting your diaphragm, while your elbows bend and your body folds forward from the pelvis? It wouldn't be a single-note response, but a symphony of movement. That's an *acute* situation. A *chronic* situation occurs slowly, over weeks, months, or years. Repetitious muscle overload, feelings of despair, or other chronic stressors, can lead to changes in respiratory function, such as shallow or rapid breathing. Breathing affects every cell. When one link in a kinetic chain becomes stuck or compressed, or holds excessive tension, the rest of the chain compensates for that dysfunction. Tissues experiencing excessive tension or compression receive blood that is less rich in oxygen and nutrients.

Suppose you've been in an automobile accident in which you were rear-ended, and you feel much of the stress in your neck. It's possible that only 20% of the problem may be in the neck; the other 80% may be located elsewhere within the myofascial kinetic chain. It could even be coming from your feet and still result in compression at the shoulders and neck. We all wear full three-dimensional body stockings of fascia. As Tom Myers (2001) puts it in his book *Anatomy Trains*, "A tug in the fascial net is communicated across the entire system like a snag in a sweater, or the pull in a corner of an empty woven hammock." He explains how patterns of strain communicate through the myofascial web, contributing to postural compensation and movement stability. Myers describes kinetic "express" trains and "local" trains: express trains cross more than one joint, while local trains cross only one joint.

Even when you stub your toe, the rest of your body reacts. You limp, your shoulders hunch down, and you may give voice to your displeasure. You may favor that foot, making the other foot work harder, and your gait may change as a result. To avoid putting extra weight on the hurt foot, your hip on the injured side lifts a little, causing less room for the tissues in the low back. The shoulder on the opposite side then compensates to balance the raised hip. So it is with any injury. Your body compensates to maintain balance, and those changes can be damaging over time, creating motion habits that give rise to other dysfunctions affecting you in ways you may not suspect. For example, you may feel fatigued and not know why. If one leg joint, such as the knee or ankle, is restricted, walking takes as much as 40% more energy. If two joints in that leg are restricted, walking can use up to 300% more energy (Greenman 1996). The resulting fatigue may be blamed on fibromyalgia or called chronic fatigue, but it may be caused by kinetic restrictions from TrPs.

Joints are just spaces where bones come close together, but they are complex spaces where many tissues converge. Many of these tissues can and do contribute to joint stiffness. The myofascia itself can stick together, causing further restrictions. During life, we accumulate traumas: some are abrupt, such as a fall; others are gradual, such as those caused by repetitive motions. Trauma can cause the myofascia to stick together in tight clumps of tissue or folded-over sheets and lines. It can also cause scars, which are a localized healthy response to tissue damage, but they can have far-reaching effects. For example, any abdominal scar can cause significant back problems. Even a small appendectomy scar can cause massive abdominal and back pain due to tissue restrictions (Kobesova and Lewitt 2000). Scar tissues that cause symptoms are called active scars and tend to have TrPs. These can generate pain that can promote or maintain FM. Even if pain has persisted for decades, studies show that scar TrPs can be effectively treated manually (Kobesova et al. 2007). This research gives patients hope, but leads one to wonder how many people now live with unnecessary pain.

Observe a healthy child or cat in motion. They flow, using full body action efficiently and effortlessly. That's how we were meant to move. Myofascia is a network for communication, as well as a source of that fluidity. Myofascia has magnetic, electrical, and crystalline properties. Many myofascial therapies take advantage of these properties, and research has begun to reveal how some microcurrent and other electrical therapies can create changes in myofascia (Hart 2009). The Chinese concept of chi meshes well with these forms of therapy. The energy flow of the body—the chi—circulates through the myofascia. Ground substance in the myofascia can change from gel to glue, transforming the texture of tissues and the movement of the body. When myofascia is stuck, it must be released before healthy function returns.

Poetry in Motion—Or Not

The body is designed to function efficiently, but pain is a promise that life always keeps. When one part of the musculoskeletal system fails or becomes weak, other parts do their best to compensate. Muscles become stiff to brace a weak muscle, or tighten to protect an area that hurts when it moves. Each part of the body has its own optimum position: for example, when your body is at rest, your tongue should be in its physiological resting position behind the front teeth on the roof of the mouth. Travell and Simons mention this in their medical texts, and Chinese t'ai chi masters teach it to their students as well, but they don't always explain why. When the tongue is in this position, the hyoid muscles can contract, which creates the proper amount of stiffness to support the neck joints. When the tongue is out of position, the sternocleidomastoid (SCM) muscles shorten more than the optimum needed, to provide additional compensating stiffness. This added SCM contraction causes the pectoral muscles to shorten, taking up the slack that the tight SCMs have caused. Other muscles follow in a cascade. This shortening is often due to TrPs. This common situation leads to the head-forward posture, including forward, rounded, slumped shoulders. Any stiffness or held tension in a kinetic chain affects the whole kinetic chain. No muscle is isolated, and the smallest dysfunction can lead to loss of stability. For example, patients with cervical TrPs have deficits in standing balance, especially when standing on foam flooring (Talebian et al. 2012); the foam disrupts sensory information from cutaneous mechanoreceptors on the soles of the feet, contributing to postural instability that increases with TrP-related neck pain. Ankle-area muscles are then recruited to compensate for postural imbalance. The extra stress on those muscles and surrounding tissues can cause TrPs to develop. This has direct application for those who exercise on foam-matted surfaces, such as those used for t'ai chi chuan, gymnastics, yoga, and other exercise in which postural balance is critical.

The figures on the next few pages show the body in ways you may never have seen before; in lines of power called kinetic chains. These chains are networks that coordinate muscular contractions in the body as a whole, providing stability and orientation. All body systems and structures work together to establish links that ultimately form a functional kinetic network. If one system fails to operate optimally, it contributes to an energy crisis in tissues along the chain. Each muscle along the chain can develop TrPs.

The Kinetic Core: Stability Central

The core system is a system of stabilization. Although **core muscles** are primarily in the center of your body, the core affects the whole. If it doesn't function at its best, other parts of the neuromuscular system must compensate. Many soft tissue and musculoskeletal injuries involving the spine and extremities are caused or perpetuated by muscle imbalances and weaknesses in the core musculature and connecting tissues. Unfortunately, many people use exercise in an attempt to develop strength and neuromuscular control only in the prime movement muscles, neglecting the flexibility and strength of the core. If the core destabilizes, ineffective and dysfunctional kinetic chain patterns become established. Stresses mount, and TrPs form. Pain, injury and FM may follow. Understanding the concept of kinetic chains will help you understand the connection between pain felt in the head or neck and a tension or spasm in muscles or fascia some distance away. You will learn a lot more about such instances in the individual muscle segments of this book. By appreciating these relationships, you can more easily identify those tissues that are short and tight. The terms associated with the kinetic chains may be unfamiliar. Get to know them. The **core muscles** will be discussed in sections of Part II, with the term "**core muscles**" being noted in boldface type to remind readers of their importance.

Core anatomy structures in the lumbar-pelvic-hip area produce dynamic forces and stabilize the kinetic chains during functional movements. Many deep muscles help support pelvic organs and maintain healthy pressure in the abdomen. **More than 29 muscles attach to the core unilaterally: rectus femoris, semitendinosus, semimembranosus, biceps femoris, psoas (major, minor), iliacus, rectus abdominis, obliques (internal, external), transversus abdominis, pyramidalis, quadratus lumborum, quadratus femoris, obturator (internus, externus), gemellus (superior, inferior), adductors (longus, brevis, magnus), gracilis, pectineus, gluteus (maximus, medius, minimus), tensor fasciae latae, erector spinae (iliocostalis, longissimus, spinalis), latissimus dorsi, multifidi, piriformis, levator ani, and coccygeus.** Deep stabilizing ligaments and tendons also can develop multiple TrPs. The primary function of the core's myofascial structures, including the fascia and ligamentous chains, is to provide postural control by keeping the center of gravity over our base of support during dynamic movements. Kinetic figures are reproduced here from the book *Fascial Release for Structural Balance*, with the kind permission of the authors, Earls and Myers (2010). The terms "line" and "chain" are used interchangeably. We ask our non-medical readers to have patience with muscle names. Some will become as familiar as friends once you get to know them in later sections. They are closer than your friends. They are part of you.

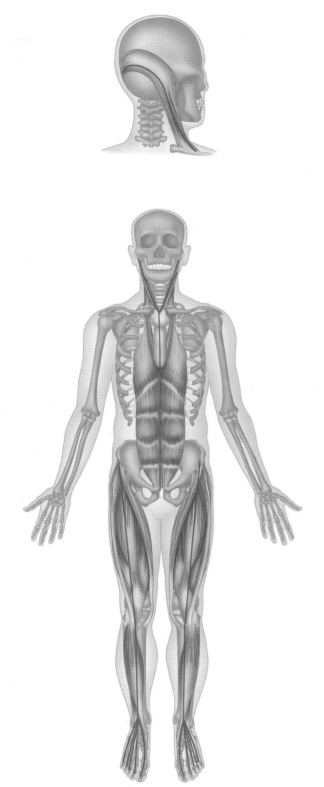

The superficial front line (SFL).

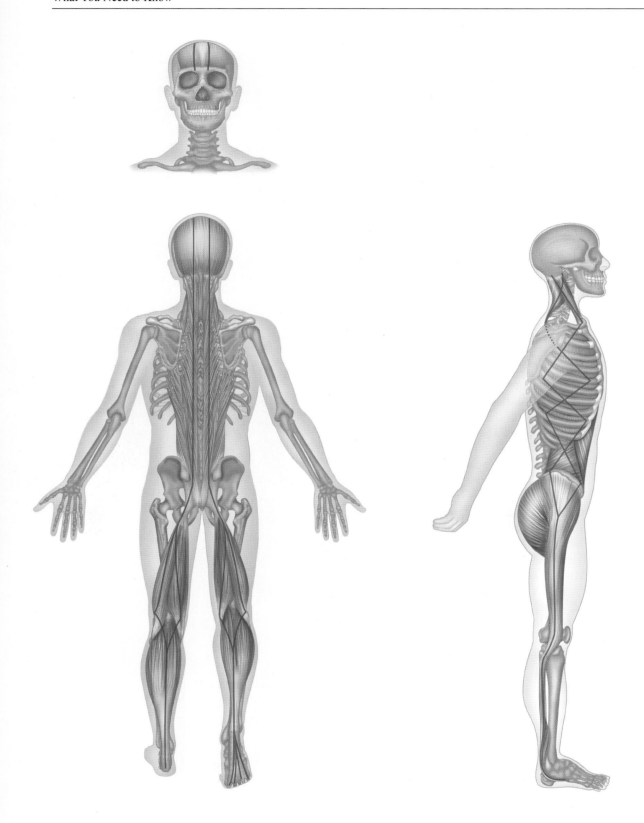

The superficial back line (SBL).   *The lateral line (LTL).*

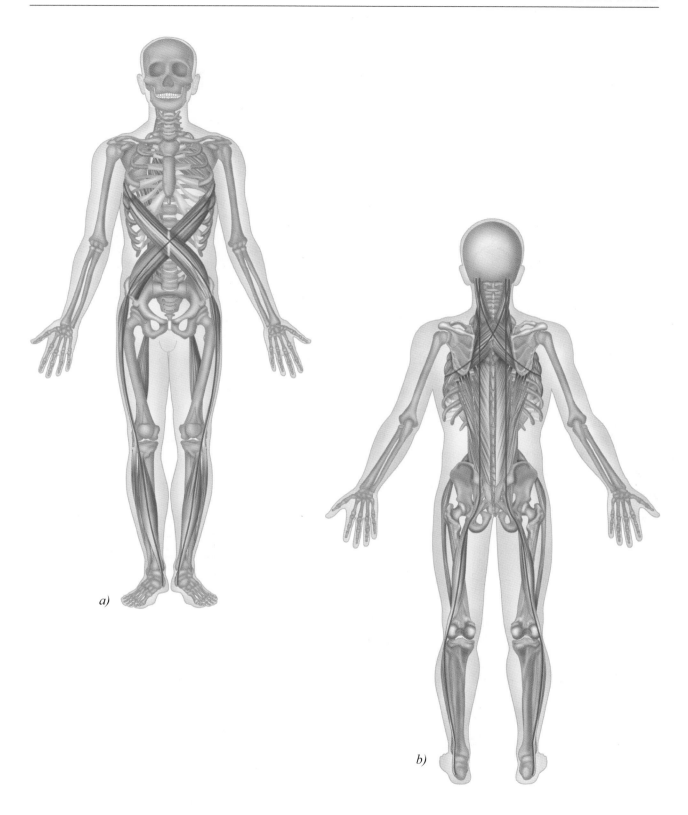

The spiral line (SPL): a) anterior view, b) posterior view.

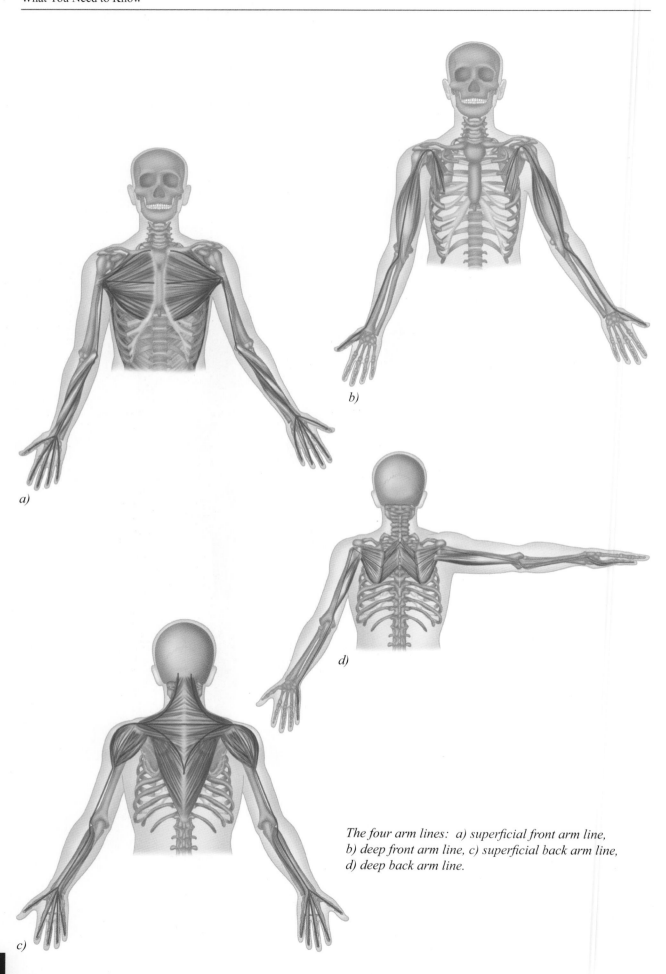

The four arm lines: a) superficial front arm line,
b) deep front arm line, c) superficial back arm line,
d) deep back arm line.

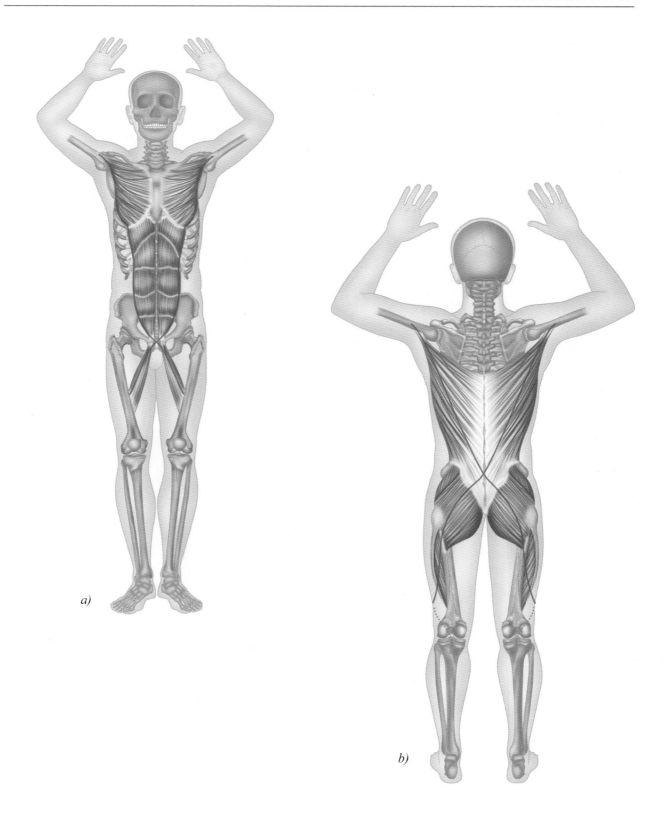

The two functional lines: a) front functional line, b) back functional line.

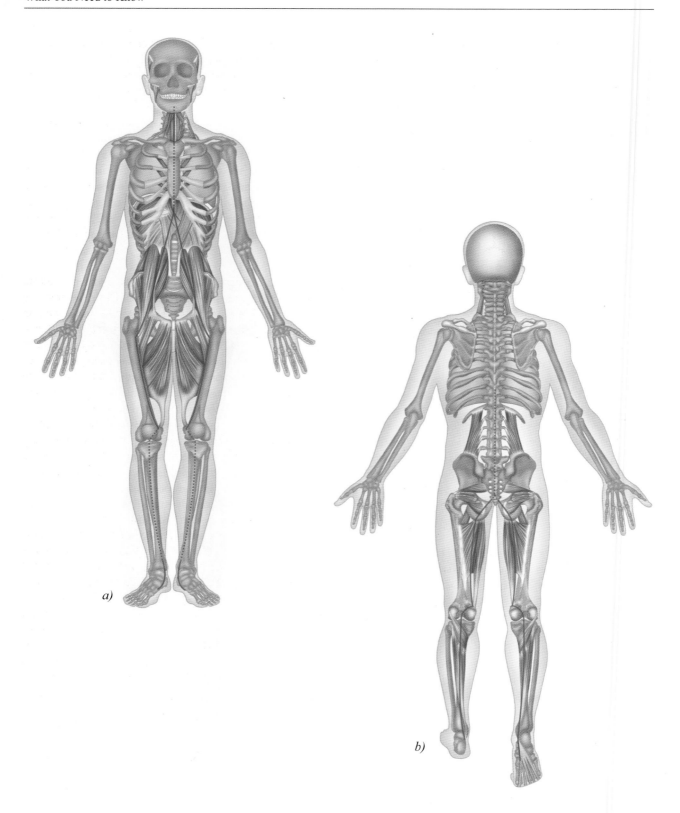

The deep front line (DFL): a) anterior view, b) posterior view.

Full-Body Kinetic Chain Implications, the CNS, and FM

We want to encourage a focus on the role of the CNS (brain and spinal cord) as it shapes and molds itself through movement experiences, to provide the individual with the most efficient selection of muscle synergies. Muscle synergies are the relationships between muscles working as a team to perform a required movement or task. One person may perform a given task more quickly and strongly, more economically in terms of using energy, and less stressfully than another person. Inappropriate synergies cause energy leaks and joint/bone stress, ultimately resulting in pain and/or injury. Inappropriate muscle responses to CNS commands can confuse the CNS, adding to dysfunction. This can be magnified by FM.

The kinetic chain works in a synergistic fashion, providing *eccentric* contractions (muscles contract but lengthen) to decelerate, *isometric* contractions (muscles contract but don't change length) to stabilize, and *concentric* contractions (muscles contract and shorten) to accelerate. To demonstrate, let's look at walking. Standing muscles are contracting to hold you upright, but they're neither shortening nor lengthening: this is an isometric contraction. You begin to walk forward by swinging your right leg forward. You must contract your hip flexors and quadriceps muscles: these are concentric contractions (muscle shortening equals acceleration). As your right leg swings forward, your hamstrings begin to lengthen immediately due to the stretch reflex. The stretch reflex occurs within the muscle being stretched—it is a CNS contraction response that helps regulate the length of the muscle. Your hamstring muscles, although lengthening, contract to slow the swing motion. Otherwise your knee could hit your chin: this is an eccentric contraction. Although this description is simplified, it helps make the point.

Any movement of one body part will have a lesser or greater effect on all other body parts within its kinetic chain. Each kinetic chain includes the fascia and all the soft tissues, as well as the periosteum of the skeletal system and the nervous tissues. If one link in the chain does not operate efficiently due to abuse, overuse, disuse, or neural inhibition, the result will involve a change in function and structure throughout the entire chain. *All* tissues contribute to joint stiffness. For example, the joint capsule comprised of associated ligaments contributes 47%, while the fascia contributes 41% and the tendons 10%. Skin provides the remaining 2%. If a joint is not in its correct alignment, tensional force is placed on the associated soft tissues, continuously changing the length of those soft tissues, and therefore changing the tension relationship those tissues have with related joints. This in turn will affect efficiency throughout the entire body.

Imagine an individual who finishes a daily workout with dozens of repetitions of sit-ups. Doing sit-ups is a common and avoidable TrP perpetuating factor, and an example of inappropriate exercise: it leads to a shortened SCM. The SCM muscles are situated on either side of your neck, and when they shorten they change the curve of your neck, resulting in a head-forward posture. Then you can stack one postural stress on top of another, until the body finds it impossible to compensate to avoid further damage and, ultimately, pain. Sit-ups also place the psoas in a shortened position, grievously stressing a muscle that is often short and spastic. With such postural aberrations, every step you take causes forces that are normally dissipated throughout the kinetic chains to focus in specific tissues such as tendons, ligaments, and bone. Muscles tighten, pulling on fascia and irritating the outer covering of bone, leading to conditions such as bone spurs and low back pain, or to more serious pathology such as stress fractures. Many joint pains originate from kinetic dysfunctions in muscles and connective tissues below or above the joint. The first step in reducing pain is to address postural problems by providing neuromuscular balance to the tissues. Combined therapies such as myofascial release, massage, TrP myotherapy, stretch and spray, and soft tissue release can help correct damaged tissues. They also prevent pain bombardment to the CNS, and thus prevent or ease FM.

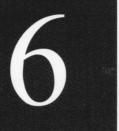

6

Keys to Symptom Management: Identification and Control of Perpetuating Factors

Initiating, Aggravating, and Perpetuating Factors

Anything that perpetuates a TrP is called a "perpetuating factor." Anything that is a TrP perpetuating factor is automatically a fibromyalgia (FM) perpetuating factor, because TrPs perpetuate FM. What initially activates a TrP may be different from what aggravates (worsens) or perpetuates (maintains) it, but they're all commonly called perpetuating factors. *The key to controlling any symptom is the control of as many perpetuating factors as possible.* A good medical history will indicate if pain patterns are stable or evolving. Neither chronic myofascial pain (CMP) nor FM is progressive. The development of satellite TrPs that worsen symptoms, or the appearance of new symptoms, are indicators that there are perpetuating factors out of control. To control symptoms, you must identify and control perpetuating factors. If you don't, then—even with the best treatments in the world—the TrPs will recur. Some people may have perpetuating factors that can't be eliminated, but their impact may be minimized; for these people, CMP can be managed but not cured. The goal is maximum function with minimum symptoms.

We can't cover all possible perpetuating factors in the space we have, but once you understand the concept, you can hunt for them. Patients may need the help of their medical team (metabolic factors) and/or family and friends (diet, postures) to track down some. A care provider will likewise need the help of the patient and his or her companions and/or other medical team members to do the same. Controlling perpetuating factors is important, though TrPs must be treated as well. Perpetuating factors include whatever impairs muscle function, such as anything diminishing the cells' access to oxygen and nutrients, hampering removal of cellular wastes, or adversely affecting the metabolism of the neurotransmitter acetylcholine (ACh). Anything that enhances the formation of TrPs is a perpetuating factor. For instance, anything that constricts the flow of blood to the area will lessen its supply of oxygen and nutrients, adding to the energy crisis. A perpetuating factor can be anything that increases energy demand (trauma, overwork), decreases energy supply (inadequate nutrition, insulin resistance), sensitizes the CNS (pain, noise), decreases oxygen supply (OSA, congestion), enhances release of sensitizing substances (allergies, infections), or increases endplate noise (increased ACh release, reduced acetylcholinesterase). Perpetuating factors are like dragons that chase you wherever you go. They singe you with fiery breath and rake you with claws. Unless you admit that they're there and identify them, you are helpless to control the symptoms they cause. Identifying them isn't always easy, and the first step is to admit they exist; denial is a common perpetuating factor. A woman came to one of the authors (Starlanyl) for a repeat consult, more than a year after the first. When asked what had changed, she replied, "I'm ready to listen now." Denial is a tough dragon to identify. In the dance of life, there are always dragons—the secret is to refuse to let them lead.

Perpetuating Factor Types: All the Colors of Dragons

Just like dragons, perpetuating factors come in different types. Mechanical stressors include paradoxical breathing, body disproportion, muscle abuse, and articular dysfunctions. Metabolic perpetuating factors include impairments to energy metabolism, coexisting conditions such as lack of restorative sleep, and pain. Environmental perpetuating factors include pollution, medications, trauma, and infections. Psychological perpetuating factors include multiple dragons of endless shapes and sizes. Lifestyle perpetuating factors are often the least expensive perpetuating factors to remedy, but may be among the most difficult to maintain. Not all dragons fit easily into one of these groups; some are hybrids, contributing to TrP formation or activation in several ways. For example, obesity may fit into or affect all groups. To further complicate life, perpetuating factors often have perpetuating factors of their own. Consider every identified perpetuating factor to be a new opportunity to gain more control over symptoms. Dragons can be great teachers. The hunt for them may be complicated, but it won't be uninteresting. How many people get to hunt dragons, anyway?

Mechanical Stressors

Paradoxical Breathing

Paradoxical breathing is a common perpetuating factor. It's easier to check for correct breathing if you lie on your back on a firm surface with a hand on your belly. As you breathe in, your belly should swell as the abdominal cavity extends after the lungs expand fully. Breathe out and your belly comes back in. When this occurs, it indicates that your respiratory muscles are relatively flexible. They can expand to accommodate the air you need and expel residual air. If your belly is going in as the breath is coming in, and out as the breath goes out, it's called paradoxical breathing. This includes mouth breathing, and is inefficient and shallow, and usually indicates that your body isn't getting the oxygen it needs. Paradoxical breathing can occur temporarily during a time of congestion, such as a cold, and then may be maintained out of habit, or because TrPs have formed in the diaphragm or other respiratory muscles, inhibiting their flexibility. Training and awareness of proper breathing technique is important, but it's just one step in the process. Is adequate air coming in through the nose, or is there congestion? If so, why? Check into the possibility of allergies, low-grade sinusitis (often caused by fungal infection), or other problems. A TrP assessment is also needed, as TrPs can cause congestion, and their presence in respiratory muscles prevents these muscles from working properly. All the breath training in the world won't help if the diaphragm is rigid with TrPs. An assessment for TrPs includes accessory respiratory muscles, such as the scalenes.

Body Disproportion

Disproportion can stress the body significantly. Effects can start in school, or even earlier due to a poorly fitting highchair. If the upper part of the arms is comparatively short, elbows can't reach most armrests, so there is a tendency to lean to one side: this stresses shoulder elevator muscles. If you usually sit on the same side of a sofa with an armrest too low for you, the side that leans to reach the armrest is compressed, and the other side is held in a static stretch. This imbalance may show up in photos. Photos can be a great investigative tool for discovering postural perpetuating factors. If the torso is proportionally long, there's more chance for compression beneath the thighs when you sit. The same is true for people of short stature or with proportionally short lower legs. When there's no room between the bottom of the thighs and the chair, circulation is impaired. These perpetuating factors may often be remedied with a footstool of appropriate height. Proportionally short upper arms may be remedied by finding chairs with arms that fit or by adding height to the armrests by taping pads to them. Parents can check to see that their baby's legs don't dangle from a high chair, or that the school desk and chair fit their child. Once you identify the dragon, bring it under control. Short upper arms, short lower legs, and a long torso can occur together.

A common TrP perpetuator is a type of Morton's foot, in which a relatively short first and proportionally long second metatarsal occur (see Chapter 12). Look for excessive wear on the outside of the heel and on the inside of the sole of the shoe above the big toe. High heels, shoes too small, tight shoe cap, or pointed-toe shoes make this problem worse. You may need boots and shoes with maximum heels at ¾" (about 1.9 cm). See what works for you. Feet that are wide in front and narrow in back can be very difficult to fit for shoes. Ill-fitting shoes cause abnormal stress. Flat feet can be a perpetuating factor, as can abnormally high arches. Anything that affects the gait can be a perpetuating factor, whether a bone deformity or a pebble in the shoe.

Overlarge breasts require the body and the brain to work harder to keep the head erect, affecting posture. It can be difficult to find an unconstricting bra with straps that don't cut into the skin. Research indicates breast reduction surgery in symptomatic individuals can bring about a "significant improvement in … pain, disability, muscle weakness and poor posture," (Chao et al. 2002), although FM is a risk factor for poor outcome (Henry, Crawford, and Puckett 2009). Obesity is linked with musculoskeletal pain (Hooper et al. 2006). Mechanically, it affects posture and hip joint placement, with decreased range of forward motion that alters posture and gait. Abdominal obesity with a lax, pendulous abdomen is often a sign of coexisting insulin resistance. It's also associated with TrPs in the rectus abdominis, TFL and other regional muscles. Causes of asymmetry include adhesions, scars, and other TrPs that restrict ROM. Problems occur when fascia sticks to other tissues in ways it wasn't designed to do, and the body must compensate. Similar compensation occurs with hypermobile joints, one-sided deafness or vision problems, contractured muscles, glare on a computer screen, and many other perpetuating factors.

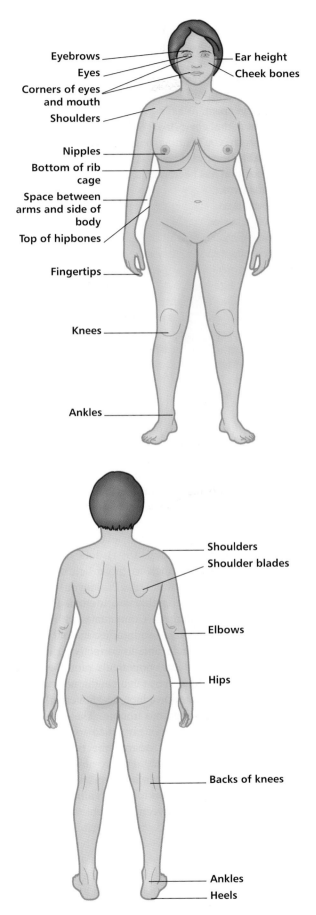

Eyebrows
Eyes
Corners of eyes and mouth
Shoulders
Nipples
Bottom of rib cage
Space between arms and side of body
Top of hipbones
Fingertips
Knees
Ankles

Ear height
Cheek bones

Shoulders
Shoulder blades
Elbows
Hips
Backs of knees
Ankles
Heels

Body symmetry check.

If your body isn't naturally balanced, it'll find a way to compensate, overworking other muscles and increasing the chance of TrP activation and perpetuation. It helps to have a professional assessment, but patients can check basic frontal symmetry in a long mirror. Check facial features for symmetry: eyebrows, eyes, corners of the eyes and mouth, cheek bones, and ear height. (Do you need an earpiece adjusted on new eyeglasses? Check for temporalis or other adjacent TrPs.) Check the shoulders, the nipples, the bottom of the rib cage, the space between the arms and the sides of the body, and the height of the fingertips. Do they match? What about the top of the hipbones, the knees and the ankles? How is the spacing between the knees and the ankles? Check out back symmetry too. Are shoulders and shoulder blades even? Do the elbows and hips match? What about the backs of the knees, ankles, and heels? Check for asymmetry from the side as well, to see if there is tilting forward or backward from the hip or neck. Any sign of asymmetry is a signal to check for TrPs. What other clues do you see? Excess weight in one area can cause stress on tissues supporting that area.

Unequal leg length can be misunderstood. A structural leg inequality of even $3/16$" (0.5 cm) can significantly tilt the body. What's more common, especially in people with TrPs, is pelvic torsion, drawing one thigh higher into the pelvis and creating a *functionally* short leg. In this case, if one adds a heel lift to the shorter leg, it compounds the problem, reinforcing the torque. It's a short-term solution causing a long-term problem. True leg length inequality is a clue to check the whole body for proportional shortness on that side and for compensation on the other side. When the horizontal core stabilizers, including deep ligaments and tendons, are not at healthy lengths, a spiral compensating effect can occur, called rotoscoliosis. This is a torque of tissues around the spinal column and can begin anywhere, but the end result may be torsion of the feet, ankles, knees, hips, and shoulders. One area twists right and the other twists left to compensate. The body seeks harmony and balance, but this compensatory twisting can create functional hypermobility or restriction in many areas.

One often-overlooked asymmetry is a one-sided small hemipelvis. Hmmmn? The knee bone's connected to the thighbone … you don't remember a hemipelvis? It rarely occurs in everyday conversation. If one or both bowl-shaped areas that make up one side of the pelvis (the hemipelvis) are smaller than the other side, it will cause body asymmetry.

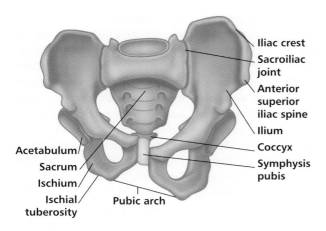

Hemipelvis.

The right and left hemipelvis should match. When the hemipelvis is smaller on one side, if you're sitting on a flat surface, the upper curve of one hip is higher than the other. Scoliosis and pelvic rotation can develop as other muscles struggle to compensate. The quadratus lumborum (QL) muscle is greatly affected by an asymmetrical hemipelvis, with the SCMs and scalenes struggling to adjust to the overload from tilted thoracic muscles. Care providers trained in TrPs can help correct this asymmetry. A properly fitted butt lift will compensate. The lift may be anything from a foam pad to a small booklet or magazine.

Muscle Abuse

Abuse of muscles takes many forms. Muscles are designed to work when warm and flexible. Pushing them to work hard when they are exhausted, chilled, or dehydrated is asking for trouble, and that's what they give you when treated this way. It can be very difficult for FM patients to learn to pace themselves, and they tend to misjudge their limits and overdo, collapsing afterwards, this repeats in a yo-yo pattern. Poor posture results in significant muscle abuse. Any postural habit that causes prolonged muscle fiber contraction can cause TrPs (Edwards 2005). Posture affects respiration, and can interact with vestibular dysfunction, compounding the symptoms (Yates et al. 2002). Become attentive to standing, sitting, and sleeping postures. Any cervical pillow must fit the curvature of your neck to support it without stressing coexisting TrPs. The size and shape of the pillow may need changing as your neck and shoulders respond to treatment. Find the bed that allows sleep in a posture that is healthy and won't perpetuate TrPs. Many bad posture habits can be identified and corrected, such as head-forward posture, bracing arms on knees, crossing legs, side leaning, and crossing arms to prop up weak muscles. These habits are often clues to locations of TrPs or other perpetuating factors such as facet pathology.

If posture is a problem, find out why. The human spine curves into a C-shape or S-shape to maintain the head in an upright position. Care providers and patients can learn to track TrP cascades from medical history. Patients—hunt for misfitting furniture, especially at work or anywhere static time is spent. What's your desk or work surface like? What's the chair like? Are they ergonomically designed to fit you? Sitting positions affect spinal and musculoskeletal stresses. As shown below, the head-forward position has been with us throughout time, from the caveman era.

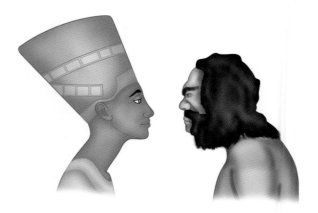

The neck angle, covered or not, indicates the head forward perpetuating factor has been with us for a long time (After Shifflett, C.M., 2011).

A job may be a key perpetuating factor, and can be a hybrid dragon with multiple claws. "Occupational exposure to muscle load should be described by three factors to indicate health risks: level, repetitiveness and duration" (Westgaard et al. 1994). Jobs that require static awkward postures such as those held by dental hygienists can be recipes for TrPs. Prolonged standing, sitting, bending, and immobility are trouble. Look for options and accommodations. Computer work is also a common cause of repetitive-use injuries, including TrPs (Treaster et al. 2006). To be able to correctly strike keys with the tips of the fingers, fingernails must be short. Material for copying must be at eye height, not lying on the desk. Repetitive motions include shoveling snow, raking leaves, vacuuming, and ironing. The old saying "If you want something done, give it to someone who is overworked" is a way to destroy the best workers. People who excel at what they do may already tend to push themselves too far. Their managers may need to intervene to lighten their workload (Davidheiser 1991). It may be the difference between being able to work and being disabled by work.

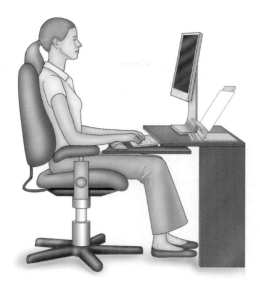

Ergonomic computer station. 1) Sufficient desk space, 2) Feet flat on foot stool or floor, 3) Adjustable chair height, 4) Thigh level on chair, 5) Chair back supporting curves, 6) Screen distance approx. 1.5–2ft away, 7) Screen slightly below eye level, 8) Wrist rest (when required), 9) Elbow bent at 90-degree angle.

Actions have consequences, no matter what the occupation or hobby. Soldiers wearing body armor suffer increased musculoskeletal pain (Konitzer et al. 2008). Children using backpacks that are poorly designed and overly stuffed with heavy items require more than better backpacks; they need education on how to wear a backpack and how to pack to minimize load. Children with TrPs may require an extra set of books to keep at home, to avoid having to carry so much weight back and forth. Patients in wheelchairs can have more compression TrPs in weight-bearing areas, but don't forget TrPs in the neck and shoulder areas from looking up and twisting to talk to standing people. Walkers are often horribly designed, improperly fitted, and cause TrPs. Poor body mechanics include putting on shoes and pants without stabilizing the body, lifting incorrectly, and leaning over sideways to lift while twisting. They include anything that can jerk the body into an abrupt correction, such as a near fall.

Sustained contraction, such as reaching up repeatedly to fold sheets or holding a power tool in a sustained position may cause arms and shoulders to scream in protest. Leaving a muscle in a shortened position can activate latent TrPs (Travell and Simons 1992, p. 19). Artificially induced stiffness has a significant effect on balance control (Gruneberg et al. 2004); thus, logically, the effect of stiffness caused by TrPs would be as profound. Immobility of a sort happens when ROM is restricted due to TrPs. We often experience this as we get older: if it hurts to move a muscle through the full ROM, we restrict the motion. Our comfortable range of motion gets smaller and smaller, like a cage with the walls moving inward. "The stiffness and the relatively painless but progressive restriction of movement that characterize decrepitude of advancing age are often due to latent TrPs" (Simons, Travell, and Simons 1999, p. 113). Lack of coordinated movement, which can cause TrPs, is often maintained by TrPs.

Constricting clothing is an enemy. This includes tight waistbands, socks, bras, heavy purses, and watches. Any restriction of fluid to or from an area contributes to an energy crisis. Nye Ffarrabas, a friend of this author (Starlanyl), says clothes for men were made to wear; clothes for women were made to be seen in. Stick the fashion police in the dragon parking lot. (Everybody needs a dragon parking lot. Don't feed the things after you park them: they're worse than tribbles.) Unsuitable shoes can be major perpetuating factors. Incorrect fit is a problem; poor design is a crime. Even heels 1½″ high can torque knee joints (Kerrigan et al. 2005). Some patients can't tolerate that. You may need to look for boots and shoes with heels at a maximum of ¾″ (about 1.9 cm). Shoe soles, including inserts, need to be *flexible*. Before buying orthotics for hyperpronation, identify the *cause* of the hyperpronation. Tailor treatment to needs. Cookbook medicine doesn't work in the myofascial world. Flexible shoe inserts themselves wear down, and must be checked periodically. As muscles respond to treatment, corrections must be adjusted accordingly.

One of the most preventable of perpetuating factors is inappropriate exercise. *You cannot strengthen muscles that have TrPs.* One of the authors (Starlanyl) heard Janet Travell and David Simons say that so many times. TrP-laden muscles are physiologically contractured. In the contraction nodule and taut band, sarcomeres are either too long or too short. The muscle must first be brought to a healthy state before attempting to strengthen. Overdoing a good exercise can also do damage. Stretching a muscle too far too fast can cause reactive shortening. Even stretch and spray therapy can be used to push a muscle too far. Care providers must understand this, or they themselves can become perpetuating factors. If you treat a patient with TrPs, you must *know* TrPs, otherwise you can do harm. For example, a podiatrist prescribing a walking cast without explaining to the patient the necessity of equal-height matching of the other shoe might cause extensive damage to the patient, requiring expensive and painful rehabilitation.

Articular Dysfunction

Joint dysfunction may interact with TrPs. Any mechanical stress affecting joint position can initiate the process of OA (Solomon, Schnitzler, and Browett 1982). Any arthritis treatment and prevention program needs to include treatment of coexisting TrPs (Cummings 2003a). Treating TrPs improves neuromuscular function and coordination. Anything that improves neuromuscular function can prevent or slow the progression of OA (Loeser and Shakoor 2003). Uneven contraction of muscles can cause or contribute to temporomandibular joint dysfunction (TMJD) and may cause bone misalignment (Koolstra and van Eijden 2005), and TrPs can cause uneven contraction. Uneven muscle contraction may be sufficient to cause jaw articular disc erosion (Liu et al. 2000). Much pain and expense may be prevented by prompt treatment of TrPs.

The spine and local TrPs interact. Active TrPs are associated with neck vertebral-disc lesions (Hsueh et al. 1998). As surrounding soft tissues are unevenly contractured due to TrPs, vertebrae may shift slightly out of alignment. Bones follow muscles. The misalignment irritates intervertebral discs. Intervertebral disc adjustments and their associated ligamentous attachment compensations cause changes in the angular motion of the body. This further stresses the inferior and superior intervertebral discs of the cervical spine (Kumaresan, Yoganandan, and Pintar 1999). It isn't unusual for one vertebral surgery to be followed by subsequent surgeries on vertebrae above and/or below the first. Soft tissue is often neglected, as it doesn't show up on imaging. Disc deterioration may further alter motion and muscle compensation, which can contribute to further pathologies in facet joints, muscles, and ligaments, resulting in a chronic pain state (Brisby 2006). Don't neglect facet joints: they can be pain-generating (and TrP-generating) dragons. In a turf battle, the turf (patient) never wins. Disc deformity or bone spurs that show on imaging may not be the *cause* of pain. Surgery performed without soft tissue evaluations can result in failed back surgery (Dubousset 2003). Subsequent surgical scars, adhesions, and TrPs, and postsurgical tightening of soft tissue, can cause added stress on adjacent vertebrae, leading to more surgeries as the pain continues. By this time, FM has often developed.

Metabolic Perpetuating Factors

Nutritional Inadequacies

You are what you *absorb*. Absorption varies from person to person, but the general principles are as follows. The stomach is lined with mucus to protect it from digestive acids. The gastric mucosa is formed of cells that secrete mucous gel, endocrine cells that secrete regulatory hormones, cells that secrete hydrochloric acid, and cells that secrete an enzyme needed to digest proteins. This is a simple description of complex processes. For example, cells that secrete digestive protein enzymes also secrete a factor allowing B12 to pass through the small intestine and do its job. Absorption of most nutrients occurs mainly in the small intestine; the small intestinal wall also has a mucosa. There are convolutions along the intestinal wall that greatly increase surface area, allowing a rapid flow of substances through the intestine into the body, and wastes from the body back into the intestine.

There are two ways in which molecules pass through the gastrointestinal barrier into the body. One way is directly through the cell. This is controlled by the integrity of the cell membrane and a variety of channels controlled by molecular gates. The other way is *in between* cells at cellular junctions. A healthy gut constitutes a barrier so tight that it forces nutrients to be converted into a form that allows them to be transported across the cell through the channels. When this barrier is damaged, a condition called leaky gut syndrome, or hyperpermeable gut, occurs. This condition is associated with chronic pain states (Jones and Quinn 2005–6). Unprocessed or partially digested nutrients, foreign substances, and large amino acids can leak through these damaged permeable junctions. The body may then mount a defense against these intruders, and allergies, intolerance, or sensitivity to them may then develop.

People in pain often consume over-the-counter (OTC) pain medications as a first-line treatment. These may be taken on an empty stomach or with acidic drinks. They can be purchased easily and are relatively inexpensive, and there are no drug police ready to pounce on doctors who recommend them or patients who take them. Many anti-inflammatory medications can damage the gastric lining, as can: excess alcohol consumption; bacterial, viral, yeast, or other toxins; or anything that affects the ability of those lining cells to heal after damage. ATP is the main cellular energy supplier; when it's depleted, more energy is needed to get inefficient systems to work, and we become fatigued more quickly. As more and more breaches in the intestinal barrier are created, the gut becomes even more dysfunctional. Nutrients that need to pass the gut lining may not be allowed through, and molecules that are not intended to pass the barrier may do so.

There is an interactive relationship between permeable bowel and chronic illness, although individual requirements of specific biochemicals for the efficient running of our metabolism can vary greatly from person to person. The medical text *Textbook of Functional Medicine* (Jones and Quinn 2005–6) gives care providers the strategies needed to manage chronic illness. Sequencing of treatment is important to the healing of the gut. First remove gastrointestinal irritants, next replace deficient digestive factors such as enzymes, then restore healthy intestinal flora, and finally begin to repair the intestinal mucosa. A healthy diet must be started and maintained. We get in trouble when we use resources faster than we replenish them. People with chronic conditions often have greater nutrient requirements than healthy individuals. We are beginning to understand more about the difference between obvious nutritional *deficiency* and a state of nutritional *inadequacy*. Warning to readers who are patients—complex but important biochemical concept approaching!

The body is a wondrous organism that takes raw substances such as oxygen and food and turns them into the biochemicals needed to maintain it. It ensures that those substances are delivered where they are needed in the proper form to be used. It removes wastes and excess materials, and sees that these residues leave the body appropriately. Each step in the processes involved is itself a complex string of biochemical reactions, and every reaction has a *rate-limiting* step.

What's a rate-limiting step? Imagine you're a traveler on a cruise ship. This ship is anchored offshore in a port that's not deep enough for the ship. A smaller ship, called a tender, must ferry passengers to shore. Once ashore, passengers spend money on goods and services for sale. Local merchants need tourist money; the tourists need, or want, goods and services for sale. Before the passenger is transformed into a purchasing tourist, the tender must ferry them and their money to shore. That tender, or another one like it, must then transport the tourists and their purchases back to the ship. The tender capacity is the rate-limiting step. Say you have 2000 people on the ship and most want to spend time ashore, and you have ten tenders that carry twenty people each trip. That takes some scheduling, but it's doable, especially if you're spending all day at dock. If you only have three tenders with a capacity of eight passengers each, and two tenders have engine trouble, you've got a "bottleneck." There can be many rate-limiting steps. What if some tender pilots have the flu? The number of working pilots then becomes the rate-limiting step. This happens metabolically too. Many vitamins and minerals function as tenders and pilots and in other roles, working to turn the cruise passengers into tourists, and allow them to complete their missions, leave port and to return to the ship. These biochemical reactions can proceed only as fast as the rate-limiting step allows.

There's wide variation in individual requirements for specific vitamins, minerals, and other necessary substances. We metabolize differently, and we absorb differently. A healthy diet is the best defense against vitamin insufficiency, but individual needs for vitamin and mineral supplements vary according to absorption ability, metabolic efficiency, and many other factors. The ability to provide wholesome meals may be affected by multiple factors such as depression, inability to create and serve wholesome nutritious meals, poverty, dietary excitotoxins (e.g. aspartame and MSG), IBS, gluten intolerance, and other coexisting conditions. Nutrient insufficiency can arise when, for a particular nutrient, there is inadequate intake, impaired absorption, impaired or increased metabolism, increased metabolic need, or increased excretion. Alcohol, oral contraceptives, and other factors, including foods, can interfere with absorption of some vitamins, and some work better when taken with other vitamins, minerals, and foods.

We are largely made up of water. We cannot live without it. Most of us take it in insufficient quantities. We consume dehydrating foods, medications, and liquids, and may live in a state of chronic dehydration. By the time thirst is evident, you are already dehydrated. High-quality water is precious. We must protect our water resources and use them wisely. Investigate your own water sources. You may need a good water filtration system; think of it as insurance, and be sure that you get the right one for your needs and that you know how to (and can) maintain it properly.

Metabolic and endocrine inadequacy and resistance are common perpetuating factors, and are often unrecognized. These include, but are not limited to, multiple hormone imbalances, hypothyroid, reactive hypoglycemia, insulin resistance and/or thyroid resistance, diabetes, and anemia (including sickle cell trait). These conditions may cause many broken or impaired links in multiple metabolic chains, and can create complicated metabolic knots to unravel. As with myofascia, everything in the body is connected to everything else: one needs to understand the relationship of growth hormone to deep sleep, tryptophan to melatonin, estrogen to serotonin, and T3 (triiodothyronine) to hyaluronic acid, as well as all the other complex interconnections. It is necessary also to understand what can happen when they don't quite connect properly due to insufficiencies, resistance, and imbalances, to treat these perpetuating factors.

As one example, thyroid hormones are part of energy production and consumption and also growth. T4 is the inactive form of the thyroid hormone, and must be converted to T3 before the body uses it. Some of us may have adequate T4 but are unable to metabolize it to T3; a condition known as thyroid resistance. That is one possible cause of hypothyroid symptoms, although in this case the thyroid hormone T4 would test just fine and the problem would be missed. There are many possible causes of thyroid deficiency or insufficiency, but commonly used blood tests for hormones often take for granted that other metabolic balances are in place. The TSH level has been used as an indicator of thyroid function, but is unreliable in chronic pain states (Tsigos and Chrousos 2002). TSH amounts are regulated through the hypothalamus in a feedback loop. In chronic pain states, as with other chronic stressors, the HPA-axis can be out of balance, and the hypothalamus feedback loop may not be functioning as expected and as needed for this test to work. The use of opioids can further impact human TSH levels (Vuong et al. 2009). Research has shown that patients with central sensitization who test normal on thyroid hormones but have hypothyroid symptoms may still require T3 supplementation (Lowe et al. 1997). Patients with low thyroid levels do better on a mix of both T3 and T4 (Eisinger 1999). Thyroid equilibrium is found by monitoring patient symptoms, not by blood tests. There are many possible causes of, and contributors to, thyroid insufficiency, and this is just *one* aspect of *one* hormone. Unraveling endocrine imbalances takes expertise, time and care.

Some care providers, especially physicians, have been trained in the art of differential diagnoses. That process presupposes that there is only one condition, and includes the elimination of other diagnoses. The patient is then labeled with that one condition, and the diagnostic work generally stops. This process has been woefully inadequate for chronic pain and other chronic conditions. Patients with conditions such as Parkinson's disease or arthritis are not treated for coexisting TrPs. Patients with TrPs too often have all their symptoms lumped under the general label of FM. Patients with chronic pain almost always have multiple diagnoses, and they often interact. This author (Starlanyl) has found that successfully treating chronic pain and many other chronic illnesses requires a new set of diagnostic skills, namely that of interactive diagnoses—the ability to identify and manage multiple interactive conditions. For example, a patient with osteoarthritis can develop weakness in her upper body due to latent TrPs in the scalene muscles. This weakness affects her ability to get around using a walker, and she becomes unable to provide adequate nutrition for herself. Nausea, gastrointestinal irritation, and intestinal permeability caused by medications taken on an empty stomach result in further food restriction. She develops IBS, GERD, and insulin resistance, with TrPs in the abdomen, hips, and back. Prescribed upper body strengthening exercises activate the TrPs, increasing pain and causing more weakness, so medication dosages are raised. Her diet worsens due to further irritation from the medications, resulting in a lack of nutrients needed to provide rate-limiting steps for a variety of metabolic functions. The IBS and GERD activate TrPs in the upper abdominal obliques and diaphragm, contributing to IBS symptoms and paradoxical breathing, further worsening the TrPs. Activity lessens because of increased pain, worsening the OA. The GERD irritates primary scalene TrPs, which have developed satellites in the upper back, shoulders, and arms, further worsening upper body weakness. Increased mucus forms to protect the nasopharyngeal area from GERD acid irritation, adding swallowing difficulty to eating problems. She is prescribed antacids and proton-pump inhibitors, further adding to intestinal permeability and digestion dysfunction, and her doctors have no clue as to why her pain and weakness keep increasing and her illness continues to "progress." This type of worsening symptom spiral is common, but often goes unrecognized in chronic illness, especially in the elderly.

Reactive hypoglycemia is a commonly missed coexisting diagnosis. With this condition, a few hours after eating a high-carbohydrate meal, the body produces excess insulin as a reaction to that meal, prompting an adrenalin response. This response can include tremors, rapid heart rate, and sweating. If this condition is not treated with patient education and dietary modification, insulin resistance usually develops. More and more insulin is produced, which prompts the production of excess glucose. The extra glucose is not used by the muscles, because the mitochondria—the energy factories of the cells—have become resistant to the insulin, whose function is normally to take glucose into the cells. So the poor, rejected glucose goes off to sulk and builds a fat pad over the abdomen, causing abdominal obesity. The muscles remain energy depleted. Insulin resistance and abdominal obesity are epidemic in some countries. Obesity may be common in chronic pain states through more than lack of exercise or faulty eating habits. Studies have linked skeletal muscle tissue and regulation of intracellular cortisol to metabolic syndrome, which includes insulin resistance and abdominal obesity (Whorwood et al. 2002). Obesity is a symptom and may have more than one cause. Obesity itself can create inflammatory changes in the body and may interact with other mechanisms in chronic pain (Wellen and Hotamisligil 2003).

Fibromyalgia

FM central sensitization can enhance symptoms of food, contact, or inhalant allergies, and may make development of sensitivities easier. Chemical intolerance (CI) is also common; even a perfumed person passing by may set off a toxic reaction (Anderson and Anderson 1998). All of this adds to the toxic environment of sick skeletal tissue and the energy crisis that promotes TrP formation and maintenance. Many patients with FM and TrPs have undiagnosed vestibular dysfunction: symptoms can include balance problems, vestibular migraine, posture control problems, and cognitive dysfunction including dizziness, memory problems, attention deficits, loss of focus, and sequencing problems. The combination of balance problems from some TrPs, FM, and vestibular dysfunction can be overwhelming. What helps one FM patient may not work for another, as different metabolic cascades are involved with each patient, and different biochemical imbalances must be corrected. Care providers and patients must understand that the healing process takes time. FM is not progressive. It may seem so, because TrPs develop satellite TrPs and new symptoms and conditions can crop up if perpetuating factors are not controlled.

Lack of Restorative Sleep

It's not normal to wake up feeling as if you haven't slept. When we sleep, our bodies and brains are still working. Much cellular repair and biochemical balancing occurs during deeper levels of sleep, and this often doesn't happen in FM. Microtrauma that occurs during the day will not be stitched up and mended by cellular construction crews if there is no deep-level sleep, or if deep sleep is fragmented or insufficient. Pain from TrPs can profoundly affect not only the quantity but also the quality of sleep, so both these aspects must be assessed. Amazingly, many studies evaluating sleep in FM patients have ignored TrPs. Research indicates an interactive connection between pain and sleep (Roehrs and Roth 2005). Lack of restorative sleep may have multiple perpetuating factors, and a sleep study is the key to help identify them, including GERD, sleep apnea, congestion, and restless legs. A good sleep study will reveal even the silent form of GERD that has no obvious symptoms but can still damage tissues and cause TrPs. GERD may activate laryngeal TrPs, and GERD episodes that occur while sleeping supine can activate jaw muscle activities, causing (among other things) bruxism (Miyawaki et al. 2004). Insomnia can contribute to loss of sleep, which perpetuates TrPs, and TrPs cause further loss of sleep. Insomnia in chronic pain patients may not be due to the pain, and must not be dismissed as such or considered to be a "normal" part of aging: it must be treated (Schneider-Helmert et al. 2001).

Pain Itself

Chronic pain is recognized as a condition in its own right. One of the body's first responses to pain is to tense the muscles. Research shows that people with low back pain develop a guarding postural rigidity that further restricts movement (Brumagne et al. 2008). Pain itself can cause major metabolic changes, such as the development of insulin resistance (Griesen et al. 2001). It can affect neural plasticity, leading to FM. Yet undertreatment of pain is common in childhood (Snidvongs, Nagararatnam, and Stephens 2008) old age (Tal, Gurevich, and Guller 2009), and in between (Galvez 2009).

Environmental Factors

Cold, heat, drafts, chilling, changes in barometric pressure—all have been reported as having effects on myofascial TrP activation and FM. Abrupt climatic changes may increase symptoms. Drafts and chill can initiate and maintain TrPs. The body is an ecosystem, but not a closed ecosystem. Our world that impacts us in many ways: we breathe, we eat, and we feel the air and what it contains touch our skins. There is a correlation between ambient air pollution and oxygen saturation, which has direct TrP ramifications. We are exposed to a variety of toxic substances that enter or surround our bodies, and only some of these are within our control.

Everyone, for their own self-interest, should become an environmentalist. There are some things we can control—to some extent. We can control some of what we put into our bodies. When most people consider high-risk behavior they think about people who free-fall skydive or bungee jump. I (Starlanyl) think about people who smoke, or eat inorganic potatoes.

Part of the environment is the weather. Patients with FM and/or hypometabolism may be more sensitive to weather changes. Many patients have reported that abrupt changes increase their symptoms. There was an interesting hypothesis put forward by Robert Gerwin MD at the Myopain 2007 International MYOPAIN Society Seventh World Congress (August 19-23) that formation of myofascial TrPs could be due to a calcium channelopathy. Perhaps it is such a disorder in the ionic calcium membrane channel of the cell that causes some of us to have difficulty adjusting to temperature and pressure changes. If so, this could be amplified by coexisting FM. It is to be hoped that more research is forthcoming in this area.

Pollution

Smoking is a direct form of pollution that affects TrPs in many ways. Nicotine causes blood vessel constriction, increases microcirculation problems, and adds to the energy crisis of TrPs. It blocks oxygen uptake in the lungs. Carbon monoxide binds to hemoglobin, so that it can't carry oxygen. Those of us with TrPs already have more than enough toxins to process, so avoid adding to the problem. Avoid substances such as high-fructose corn syrup, margarine, or aspartame. Eat as organic and as local as possible. Don't let more toxins into the body than can be metabolized and removed. The bug repellant DEET inhibits acetylcholinesterase, the enzyme that breaks down ACh (Corbel et al 2009), and could enhance TrP formation or chronicity.

Allergy

When you think of allergy, you may think of a runny nose or an itch, but allergies can also target muscles or the brain. Allergy and pollution decrease oxygen saturation in the blood (DeMeo et al. 2004). Allergies add to histamine levels, and histamine is a substance released by TrPs when they twitch (Shah et al. 2005). "… TrPs are aggravated by high histamine levels and active allergies" (Simons, Travell, and Simons 1999, p. 105). Allergies can add to conditions such as congestion, swelling, and nerve impingement, all of which can intensify difficulty falling asleep. Allergy skin testing may not give valid results if the area tested is riddled with TrPs, and the skin and underlying areas are tight and stuck together. After a time of successful TrP treatment in an allergy skin test area such as the upper arm, there may be an increasing response to allergens in testing. This doesn't necessarily mean that the allergies are worsening; it may indicate that microcirculation is improving. We all must learn to balance risk and benefit. For example, I (Starlanyl) have three furpetuating factors. I am allergic to cats, but the benefits I derive by being owned by them (I'm not in denial) outweigh the risks, and this opinion is shared by the cats.

Medications

Many medications have muscle pain and tightness as side effects. Check before adding any new medication, including OTC preparations. Don't depend on the manufacturer for information. For example, the risk of statin use for patients who already have oxygen-starved areas must be weighed carefully (Tomlinson and Mangione 2005). Increased release of calcium ions Ca^{2+} is an essential part of the TrP formation hypothesis as we understand it today. Statins may cause TrP cascade activation that doesn't abate until statins are discontinued (Sirvent et al. 2005).

Trauma

Trauma includes cumulative repetitive trauma such as keyboarding, orchestrated trauma such as surgery, and many aspects of daily life that you may not suspect, such as walking untrained dogs. There are low back pain TrPs that appear during late pregnancy, and postpartum cervical TrPs from straining during labor. There are falls off ladders and chairs, and slips and slides on mud, ice, and snow. Furniture and other obstacles that are within frequent travel paths are perpetuating factors waiting to happen. During surgical procedures, medications can obliterate normal muscle tone. If there is a lack of adequate support during surgery, the immobile patient in the chilly operating room may be in trouble (spelled T-r-P-s). This can be compounded because of neck hyperextension during intubation and failure to adequately relieve pain before, during, and after surgery. Patients may develop TrPs covered with a geloid mass in areas where corners of tables or other furniture have repeatedly impacted. The body forms what protection it can.

Infections and Infestations

Any kind of infection or infestation, including viruses, bacteria, molds and yeasts, mycobacteria, mycoplasmas, and/or parasites can initiate or perpetuate TrPs. They may initiate new TrPs or perpetuate ones already active, starting from a few days before symptoms manifested and lasting for weeks after the symptoms have gone. Most of those little buggies deplete your oxygen, and cause havoc among the systems of the body.

Psychological Factors

No amount of cognitive behavior therapy will cause a physiologically contracted muscle to relax (although it may soothe other muscles). It takes physical intervention.

That being said, having a chronic illness is difficult. When the illness is invisible and poorly understood, it can be overwhelming. When there are no objective findings, such as blood tests, there can be misunderstandings that lead, among other things, to lack of support. Patients with TrPs can lose resilience through the grind of coping with a seemingly endless series of doctors and diagnoses, symptoms and promises, and procedures and medications, until they are financially, mentally, emotionally, spiritually, and physically exhausted. Patients look fine and are expected to act accordingly. If patients feel guilty about having symptoms that nobody understands, they may push themselves to keep up; coworkers and family members may push them even more. This can contribute to the "good-sport syndrome," also called invincible ignorance. Patients often don't want to be singled out and they want to feel useful, so they volunteer and help others, over and over, hurting themselves in the process. This can be especially dangerous if they have toxic relationships with people who disbelieve their symptoms. When they can no longer perform up to expectations, they may be ridiculed. No matter how well adjusted the patient is when chronic pain begins, it causes a psychological burden. This may be greater if the patient has suffered in silence, trying to perform at work or school, and has missed time that was unexplainable or has been unable to complete assignments. This may be compounded by expensive and sometimes painful therapies and procedures that may have resulted in even more extensive symptoms. There is no failure or guilt involved in needing help to cope with this reality.

> Added burdens of invisible illnesses
> If I had no legs, you would not ask me to bear your burden.
> If I had no eyes, you would not ask me to be your guide through treacherous paths.
> If I had no hands, you would not ask me to bake your bread.
> My handicaps are invisible, so you ask this all of me, and more.

Do your best to keep positive. Living with chronic invisible pain can be a relentless challenge. The grind can wear you down. It's all well and good to say that if Plan A doesn't work, switch to Plan B, but when you are already trying Plan Z and seeing double letters ahead and it's not yet time for lunch, frustration can be a daunting dragon. There are always options. You have chronic pain—it doesn't have you. Finding and maintaining a positive attitude is a big step towards improving quality of life. It isn't easy, but it's possible. Events that once caused frustration can become educational opportunities. Positive choices are available if you start looking for them. You may have to look "outside the box," meanwhile paying attention to who has built that particular box that restricts your choices. Learn that "No" is a complete sentence. Be attentive to anything that causes an increase in tension and leads to tightening muscles.

Some "psychological" dysfunctions connected with chronic pain may actually be dysfunctions in the perception and understanding of TrPs. "Many patients have suffered grievously and needlessly because a series of clinicians unacquainted with myofascial TrPs erroneously applied the psychogenic label to them covertly if not overtly" (Simons, Travell, and Simons 1999, p. 31). Hopelessness and helplessness are twin dragons that love to hang around people with chronic illness. They congregate with other dragons to create huge dragon feeding-grounds, munching on and causing more negativity. Avoid negativity generators such as toxic people and situations at all costs: they can create a perception of total lack of control. Everyone has some lack of control in life—it's part of living. Every patient (and every care provider) needs a network of companions where there is sharing of mutual support. We need to learn to balance patient and care-provider limits with the patient's needs and ability for self-help. No one can expect another person to fix all the problems in life. Yes, there is a need for educated medical support, but the patient must be empowered to do her or his part and act as a responsible consumer of health care. Boundary control is a big task, both for the health care professional and for the patient. Learn to respect the boundaries of others and your own boundaries as well. It is a huge task. Sometimes the dragon isn't the perpetuating factor itself; the dragon is your response to it. Denial is one of the toughest of dragons. Expecting someone else to be your dragon tamer is another. No matter what the dragon, you are ultimately responsible for how you handle it: it's your life, and your responsibility. All actions have consequences. Sometimes TrPs are the consequences of our actions, and sometimes they aren't. We learn to control what we can, and to avoid fretting about the rest.

Lifestyle

Sometimes when you have many perpetuating factors, you may feel as if you've fallen into a deep hole and there is no getting out. The first step in getting out of a hole is to stop digging the hole. Take a look in the mirror. Is that a shovel in your hand? Or are you driving a backhoe? Is there a denial dragon grinning toothily next to you? Do you ignore pain and tough it out, pushing yourself too hard and then collapsing for a few days? This can also occur with overenthusiastic home therapy, and is known as the "yo-yo effect." Listen to your body and tend to its needs. This can be much different than what you want. Become attentive to habits such as jaw or hand clenching, gum chewing, mouth breathing, and/or habitually leaning. Check your posture in photos. Lifestyle changes can involve more than bad habits.

Does your lifestyle include being the caretaker of someone who is critically ill? Maybe you need to recruit some help and take some time to take care of you. Does modern dance bring you excitement as it ruins your health? Perhaps you can change routines, teachers, or schedules so that you can still enjoy the dance without a dragon stepping on your feet. Look at your limits. Maybe you can stretch them a little, but you can't deny that they are there. Focus on what you can do. Find ways to bring joy into your life while avoiding perpetuating factors. There are always choices and always possibilities. We all have limits. You may not be able to fly like a bird, but you may be able to ride a dragon.

Perpetuating factors! How to deal with them all! Don't be overwhelmed if you realize that you have a whole dragon pack following you, or even riding on your shoulders. Tame those dragons, one at a time if need be. Make a list of things you can change. Find a way to function without causing yourself harm. Don't push to work in spite of the pain. Become function-oriented: medications and therapies are needed to function—not to avoid function. Patients and care providers need to be aware of this. If you have pain and dysfunction now, things must change if you want to ease the symptoms. This includes being attentive to diet, sleep habits, excess alcohol consumption, smoking, and the quality of the environment at home and at work. Think about relationships. Think about posture. Learn to live mindfully. Patients, if there is a need for lifestyle changes, you have control over your choices. They are challenges, not obstacles. Life as you know it will change, but life as you know it includes pain and dysfunction. Change is inevitable in life; make your changes positive ones.

7 Symptom List

Many people have difficulty discerning if a symptom is caused by FM or TrPs, although some symptoms may have components of both, or may be due to other reasons such as medication side-effects. Here is a TrP-symptom list with the most common locations of TrPs that can produce them. We only have space to give our readers a general idea of the scope of TrP dysfunctions, as well as some specific types of TrP pain. Pain is the symptom most often associated with TrPs. TrPs can mimic angina, bursitis, prostatitis, appendicitis, cystitis, arthritis, esophagitis, carpal tunnel syndrome, pelvic inflammatory disease, pain of a heart or gall bladder attack, diverticulosis,

costochondritis, or sciatica. They can also cause or contribute to many bewildering symptoms including sweating, skin blanching, coldness, gooseflesh, redness, excessive sweating, dizziness, dysmenorrhea, voiding dysfunctions, muscle stiffness, earache or stuffiness, frozen shoulder, gait abnormalities, clumsiness and loss of fine motor control, difficulty breathing, and difficulty raising arms. The following list is just a sample; you will find much more in the individual muscle chapters. Rule out any associated medical condition, and always follow medical advice.

Signs and symptoms	Possible site(s) of TrP(s)
abdominal cramping/colic	lateral border periumbilical
abdominal fullness/bloating/nausea	abdominals, especially upper rectus abdominis paraxiphoid
ankle weakness	tibialis anterior, peroneus
anorexia	rectus abdominis
bed wetting	active TrPs in lower abdominal wall
belching	abdominals (especially rectus abdominis), upper thoracic paraspinal
bladder pain	upper adductor magnus
bloating	transversus abdominis, rectus abdominis
blocked ears/hearing loss/ hyperacusis/hypoacusis	pterygoids, masseter
blurred vision/visual disturbance	splenius capitis, eye muscles, sternal SCM, upper trapezius, orbicularis oculi, masseter (near vision)
bruxism (grinding and/or clenching of teeth)	temporalis
buckling ankle	peroneus
buckling hip	extension of both rectus femoris and upper vastus intermedius
buckling knee	vastus medialis, vastus lateralis
calf cramps	gastrocnemius
cardiac arrhythmia	pectoralis major between fifth and sixth ribs, midway between nipple and sternum right side (inactivate sternal TrPs first); pectoralis minor
carsickness/seasickness	SCM
choking sensation swallowing saliva	laryngeal muscles, digastric
clumsy thumb (difficulty writing, buttoning)	adductor pollicis, opponens pollicis
colic	transversus abdominis, rectus abdominis
congestion/sinus pressure/sinus obstruction	masseter, pterygoids, internasal and sinus areas
constipation	abdominal, possibly mesentery, obturator internus
cough, dry hacking	convergence of sternal SCM, pectoralis, and sternalis

Signs and symptoms	Possible site(s) of TrP(s)
diarrhea	lower abdominal area, right lower rectus abdominis, transversus abdominis
difficulty climbing stairs	erector spinae, QL, tibialis anterior, soleus, long toe flexors
difficulty swallowing	longus capitis, longus colli, medial pterygoid, buccinator, omohyoid, digastric
diffuse abdominal/gynecological pain	lower rectus abdominis, upper adductor magnus
dimming of perceived light intensity	SCM
disturbed weight perception of objects in hand	SCM
dyspareunia (pain on intercourse)	bulbospongiosus, piriformis, upper adductor magnus
elevated first rib	anterior scalene (can cause or contribute to costoclavicular syndrome), omohyoid
entrapped carotid artery	stylohyoid
erectile dysfunction	multiple pelvic TrPs (especially ischiocavernosus)
eye, explosive pressure in	splenius capitis
eye, inability or slowness to raise upper lid	sternal SCM with spasm of orbicularis oculi
eye, redness	frontalis, superior orbicularis oculi, sternal SCM
eye irritation, redness	SCM, extrinsic eye muscles
eye pain	SCM, occipitalis; longus capitis
eye pain, behind the eye	temporalis, occipitalis, trapezius
eye pain, coming from back of head	obliquus capitus inferior, upper nasal septum, frontonasal duct, frontal sinus
eye pain, deep	sternal SCM
eye tear production, excessive	front area temporalis, mid temporalis, sternal SCM, frontalis, superior orbicularis oculi
female sexual dysfunction	piriformis and other short lateral rotators, pelvic floor
flatulence	abdominals
food intolerance	transversus abdominis
foot drop; foot slap	tibialis anterior
full sensation in rectum	obturator internus
genital pain	ischiocavernosus, bulbospongiosus, upper adductor magnus, transversus abdominis
grip strength, loss of	infraspinatus, scalenes, hand extensors, brachioradialis, abductor pollicis brevis
heartburn	upper abdominal external oblique, upper rectus abdominis paraxiphoid, transversus abdominis
hiccups	reflex contraction diaphragm, uvula
hoarseness	laryngeal TrPs
hyperacusia (hypersensitive hearing)	temporalis, medial pterygoid
IBS	rectal TrPs, abdominals (especially obliques), mid and low back multifidi, pelvic floor, upper adductor magnus
impotence	bulbospongiosus, ischiocavernosus, piriformis and other short lateral rotators, pudendal nerve and blood vessel entrapment
inability to stand up straight	psoas
inability to sit still	gluteus maximus, obturator internus, gluteus maximus, upper adductor magnus
incontinence, urinary and fecal	pelvic floor, pyramidalis (urinary), obturator internus (both)
indigestion	rectus abdominis

Signs and symptoms	**Possible site(s) of TrP(s)**
jaw opening, restriction of	masseter, many area TrPs; the zygomaticus major alone may cause restriction of the opening by 10–20 mm
knee weakness	rectus femoris
kneecap, locked	vastus medialis, vastus lateralis
light sensitivity	frontalis, superior orbicularis oculi, sternal SCM, rectus capitis
loss of ability to empty bladder fully	pyramidalis
loss of attention or focus	rectus capitis anterior and lateral
lumbago	iliocostalis lumborum, longissimus thoracis, piriformis and other short lateral rotators, erector spinae, quadratus lumborum, gluteus medius, psoas major
lump in throat	longus colli, longus capitis, digastric
nasal and sinus congestion	SCM, lateral pterygoid
nausea	abdominals, upper thoracic paraspinals, transversus abdominis, temporalis
nipple hypersensitivity/intolerance to clothing	pectoralis major (check both sides)
pain during orgasm	pubococcygeus
painful bowel movements	levator ani, obturator internus
palpable rigidity and deep tenderness of lower abdominal wall	T9 level of erector spinae
petit mal seizure-like symptoms	rectus capitis major and minor
phantom limb pain	after removal, TrPs in the flesh surrounding the missing leg, arm, breast, or organ cause pain in the area of the removed tissue
plantar fasciitis	superficial and deep intrinsic foot muscles
postnasal drip	pterygoid, SCM
premature ejaculation	bulbospongiosus, ischiocavernosus
projectile vomiting	"belch button" TrP on either side, at or just below angle of twelfth rib
radial artery entrapment	pectoralis minor
reflux	upper external abdominal oblique
restless pain on prolonged sitting	pelvic floor, gluteus maximus, piriformis, ischiocavernosus, transverse perineal, inguinal ligaments, sacrotuberous ligament
retraction of the testicle	multifidi
ringing in ears	pterygoids, masseter, medial pterygoid, splenius capitis, SCM, temporalis
salivation, intense	mid temporalis
sensation of a full bowel	coccygeus
sensitivity to sound and light	occipitalis
shin-splint-type pain (anterior)	extensor digitorum longus, tibialis anterior
shin-splint-type pain (posterior)	flexor digitorum longus, tibialis posterior
shortness of breath	levator scapulae
shoulder impingement syndrome	serratus anterior
sore throat	TrP area at base of tongue, laryngeal muscles, omohyoid
spasm of urinary sphincter muscles	pyramidalis
stitch in side	serratus anterior and/or external oblique, diaphragm

Signs and symptoms	Possible site(s) of TrP(s)
swallowing, sore and/or painful	pterygoids, digastric, mylohyoid, stylohyoid, cricoarytenoid, omohyoideus, longus capitis, SCM
swelling, foot and ankle	piriformis, soleus
swelling, hands	scalene
swelling, throat	digastric TrPs (mimics swollen lymph nodes)
swelling, leg	piriformis and other short lateral rotators, adductor longus and brevis
swollen glands sensation	digastric, SCM, pterygoids, anterior neck
tachycardia, arrhythmia (including auricular fibrillation)	pectoralis major, intercostals, autonomic concomitants
testicle, retraction	erector spinae
thigh and leg weakness	rectus femoris
thoracic-outlet-syndrome-type pain	scalenes, pectoralis major, latissimus dorsi, teres major and subscapularis, pectoralis minor, trapezius, levator scapulae, triceps brachii
throat drainage	pterygoids, anterior neck muscles, digastric
thumb cramps	abductor pollicis longus
tidal volume reduction	serratus anterior, intercostals
TMJD	lateral pterygoid, deep masseter
toe cramps	long extensors of toes
tooth pain and sensitivity (cold, heat, pressure)	clavicular SCM, trapezius, masseter, temporalis, upper trapezius, digastric, hyoids, longus capitis, lower nasal turbinate, maxillary sinus ostium, buccinator
trigger finger	hand and finger flexors, finger flexor tendon sheath
trigger thumb	flexor pollicis longus tendon sheath
upper respiratory dysfunction	pectoralis major (bronchi), intercostals
vaginismus	pelvic floor and related areas
vascular thoracic outlet syndrome	subclavius TrP vascular entrapment
vertigo	SCM, upper trapezius, splenius capitis, semispinalis cervicis, temporalis
vocal dysfunctions	pterygoids, anterior neck muscles, digastrics, laryngeal muscles
vomiting	abdominals (especially rectus abdominis)
vulvodynia	pelvic floor (especially anterior inferior levator ani, vaginal wall, obturator internus), psoas, rectus abdominis, obturator internus
writer's cramp	brachioradialis, forearm extensors

These TrPs with these symptoms are listed in the following references: Bezerra Rocha, Ganz Sanchez, and Tesseroli de Siqueira (2008); Doggweiler-Wiygul (2004); Funt and Kinnie (1984); Qerama, Kasch, and Fuglsang-Frederiksen (2008); Sharkey (2008); Simons, Travell, and Simons (1999); Starlanyl and Copeland (2001); Teachey (2004); and Travell and Simons (1992).

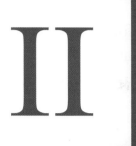

II

THE GALLERY:
IDENTIFYING THE SYMPTOM SOURCE

This section will teach you how to identify and deal with individual TrPs. Some muscle sections have two segments called **Hints for Control:** one for the care provider and one for the patient. Readers may find it enlightening to read both sections. There are stretches, but not all muscles are designed to be stretched the way one ordinarily thinks of the term, and that will be explained too. Each muscle or muscle group has an anatomical drawing (sometimes more than one), showing muscles in deep red, and indicating the direction of the muscle fibers; the fiber direction can help identify and treat individual muscles. The muscle-connecting tendons are in white. Other body structures are illustrated and labeled when they are important for TrPs or are helpful for locating the muscle. The referral patterns are shown separately: dark red in those figures indicates the most intense pain. The lighter and less dense red areas indicate spillover pain. Such expansion of the referral pattern is an indication that the TrPs are very active and exceedingly annoyed, and may indicate accompanying FM. Muscles and referral patterns can occur on both sides of the body, but we often show only one. If there are different referral patterns for the same muscle, depending on the location of the TrP, we at times will show one pattern on one side of the body and another on the other side. Referral patterns may vary from patient to patient, especially when there are multiple overlapping pain patterns and FM.

Those of you familiar with myofascial TrPs will notice something different here. You will not see "X"s marking guideline locations of TrPs, because TrPs can occur in any place in any muscle. This depiction was first pioneered by John Sharkey (2008). Others who have shown TrP "X" guidelines have had them misunderstood. People check "X" spots and, finding none, erroneously assume that the muscle has no TrPs. They may not even examine the associated attachments. Instructions for finding

TrPs by palpation (exploratory touch) and a blank chart are found in Chapter 14. Differences in referral patterns are important clues to TrP locations. Accuracy and completeness are important. For example, many referral patterns include part of the shoulder blade.

Eventually, readers with multiple TrPs will be drawing their own patterns. Pain areas and non-pain areas help to identify the TrPs. Our figures are depicted as if they were the only TrPs, because that's the best way to learn the individual referral patterns. In reality, TrPs enjoy the company of their own kind. They rarely occur alone. Each part of the gallery segment begins with a regional overview of that segment, including an example of a patient who has overlapping referral patterns. The overviews will help patients and care providers begin to think in terms of multiple TrPs and interactions among tissues of the body.

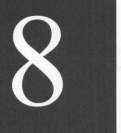

8 Muscles of the Face, Head, and Neck

Introduction

This book is divided into specific segments. Please understand that this separation is artificial, and that there's nothing unusual about a calf TrP referring pain to the jaw. Also, different areas of the head and neck interact, as do different tissues. For example, a runny nose may be caused by a variety of conditions, including TrPs, and the mechanical irritation of the drip itself may activate a number of nose and throat TrPs. Each of these TrPs may set up other TrPs. These TrP cascades can develop slowly or quickly. Once each of the TrPs is active and generating pain, healthier muscles attempt to compensate by taking on some of the workload for the painful weakened ones. The ground substance of tissues hardens, guarding the TrP-laden muscles and minimizing their pain-generating movement. The brain sends out signals to prevent full ROM because of the pain, and the muscle shortens even more. Welcome to the downward spiral. Fortunately, education can prevent this scenario, and that's what you'll find here.

Regional Kinetics: The head and neck region is open to attacks from allergens, infectious agents, and the trauma of dental work, and eye, ear, and throat conditions. This region of the body is most impacted, literally, by whiplash. The often-excessive response to collisions and other whiplash incidents can be explained by the startle response that provokes extreme muscle contraction (Blouin, Inglis, and Siegmund 2006). This response can even be provoked by abrupt loud noise. Extreme muscle contraction often translates into TrPs. Many headaches of many varieties, including migraines, have treatable TrP components. Instead of the term "tension headache," we often use the term "myogenic headache," because these headaches originate in the muscles. Tight muscles can have many causes other than psychological stress, and psychological stress is often the first thing we think of when we hear the word "tension." Many temporomandibular complaints have treatable TrP components. The child's earaches and unexplained toothaches, the senior's dizziness, and the teen's inability to listen may all have a common cause in myofascial pain. Many head and neck TrPs have symptoms often considered to be neurological until tests indicate otherwise. They are then often erroneously regarded as psychological.

When emotional and physiological stressors cause the shoulder position to creep upward to the ears, the head goes forward and the shoulders curl round and inward. The head-forward position can set up the body for increased trauma from subsequent abrupt muscle movement. If the tongue is out of its normal position of rest at the roof of the mouth, the hyoid bone is not in its healthy position and many muscles are out of alignment, setting them up for further injury. When the hyoid bone is out of alignment, the carotid artery may be entrapped, causing false-positive test results and diagnostic confusion (Kolbel et al. 2008). TrPs are often the reason that structures are not in healthy alignment. It's critical that diagnosis and treatment are prompt and sufficient, or permanent tissue changes could result. A high percentage of patients with TrPs in the posterior neck also have FM (Sahin et al. 2008). This state of central sensitization may erroneously be considered "functional," psychological, or "somatoform," by those who don't know any better.

Regional TrP Comments: Headaches, even migraines and one-sided cluster headaches, are often associated with TrPs. The TrPs can be initiating, contributing or maintaining factors and can lead to central sensitization. (Calandre EP, et al. 2006.) The central sensitization may begin with migraines or other localized manifestations but can often develop into generalized FM. Even in children, TrPs are a common cause of headaches (Fernandez-de-las-Penas et al. 2011). Although migraines may have persisted for years, some may be resolved or minimized with TrP treatment (Nelson, Fernandez-de-las-Penas, and Simons 2008). TrPs in any muscle, ligament, or tendon that can pull the jaw out of alignment could be involved in contributing to TMJD pain. They also can prevent muscles from performing integrated, efficient movements, thus adding to fatigue.

Regional CMP Comments: When CMP has developed in this region, it may be difficult to find the source of the symptoms, even if the care provider understands individual TrPs, because so many muscles may be participating in symptom generation. Justine Jeffrey, my (Starlanyl) TrP myotherapist, has invented words such as "shnead" to indicate a shoulder/head combination of symptom generators, and "shneck" for a shoulder/neck combo. Misleading symptoms of multiple TrPs can cause use of unneeded antibiotics, initiating fungal overgrowth. Primary insomnia and sleep apnea are often related to TMJ pain (Smith et al. 2009), and that often involves TrPs.

What does CMP look like? Here's a simple example: A 20-year-old college student came with a headache that had persisted for several months. The headache was located predominantly in the temples, although on questioning he admitted to intermittent tooth and jaw pain and eyestrain on the right side.

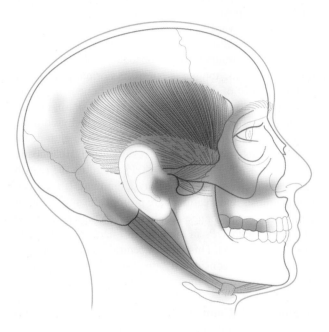

CMP patient pain pattern.

History revealed he'd had a root canal on a right upper tooth a month before the headache started, and the procedure was prolonged due to an interruption. Several weeks afterward he developed a sore throat and swollen glands, and earache on the right side. Later his jaw started to ache again, but a return trip to the dentist found no other tooth problems. Recently he experienced difficulty sleeping, and trouble concentrating during the day. He'd been taking OTC anti-inflammatory medication for two months. On examination, TrPs were found in the front of the right temporalis, posterior digastric, and lateral pterygoid. He recognized their pain patterns as his own. Treatment with stretch and spray was successful. He was taught finger pressure technique and given home stretches. During a follow-up call a week later, he reported no symptoms, and that he had discontinued the anti-inflammatory medication.

Regional Perpetuating Factors: Interactive conditions such as TMJD, allergies, osteoarthritis, trauma or other muscle overload, hormonal or vascular imbalances, chronic infections, and poor posture (especially head-forward posture and forward rotation of the shoulders) are common initiating and perpetuating factors in this region. Use of CPAP (pressure from head straps and a face mask) can cause TrPs in the head and neck, as can the weight of heavy eyeglasses, vision impairment, paradoxical breathing, immobility, sustained computer use, psychological stress, and/or sustained dental work. Perpetuating factors must be brought under control for successful head and neck TrP treatments to last.

Note for Dentists: If you have patients with TrPs, equilibration on these patients must be accompanied by TrP assessment and treatment, because the bite will change as the TrPs release. You can often prevent disc deterioration with TrP assessment, treatment, and control of perpetuating factors. Stretch and spray, ice stroking, hot moist packs, and/or topical anesthetics can be useful (see Chapter 14). You can assist your patients by giving them frequent breaks and encouraging dynamic jaw movement during those breaks, coupled with the application of moist heat packs or stretch with spray, to avoid TrP formation during long dental procedures.

Regional Hints for Control: Check for mouth breathing and other types of paradoxical breathing, and for head-forward position and other posture deviations. Check photos and assess postures. The history or exam may give clues to the primary or key TrP. Successful treatment of one or two areas in the neck may give symptom relief in vast areas of the head and face (Mellick and Mellick 2003). Perpetuating factors must be brought under control or the treatment results will not last.

Buccinator
Latin *bucca* means "cheek."

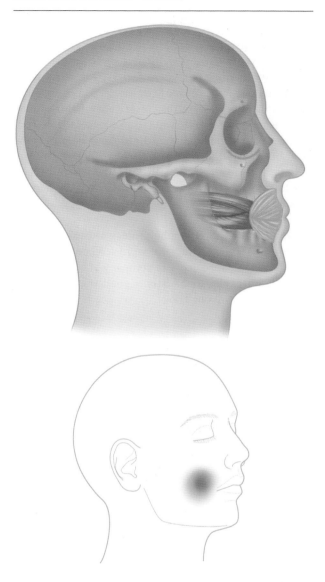

What It Does: Aids the chewing process by keeping food between the teeth, and forms a substantial part of the cheek. It has lower fibers running to the upper lip and upper fibers running to the lower lip in a crossing pattern. It's involved in sucking, whistling, swallowing, blowing a wind instrument, pursing the lips, and producing facial expressions.

Kinetics Comments: Whenever you blow a balloon up or suck a liquid through a straw, you are exercising the buccinator. If you have fangs, this is the muscle you use to bare them.

TrP Comments: TrPs in the buccinator cause pain locally that may spill over to the teeth. These TrPs may give the sensation that swallowing is impaired, because the buccinator attaches to the superior pharyngeal muscle. Tightening of one muscle by TrPs stresses surrounding muscles. These TrPs can cause mouth twitches, and may entrap the parotid salivary duct. They may contribute to proprioceptor dysfunction, resulting in tongue or cheek biting. We believe that buccinator TrPs may be involved in nocturnal drooling or dry mouth. These TrPs may be responsible for nonverbal miscues, as they contribute to misleading facial expressions. Deep nodules felt at the side angles of the mouth may not be TrPs: they are the locations of the interlacing of buccinator and orbicularis oris fibers.

Notable Perpetuating Factors: Extended chewing of tough substances, ill-fitting dental appliances, poor bite, and lack of smiling. Come on—give us a smile.

Hints for Control: Try to avoid lengthening the muscle and holding it for several seconds, as this, believe it or not, may actually compound the excessive tension and stiffness in the muscle. Dynamic range of motion stretching can be accomplished by blowing air out through pursed lips, and allowing it to escape gently and slowly over three or four seconds in a controlled fashion. If you place your finger between your cheek and teeth and then purse your lips, you can feel the buccinator contract as it presses the finger against the teeth. You may be able to feel TrP contraction nodules, and press them between your finger and thumb. Topical anesthetic safe for use inside the mouth may minimize pain: apply the anesthetic to the TrP pain source, not to the area of referred pain. Moist heat compresses on the outside may be soothing. We recommend finishing with a cool compress to avoid encouraging swelling.

Zygomaticus Major and Minor
Greek *zugoma* means a "bar" or "bolt."

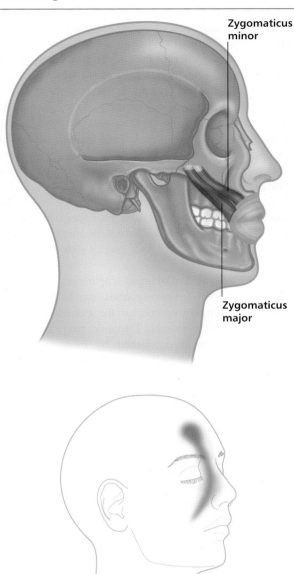

Zygomaticus minor

Zygomaticus major

What They Do: Draw upper lip upward and sideways when you smile or laugh.

TrP Comments: TrPs here cause pain reaching upward in an arc along the side of the nose. This pain extends over the bridge of the nose to the mid forehead. These TrPs may restrict the opening of the jaw by as much as 20 mm, so if you can't open your mouth wide enough to fit in a sandwich, TrPs may be the reason why. One of the authors (Starlanyl) has found that TrPs in this muscle can contribute to drooling, especially during sleep. TrPs occurring in the zygomaticus, orbicularis, and levator labii muscles can produce symptoms of trigeminal neuralgia (Yoon et al. 2009).

Notable Perpetuating Factors: Habitual frowning, squinting, poor vision, poor lighting, TMJD, and TrPs in the sternal division of the SCM.

Hints for Control: A good stretch for these muscles is the pursed-lips kiss, but avoid holding the kiss for too long. That said, repeating this particular stretch can be very enjoyable. You may be able to feel TrPs in this muscle by placing one finger inside your mouth and your thumb outside. Gentle pressure on the TrP may help, as may moist heat or cold. Rolling and squeezing available TrPs between your thumb and your finger may help treat the TrPs, but be gentle—it hurts. Check jaw opening before and after treatment. If it is effective, the jaw restriction should ease substantially, and thick sandwiches may be back on the menu.

Stretch: Smiling and laughing are good exercises for this muscle, as is saying the word "Whee!" *Caution*: saying "Whee!" repeatedly in company at odd moments may require explanation. It is a good opportunity for educating others about TrPs.

Occipitofrontalis
Latin *occiput* means "the back of the head"; *frontalis*, "relating to the front of the head."

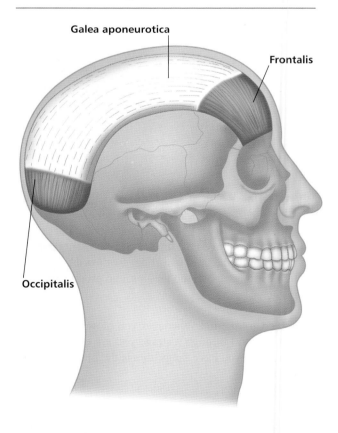

Galea aponeurotica

Frontalis

Occipitalis

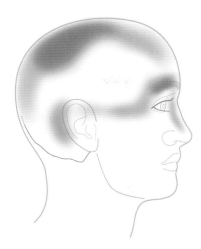

Occipitofrontalis.

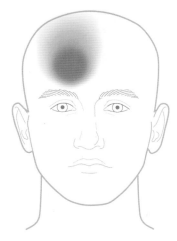

Frontalis.

These are two muscles, jointed together by a fibrous tendon area.

What It Does: The occipital and frontalis segments of this muscle work together. The occipitalis moves the scalp backward and helps the frontalis to raise the eyebrows and wrinkle the forehead. The frontalis moves the scalp forward and wrinkles the forehead skin horizontally.

Kinetics Comments: Tension in the posterior back-line kinetic chain can shorten this area. Muscle spasms in the hamstrings or plantar fascia, for example, can result in occipitofrontalis tightness. This adds to head and neck tension, contributing to headaches and a hyperextended neck. The body then compensates with a posteriorly rotated pelvis to keep the eyes level during walking and running motions. all of these reactions contribute to TrP formation and are major perpetuating factors.

TrP Comments: Upwardly referred pain over the forehead is common. Pain can be referred inside the head, behind the eye, into the eyeball, behind the ear, or into the nose, with occasional referral to the eyelids.

Sound and light sensitivity can occur with these TrPs, with accompanying pain increase. The patient may be unable to bear the weight of the head on a pillow. Hats and headbands are unendurable. The deep ache of these TrPs must be differentiated from the hot prickling pain of entrapment of the greater occipital nerve by posterior cervical TrPs. Sharp or searing pain originating on one side but spreading across the forehead can be due to entrapment of the supraorbital nerve by frontalis TrPs. Frontalis TrPs can cause excessive tear production. Occipitalis TrPs are more common in patients with decreased vision and/or glaucoma; frontalis TrPs are more common in patients who use computers. Pain occurs on the same side as the TrP, although TrPs can occur on both sides with overlapping pain patterns. It is suspected by this author (Starlanyl) that TrPs form in the galea aponeurotica along either side of the suture line on the skull, and that they can have quite distinct referral patterns. In general, ice is more helpful for nerve pain, and hot moist heat is more beneficial for muscle pain.

Notable Perpetuating Factors: Direct trauma, habitually frowning or otherwise wrinkling the forehead, chronic computer use, poor vision, and other TrPs.

Stretch: Gentle massage of the scalp with the tips of the fingers is the ideal way to keep this area supple. Raise the eyebrows, and then lower them. Or do it one at a time. Live long and prosper.

Orbicularis Oculi
Latin *orbiculus* means "small circular disk"; *oculus*, "eye."

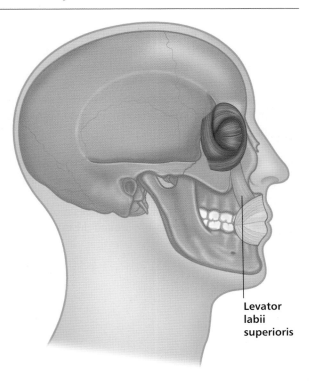

Levator labii superioris

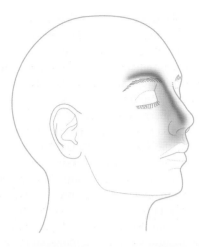

What It Does: Pulls down the upper eyelid and raises the lower lid to wash the eye with tears. Enables squinting to protect the eye from sudden or over bright light. One part of the muscle dilates the tear sac.

Kinetics Comments: This is a multipart and extremely complex muscle. It slows the act of blinking and returns the eyelid to "open." It's part of the "crow's feet" wrinkle effect of aging at the lateral corner of the eye. The orbicularis oculi plays an important part in the nonverbal communication of body language, and can send the wrong signals if burdened with TrPs.

TrP Comments: TrPs in the orbicularis oculi refer pain above the eyebrow and along the nose, to the nose and just below. They are frequently misdiagnosed as sinus pain, and can be activated by sinus problems. They can be involved in eye twitching. Myofascial entrapment from these TrPs can affect tear ducts. If the levator labii muscle is involved, these TrPs can cause symptoms that mimic trigeminal neuralgia (Yoon et al. 2009). These TrPs can cause the print on a page to jump around when reading, especially if the print is in a strong contrasting color. These symptoms may be blamed on FM.

Notable Perpetuating Factors: Sinus and eye infections, eye irritation, uncorrected eyesight, and prolonged computer use.

Hints for Control: Jumpy print can sometimes be subdued by placing a piece of plastic wrap over the page before reading, to diminish the contrast. The TrPs still need to be treated. Self-treatment includes moist heat or cold, and gentle finger pressure around the eye.

Extrinsic (Extraocular) Eye Muscles
(medial rectus, lateral rectus, superior rectus, inferior oblique, superior oblique, inferior rectus)
Latin *extrinsecus* means "on the outside."

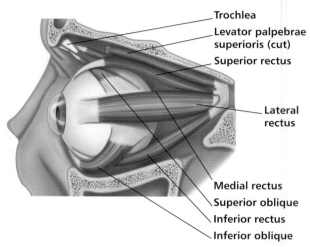

Trochlea
Levator palpebrae superioris (cut)
Superior rectus
Lateral rectus
Medial rectus
Superior oblique
Inferior rectus
Inferior oblique

What They Do: These are the six muscles that move each eyeball in vertical, horizontal, and rotating motions. The medial and lateral rectus muscles enable the eye to move horizontally, from the center to the side and back. The rectus muscles pull the eye centrally as well as horizontally. The superior rectus also pulls the eye up; the inferior rectus also pulls the eye down. The anatomy of the oblique muscles causes them to pull to the side as well as up and down. The superior oblique pulls the eye down and to the side; the inferior oblique pulls the eye up and to the side. The trochlea (Latin for "pulley") is a common TrP site. When functioning well, these eye muscles move together in harmony, with each movement of the eyeball requiring the coordination of at least three different eye muscles, directed by the brain. Pretty spectacular.

Kinetics Comments: Changes in positioning of these muscles will affect the suboccipital muscles. Thus, easing the TrP tightness of the extrinsic eye muscles through exercise may help the muscles in the back of the neck, easing headaches and other symptoms.

TrP Comments: TrPs in these muscles can contribute to headache, eye twitching, blurry vision, eye irritation, or sinus pain, depending on which muscle is affected. TrPs in any of these muscles can contribute to proprioceptor dysfunction. For the eyes to work together, the muscles must be contracted to their normal length. If one or more of them is shortened by TrPs, this can affect stereoscopic vision, contributing to visual disturbances, including dizziness, when moving rapidly forward, backward, or sideways, or looking up or down. This variance can alter the brain's perception of where one is in relation to the world. TrPs in these muscles may be responsible for changing the vision, but, once eye exercises are a part of the healing routine, this problem often ceases. Starlanyl and Copeland (2001, p. 83) previously noted extrinsic eye TrPs, and the presence of TrPs in at least one of the extrinsic eye muscles has been confirmed by Fernandez-de-las-Penas et al. (2005). There are also intrinsic eye muscles that control the lens and the pupil dilation. TrPs are suspected there as well, but have not been verified, although vision exercises to stretch them have improved those functions in several patients.

Notable Perpetuating Factors: Muscle fatigue caused by long hours of holding the gaze in one position, such as with computer use, sewing, or reading. Allergies and irritating fumes can also stress the eyes and these muscles, as can nearby sinus infections or eye infections. Many OTC eye drops dry the eyes and should not be used continually: talk to your eye doctor for a recommendation. Avoid eye irritants such as chlorinated pools. If you use a CPAP, ensure that the air isn't blowing into your eyes.

Self-treatment: This includes eye exercises, looking to each corner, with special attention looking upward. Even eyes can do push-ups! Remember how an eye doctor has you follow her or his finger around in a circle? Do that eye circling now, using your own finger, and you can find the probable location of TrPs, as well as stretching those muscles that have the TrPs. They will let you know exactly where they are. Ouch! Start slowly, just one eye circle each time, but do that one circle each way several times during the day. If you feel eye pain, or signs of a headache developing as you do this, stop temporarily—understanding that it's a signal that you need to do this stretch. The next time you try the exercise, bring your finger in closer and don't stretch so much, so fast, or so often. Move your eye muscles more during the day. Eventually, you will be able to do several repetitions each way, several times a day. That will help keep these muscles supple. Become attentive to how you use your eyes: are your neck muscles doing a lot of the repositioning for you? Make sure that your lighting for close work is sufficient and without glare. Talk to your eye doctor about the use of a gentle gel eye-drop, especially one that can be kept in the refrigerator for added mechanical cooling to help ease these muscles. The application of cool moist cloths to the eyes may help ease muscle tightness in this area.

Procerus and Corrugator Supercilii

Latin *procerus* means "long" or "stretched out"; *corrugare*, "to wrinkle up"; *supercilium*, "eyebrow."

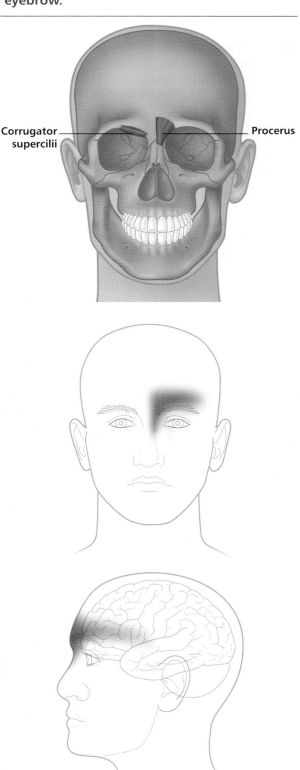

Corrugator supercilii

Procerus

What They Do: The procerus attaches to a membrane covering the roof of the nose and forming a bridge between the nose and the forehead, pulling the middle of the eyebrow down. It wrinkles the nose, and also helps the actions of the frontal bone. The corrugator supercilii muscles pull the eyebrows together and downward when you frown or intensely concentrate.

Kinetics Comments: These TrPs can contribute to deep vertical wrinkles between the eyebrows. The wrinkles may offer clues to facial (and fascial) asymmetry. Sunglasses can help to reduce muscular tension on particularly bright days. Tension from further down the kinetic chain, all the way down to and including the foot, needs to be "freed up." Wrinkles between the eyes are also a sign of vagus nerve irritation in some forms of Traditional Chinese Medicine (Dr. Yun Hsing Ho, personal communications).

TrP Comments: These TrPs usually occur in conjunction with other facial TrPs. They produce a dull headache referring deep into the front of the brain, with dull pain behind the eyes. They may contribute to eyestrain. These TrPs may contribute to droopy upper eyelids (Ghalamkarpour, Aghazedeh, and Odaaei 2009) or to migraine (Smuts, Schultz, and Barnard 2004).

Notable Perpetuating Factors: Frequent contracting of the muscles during frowning or intense concentration. Some CPAP masks and their outflow can perpetuate these TrPs, as can heavy eyeglasses or long-duration viewing of a computer monitor or television. Holding a cigarette between the lips for several seconds as the smoke trails past the face irritates the eyes and these muscles. Our tip: avoid smoking, and don't spend so much time watching television or looking at computer screens. Be an active participant in life.

Hints for Control: Avoid wrinkling the brow. A light pinching of the tissue along the eyebrow area, gently pulling the skin away from the face, may help release these TrPs. It is important to hold this gentle "pinching" or "lifting" of the tissue for at least 90 seconds. Avoid letting the tissue "spring back." Release it slowly to its starting position. Treatment of TrPs in local muscles, including eye exercises, may ease the stress on these muscles. Take frequent breaks during close work, and use adequate magnification. Ensure eye correction is current. Cool compresses, ice sweeps, or chilled eye-drops may relieve pressure from these TrPs. To our knowledge, these TrPs have not previously been described; it is hoped that more research will be done concerning them.

Masseter
Greek *maseter* means "chewer."

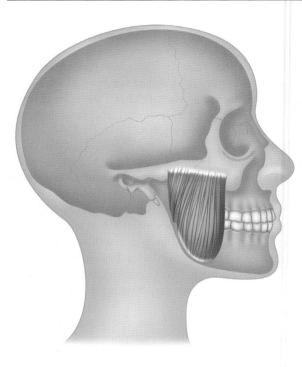

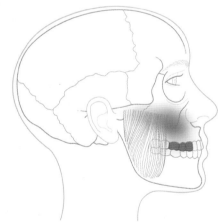

Superficial masseter upper attachment TrPs.

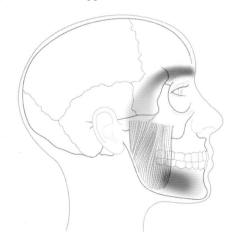

Superficial masseter lower attachment TrPs.

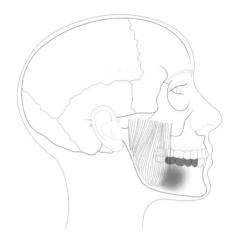

Superficial masseter central TrPs.

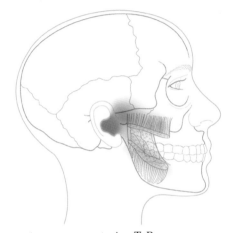

Deep masseter upper posterior TrPs.

What It Does: Elevates the lower jaw enabling upper and lower teeth to meet; the superficial masseter helps move the jaw forward.

Kinetics Comments: A head-forward posture stresses the masseter. Overtraining the abdominals stresses the anterior throat muscles, which, in turn, stress the masseter. Tightening the posterior neck muscles will also stress the masseter.

TrP Comments: If you can't open your mouth fully, this muscle is most likely the culprit. These TrPs also increase muscle tension in the area, contributing to headaches. Their referred pain can be accompanied by tooth pressure and temperature sensitivity. Masseter TrP symptoms can include earache, and may be mistaken for sinusitis. TrPs in the interior masseter may refer pain deep into the ear on that side. Interior TrPs may also cause tinnitus (ringing or other noises, including a low roaring); these noises may be constant, or may be set off by TrP pressure, and may be severe enough to be life-altering. Masseter TrPs are frequently overlooked in young children who have poor dental hygiene or have had long periods of dental work. The pain caused by these TrPs alerts patients to their presence, but they may be totally unaware that TrPs are restricting mouth opening. A healthy, relaxed mouth can open wide enough to allow the first two knuckles of a hand to enter between the teeth. Try it.

Notable Perpetuating Factors: Poor bite, paradoxical breathing, nail biting, pipe smoking, jaw clenching, teeth grinding, emotional stress, constant gum chewing, long periods of dental work, temporomandibular dysfunction, and poor posture (including tongue posture). With the mouth closed, the tongue should rest on the surface of the roof of the mouth, with the tip of the tongue in front of the ridge. Biting on hard objects, or chewing aggressively on tough meat, can also perpetuate these TrPs.

Hints for Control (Patients): Correct a head-forward posture. Work with your health care team to find the cause of bruxism and bring it under control—it's not always stress related. Nighttime bruxism can be caused by sleep disturbances. Check with your dentist to see if your upper and lower jaws match. Ensure that TrPs are treated before the bite is corrected, and that your dentist is aware of coexisting TrPs and their ability to contract muscles.

Hints for Control (Care Providers): Masseter TrPs are found most easily by pincer palpation, and can be treated with that same movement. The masseter and other chewing muscles may correct themselves as neck TrPs are released. Chewing muscles are often involved on both sides. Unilateral tinnitus may be a referred sensory stimulus, or may be due to referred motor unit activity of the tensor tympani and/or stapedius muscle, which lie within the reference zone. The maxillary vein may be entrapped by masseter TrPs. Earaches of unexplained origin are often due to deep masseter or clavicular SCM TrPs.

Self-treatment: You can learn to work these TrPs using a topical OTC anesthetic. Gently through. Interior mouth work hurts! Before any stretching program is started, speak with your dentist to ensure that there is no disc problem or other joint condition that could be aggravated by stretching. When you know it is safe to stretch, try ice sweeping as you slowly open your jaw.

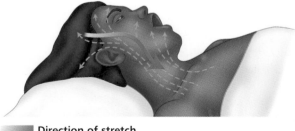

▬▬▬ **Direction of stretch**
╌╌╌╌ **Direction of ice strokes**

Ice stroking: both sides of the face must be treated before any stretching, because these paired muscles need to work together. Follow stretching with moist heat.

Temporalis

Latin *temporalis* means "relating to the side of the head."

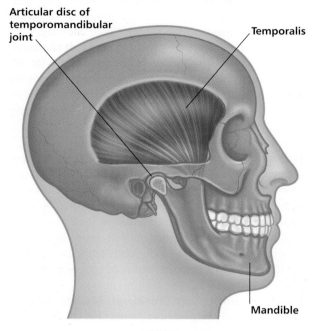

Articular disc of temporomandibular joint

Temporalis

Mandible

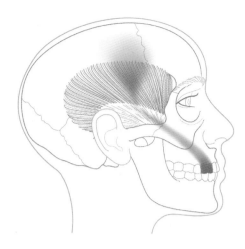

Lower center attachment TrP.

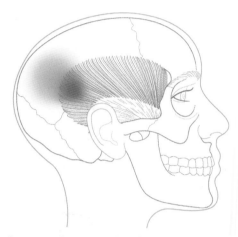

Central temporalis TrP (behind ear point).

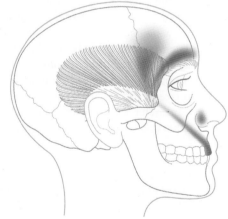

Lower front attachment TrP.

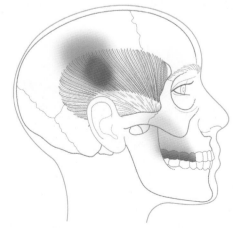

Lower rear attachment TrP (in front of ear area).

What It Does: This muscle helps chew; its contraction elevates and retracts the mandible.

Kinetics Comments: The temporalis works with the masseter to control mouth opening. If TrPs are present in either, these muscles may have a difference of opinion, adding to dysfunction. Overdeveloping the trapezius can lead to temporalis shortening, TrPs, and TMJ dysfunction. A shortened temporalis can contribute to teeth clenching, which in turn can damage the proprioceptive tooth surface. Temporalis shortness can cause restricted and/ or uncoordinated mouth opening. Reflex temporalis shortening is often caused by TrPs and may be secondary to any chronic infection or inflammation. TrPs caused by these conditions may persist long after the initiator is treated.

TrP Comments: TrPs in this muscle, depending on where they are and on associated TrPs, can cause myogenic ("tension") headache. This aching pain can extend to the upper teeth and include hypersensitivity to cold, heat, and pressure. If these TrPs are present, the teeth may not meet correctly, and there may be uncoordinated chewing and opening and closing of the jaw. These TrPs can contribute to teeth grinding. Associated temporalis

TrP proprioceptive dysfunctions include vertigo, nausea, and hearing irregularities such as hypersensitive hearing, tinnitus, and/or inability to tell from which direction a sound is coming. These TrPs can mimic trigeminal neuralgia and cause visual dysfunctions. They can contribute to tension headaches and eyestrain, and interact with TMJ disc problems. The TrPs shorten the muscle, pulling the disc area out of alignment and contributing to disc degeneration. Pain and inflammation at the disc site stress the surrounding muscles further, causing more TrPs. Eventually, if the TrPs are not treated, the disc may need replacement.

Notable Perpetuating Factors: Habitually chewing gum, head-forward posture, teeth grinding, jaw clenching, long periods of jaw immobilization, a cold draft over fatigued muscles, direct trauma such as an accident, and pressure from too-tight earpieces of eyeglasses.

Hints for Control (Patients): The temporalis can be more easily palpated and treated manually if the mouth is three-quarters of the way open. Moist heat packs may help ease TrPs, especially before sleep, as may exaggerated yawning if there is no contraindicative disc problem. Break up long dental procedures with several ROM stretches that involve gently opening and closing the mouth and moving the jaw from side to side. Avoid cracking ice or hard foods with the teeth.

Hints for Control (Care Providers): Tightness in this muscle may contribute to possible cerebrospinal fluid disruption, lateral kinetic chain disruption, and myokinetic chain involvement via the posterior cervical muscles. Check for reduced thyroid function, metabolic disorders, and nutritional deficiencies. A true tooth or TMJ disc problem may perpetuate TrPs in this muscle. Multiple conditions may be bidirectionally interactive.

Self-treatment: Massaging the area with light finger pressure will help release the tension that this muscle can accumulate. Gently opening and closing the mouth while massaging adds to the release. Experiment with moist heat and cool compresses, but avoid overheating or over chilling this area. Discover what works best for you.

Internal Mouth and Nose Muscles
(nasal septum, turbinates, frontonasal duct, frontal and maxillary sinuses, uvula, genioglossus, hard palate, back of tongue)

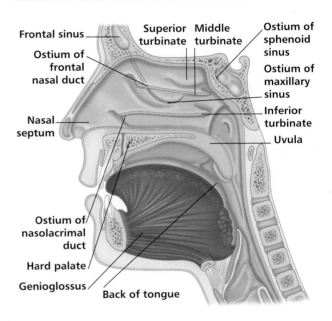

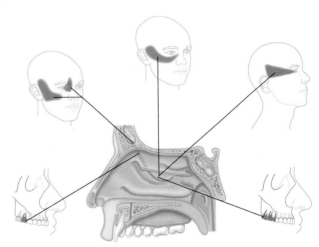

Frontal sinus, frontal sinus duct, and the osteum of the maxillary sinus.

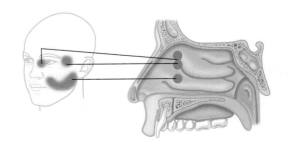

Nasal septum.

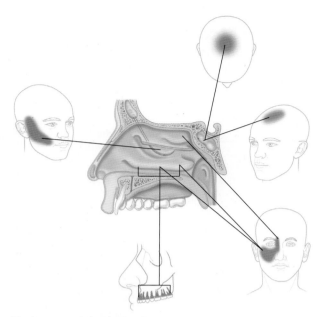

Turbinates and sphenoid sinuses.

Referral pattern figures are furnished with permission from Dr. Lawrence A. Funt, after McCauliff GW, Goodell H, Wolff HG. 1943.

What They Do: TrPs in this area cause many baffling and misinterpreted symptoms. The palatine uvula is more than a blob of soft tissue hanging from the soft palate: its connective tissue containing muscle fibers and branching grape-like glands. The genioglossus muscle is the largest upper-airway dilator muscle, moving anteriorly during inward breathing, and posteriorly during outward breathing.

Kinetics Comments: The interior mouth and nose affect breathing, speaking, digestion, and fluid drainage. Much of this area is empty space, but important space. The sinuses give lightness to the head, allowing us to walk upright. The structure of the nose and mouth allows air to be warmed and breath to be somewhat filtered. Glands empty into this area, and it is here that digestion begins. Irritants, such as pollutants and allergens, can enter from the environment through the nose and mouth, and affect the body: so can medications such as nose sprays and oral preparations. Tender, sore areas of the mouth and nose can cause headaches and add to eyestrain. Teeth and gums play an active part of this region, as does the health of the tongue.

TrP Comments: There is a trigger area in the back part of the tongue that can cause or contribute substantially to sore-throat pain and/or to headaches. Sometimes it may be phantom pain from removed tonsils, and will respond to FSM treatment. Trigger areas in the nose can cause chronic headaches (Abu-Samra, Gawad, and Agha 2011). Triggers in the nasal-oropharyngeal areas can increase congestion, adding to sleep apnea problems. They may be associated with increased tear production and/or

redness of the eye, as well as sensitivity to light and pain. The posterior tongue area is often affected by postnasal drip, causing referred throat and frontal head pain. These TrPs like to play with each other—to our detriment. For example, a patient with a runny nose from SCM TrPs is mistakenly given a course of antibiotics that do not help the symptoms. Another course of antibiotics turns the area into a penthouse suite for fungus, worsening the postnasal drip. Suddenly there is a big problem, including CMP with multiple perpetuating factors. Central sensitization of the gut and head can occur, and FM may not be far behind.

A TrP in the right tonsillar area has been documented in glossopharyngeal neuralgia (Kandt and Daniel 1986), and a TrP in the uvula associated with hiccups (Travell 1977). The uvula TrPs can be treated with pressure from the back of a cold spoon. One of the authors (Sharkey 2008, p. 219) discovered that resistant knee pain is often relieved by working TrPs in the interior mouth; the other author (Starlanyl) found that TrPs in this area could cause inability to articulate the rolling "R" common to languages such as French and Spanish. That author (Starlanyl) has also traced other speech impediments to TrPs in this area, mostly in the anterior genioglossus. TrPs in some related anterior neck muscles cause these muscles to tighten and pull on the genioglossus, contributing to restricted air flow, especially when one is lying down. It is suspected that the inner ear can be involved in TrPs of this region. The turbinates, ducts, and ostia are most sensitive to pain and most easily irritated in these areas; they're most likely to cause reactive constriction and head, neck and shoulder pain. (McCauliff, Goodell, and Wolff 1943).

Notable Perpetuating Factors: Irritation from postnasal drip can greatly aggravate some of these areas. When the back of the tongue and throat is sufficiently irritated, this area provides an excellent home for organisms, and if these buggies take up housekeeping long enough, they often form biofilms. A biofilm is a microscopic life form's way of protecting itself. Once the biofilm is in place, it is difficult to reach the organisms living in the inner layers surrounded by the biofilm. The biofilm forms a protective coating that shields organisms from antibiotics, antifungals, or whatever else we try to use against them. The organisms are protected by the outer layer and multiple defense mechanisms as they slowly build resistance to whatever we throw at them. These multilevel mats or masses of organisms may lurk in many nose and throat areas. Perpetrators of runny nose, including allergies, irritants and other TrPs, should be aggressively controlled. Any infection—bacterial, viral, or fungal—can activate these trigger areas, as can acid fumes from gastric reflux. Patients with TrPs are not good candidates for sinus or obstructive sleep apnea surgeries. Interior nose and mouth trigger areas often interact with TrPs in surrounding areas, each worsening the others and making us generally miserable.

Hints for Control (Patients): Identify and control perpetuating factors, including tooth problems, allergies, irritants, and other interactive TrPs. Avoid smoke. Be attentive to dental hygiene. The posterior tongue trigger area responds well to the use of a tongue scraper. A cold pack on the back or front of the neck may soothe the throat. Please don't add heat to an already inflamed area. Postnasal drip can sometimes be helped by controlling mucus secretion with warm saltwater irrigation, but don't use this (or Netti pot irrigation) if infection is suspected, to avoid spreading germs. If the nasopharyngeal areas have been irritated for a while, be kind to yourself. Use a *very* weak salt solution and *lukewarm* water. When you irrigate, you may find that the areas are extremely raw. FM can amplify this sensation. Running a flat electronic massager over the sinus areas may relieve pressure. This should not be done if infection is suspected, as use of such a device often provokes sneezing, which can spread infection to other parts of the area, such as the inner ear. Keep the tissues as supple as possible so that drainage can occur in a healthy manner. Drink ample fresh water, and avoid anything that adds to congestion.

Hints for Control (Care Providers): Some interior nasal and mouth trigger areas respond to topical anesthetic on a cotton swab. Finger pressure may work on interior mouth areas, using topical anesthetic, but they may be sensitive. Work gently and only on a small area for a brief time. Start with gums and eventually proceed to other mouth areas. A typical session with a trained massage expert may be far too painful and far too long, enhancing FM. A few minutes' gentle exploration will tell what can be endured for how long, with awareness that aftereffects may be delayed. Tongue-depressor exercises to strengthen floor-of-mouth, tongue, genioglossus, mylohyoid, anterior digastric, medial pterygoid, and intrinsic tongue muscles should only be used if, by palpation, these muscles are cleared of trigger areas. The prescription nasal spray ipratropium bromide is an acetylcholine inhibitor. It may be of more help for TrP-mediated runny nose than other sprays, but allergies require additional spray as well.

Be vigilant against overuse of antibiotics, and aware that many chronic sinus and ear infections are caused by fungus.

Medial Pterygoid
Greek *pterygoeides* means "wing-like."
Latin *medialis* means "middle."

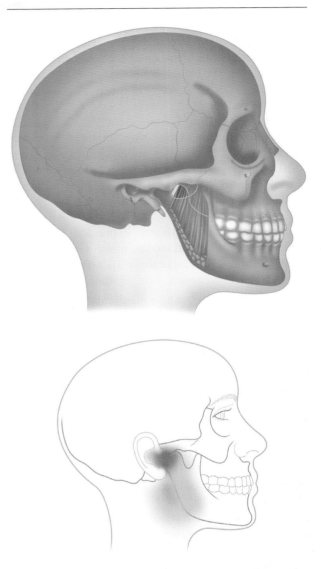

What It Does: Opens and closes the mouth and helps to move the jaw from side to side. This action also involves the infrahyoid muscles that act to stabilize the hyoid bone. The medial pterygoid fibers run up and down. And you didn't even know they exercised!

Kinetics Comments: If this muscle and surrounding fascia are tight with TrPs, the tensor veli palatine muscle may not be able to fully dilate the Eustachian tube, producing a feeling of stuffiness in the ear on the same side as the TrP. Pain from this TrP may increase when the mouth is open wide, during chewing, or when teeth are clenched. TrPs in this muscle may entrap the chorda tympani portion of the lingual nerve, resulting in a bitter and metallic taste.

TrP Comments: TrPs here cause pain locally and can refer pain deep into the TMJ and maxillary sinus, tongue, back of mouth, throat, hard palate, floor of the nose, and ear, and below and behind the TMJ. Swallowing may be painful or difficult. *These TrPs are more often the cause than the result of bite irregularities.* These TrPs may contribute to hypersensitivity to sound, hearing loss, "blocked ears," gum pain, or earache. Maxillary sinus congestion may be caused by blood vessel entrapment by these TrPs.

Notable Perpetuating Factors: Head-forward posture, excessive thumb sucking after infancy, excessive gum chewing, clenching or lateral grinding of teeth, GERD, anxiety and emotional tension, local cellulitis, and infection in the region. Check for tight pectoralis muscles.

Hints for Control (Patients): Work the TrPs from inside the mouth, behind the last molar. Go slowly and carefully—when you finger those TrPs, they hurt! Oral anesthetics help to endure working these TrPs. Ensure that your sleeping pillow fits, and that sleep position is not a factor. If swallowing pills is a problem, place the tablet or capsule under the tongue behind the front teeth. *Then* swallow water: it may help get the pill down.

Hints for Control (Care Providers): Electrical stimulation and ultrasound may be useful for these TrPs. If there is difficulty swallowing, also check the SCM, digastric, longus capitis, and longus colli for TrPs. Be very gentle when working the mouth area internally. Use oral anesthetic: the patient will still be able to feel the treatment, but it won't hurt as much. You also have a much greater chance of keeping your fingers.

Stretch: Sit comfortably, keeping your head upright and still. Place the web of your thumb and forefinger against the front of your lower jaw. Keep the tip of your tongue behind your top teeth, on the roof of your mouth. This will help to stabilize your neck and offer general support to the area. Gently push your jaw downward until you feel a nice gentle stretch. You can repeat this several times as long as it feels good. Stay within the normal ROM.

Lateral Pterygoid
Greek *pterygoeides* means "wing-like."
Latin *lateralis* means "relating to the side."

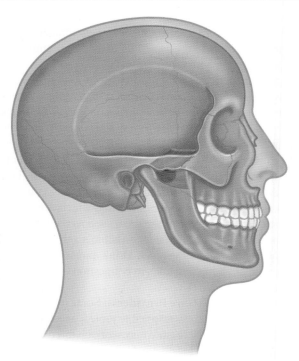

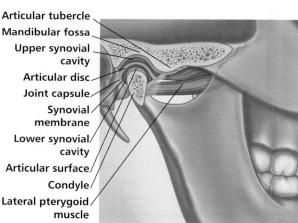

Articular tubercle
Mandibular fossa
Upper synovial cavity
Articular disc
Joint capsule
Synovial membrane
Lower synovial cavity
Articular surface
Condyle
Lateral pterygoid muscle

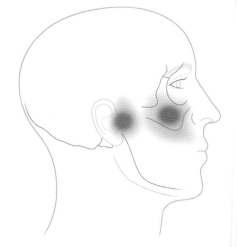

What It Does: Pulls the head of the mandible, the disc, and the joint capsule forward, opens the mouth, and moves the jaw from side to side. This is the muscle that is responsible for you sleeping with your mouth open.

Kinetics Comments: These muscles are not very strong, and are susceptible to strain as they attempt to slow and control jaw closing. Each lateral pterygoid has eight tendinous layers that can affect many other structures to which they attach. Tightness of this muscle affects speech, singing, and playing of musical wind instruments. Maxillary sinus congestion could be aggravated by blood vessel entrapment and drainage constraints due to TrPs in this muscle.

TrP Comments: TrPs in this muscle can cause deep TMJ and maxillary sinus pain, crackling noises from the TMJ on movement, tinnitus, and/or soreness or pain in the back of the mouth. There may be difficulty swallowing and excessive secretion from maxillary sinuses. Symptoms may include dizziness, earache, ear pain, and gum pain. This muscle is attached to the TMJ disc; TrPs can therefore cause disc displacement, eventually leading to disc erosion. Muscle accommodation to TrPs during chewing action can cause distortion of the incisor and cuspid teeth, changing the cutting path and causing malocclusion. This may be worsened by TrP-associated proprioceptor effects, resulting in tongue and/or cheek biting.

Notable Perpetuating Factors: TMJ degenerative changes or bruxism may be caused by TrPs in this muscle. TrPs in this muscle can be caused by stress from unequal leg length, unequal hemipelvis, and contractured neck muscles. Head-forward posture, poor tongue posture, B vitamin insufficiency, nail biting, excessive gum chewing, thumb sucking, or playing a wind instrument or violin can also activate or perpetuate these TrPs.

Hints for Control (Patients): These TrPs are often misdiagnosed as TMJ arthritis or sinusitis. A thinned cotton applicator (Q-tip) with topical anesthetic artfully applied to this muscle inside the mouth, followed by three full ROM movements, can be helpful. Finger massage of this muscle inside and out may ease joint clicking and pain.

Hints for Control (Care Providers): Some of these TrP symptoms may be due to the connection with the sphenoid bone and the lateral and medial pterygoid plates. If the buccal nerve is entrapped, these TrPs may be mistaken for tic douloureux. Treat by TrP release, electrical stimulation, ultrasound, and stretch and spray.

Platysma
Greek *platus* means "broad" or "flat."

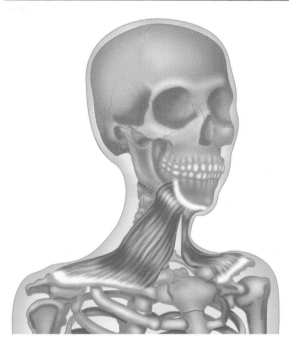

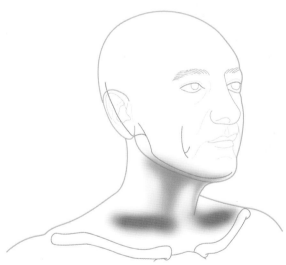

What It Does: Aids mouth opening, especially in producing expressions of horror. It pulls the lower lip from the corner of the mouth down and out to the side. The platysma is in fact a muscle of the integumentary (skin) system and technically not skeletal muscle at all!

Kinetics Comments: This is a broad, flat, thin muscle that horses use to shake off flies. It stands out when weightlifters strain to raise their weights. Platysma tightness can pull down on the facial muscles and pull up on the chest muscles. This muscle is inhibited by masseter tightness, so platysma TrPs may be satellites of masseter TrPs. This muscle overlies the thyroid gland and many small muscles, and TrP-caused tightness here could possibly affect them.

TrP Comments: This muscle is superficial. Platysma TrPs can refer pain to the chin or cause prickles that cover the cheek and/or travel across the shoulder blades and neck. Platysma pain is unusual: if you have platysma TrPs, there is a sensation of a small, angry porcupine (with quills out) rolling across your neck. It feels like multiple and relatively shallow pin-pricks of hot pain, but not like the tingling of nerve pain. The referral pattern depends on the location of the TrPs: TrPs low on the platysma cause referred pain in the upper chest, while mid and low bilateral platysma TrPs send pain to two areas above the collarbone, without characteristic platysma pain between them. Platysma TrPs may contribute to nighttime teeth grinding. Associated symptoms can include stiffness in the front of the throat. Because some of the platysma fibers interlace with the orbicularis oris muscle see interlacing of buccinator and orbicularis oris fibers, TrPs in this muscle may cause increased blinking.

Notable Perpetuating Factors: Sternal SCM, masseter and/or scalene TrPs, and nocturnal teeth grinding.

Self-treatment: Sweep the muscle with an ice cube covered with a thin wet cloth. Open your mouth through its full ROM while you sweep the covered ice cube over the skin. After closing your mouth gently, stick your chin forward as far as you comfortably can, and, if appropriate, take your head back so as to hyperextend your neck. Avoid moving your chin from side to side while you do this. Repeat this process once or twice, but rewarm the muscle in between each repetition to prevent chilling the underlying muscles (see Chapter 14). Avoid holding the stretch. Controlled movement is the key.

Laryngeal Muscles
(cricoarytenoid, cricothyroid, aryepiglottis, thyroepiglottis, thyroarytenoid)
Laryngeal means "relating to the larynx." Greek *larugx* means "upper part of the trachea containing the vocal cords."

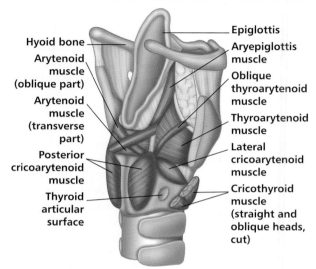

Muscles of larynx (posterolateral view).

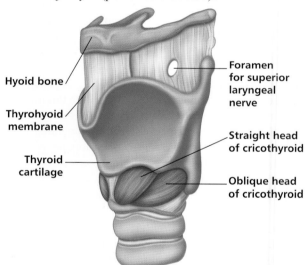

Muscles of larynx (lateral view).

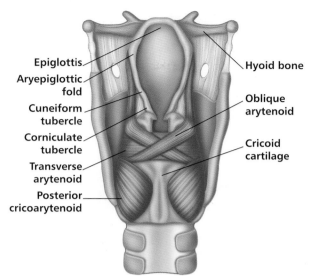

Muscles of larynx (posterior view).

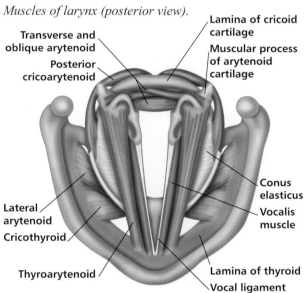

Muscles of larynx (superior view).

What They Do: Control tension on the vocal cords, affecting the ligaments and cartilage attached to them. The aryepiglottis, thyroepiglottis, and thyroarytenoid move to block passing food from entering the laryngeal space by pulling the epiglottis down and back like a trap door. They are assisted in this action by the backward movement of the tongue. Arytenoid muscles control the degree of opening of the vocal cords. Cricothyroid muscle tension affects vocal cord length and tension. Cricoarytenoid muscles abduct and adduct the arytenoid cartilages, so be aware of any changes to vocal tone, as this may be a useful diagnostic sign. The hyoid is not part of these muscles, but is a useful landmark.

Kinetics Comments: Abnormal tightness in these muscles can affect the way the voice sounds, including pitch and volume. The ability to form some specific language sounds, called glottal consonants, is affected by laryngeal muscle tightness. Tightness in these muscles can significantly affect cricoarytenoid joint mobility, causing speech problems and even loss of voice.

TrP Comments: Laryngeal muscle tension is present in a number of voice disorders. As far as we know, nothing has been published yet on TrPs as a common cause of this tension. Active TrPs in any of the laryngeal muscles can cause hoarseness, frequent throat clearing, cough, strained or strangled voice, loss of voice, and/or sore throat. TrPs in the aryepiglottis, thyroepiglottis, or thyroarytenoid can interfere with the normal closure of the epiglottis, causing a choking sensation, even with swallowing saliva.

Notable Perpetuating Factors: These include tension and head-forward posture. Exposure to toxic gases, including those from smoking, can activate these TrPs, as can excess alcoholic intake, prolonged screaming or yelling, or the mechanical irritation of intubation. Avoid very hot or very cold drinks. Do your best to avoid clearing your throat, as each time you do this you are slapping your vocal cords together, causing more irritation, swelling, mucus production, and congestion. This adds to your sense of urgency to clear your throat, which slaps your vocal cords together again, causing more irritation. Laryngopharyngeal reflux bathes these tissues in acid fumes, activating TrPs and causing posterior laryngeal mucosal thickening, edema, and redness.

Hints for Control: Hoarseness that persists for over two weeks requires investigation. Control of these TrPs depends on the causes and perpetuating factors, but must include assessment of the hyoid muscles and related structures for associated TrPs. Check for paradoxical breathing (especially mouth breathing), allergies, postural compensations, pollution, and other causes of inhalant toxic exposure. Avoid noisy areas in which one must speak very loudly to be heard. A speech therapist who knows TrPs may be necessary for instruction on the use of good vocal hygiene. Laryngopharyngeal reflux is often treated with medications to bring GERD under control, but many of these can have serious side effects. Seek the *cause* of the GERD, such as permeable gut, poor diet, lack of proper chewing, and/or insufficient enzymes. Check for coexisting conditions, such as insulin resistance. If the cause of the reflux is found and can be brought under control, medication may no longer be necessary.

Self-treatment: Cool compresses may relieve some of the tightness and subsequent pain from these TrPs, allowing gentle finger pressure to work them. Spontaneous laughter is a wonderful way to exercise these muscles. *You definitely do not want to try to stretch these muscles yourself.* Find a well-qualified and experienced therapist who can safely displace the larynx to allow for soft tissue release of the anterior neck muscles. Vapocoolant spray and vibratory massage can often release these TrPs and restore a voice within minutes.

Note: The successful use of a botulism toxin injection into the bilateral thyroarytenoid or posterior cricoarytenoid muscles for spasmic dysphonia indicates the possible presence of TrPs. Supraglottic contraction, which can also be caused by TrPs, is a critical factor in conditions previously described as "primary muscle tension dysphonia" or "muscle misuse dysphonia." Secondary TrPs from rheumatoid arthritis may significantly contribute to glottis dysfunction. We suggest that TrPs often cause or contribute to these conditions, while acknowledging that more research needs to be done on this subject.

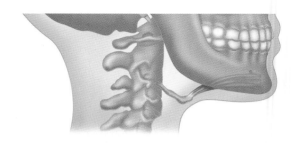

Geniohyoid.

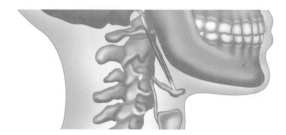

Stylohyoid.

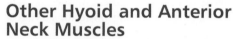

Other Hyoid and Anterior Neck Muscles
Greek *huoeides* means "shaped like the Greek letter upsilon."

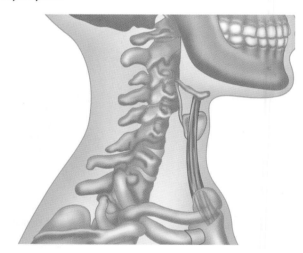

Sternohyoid.

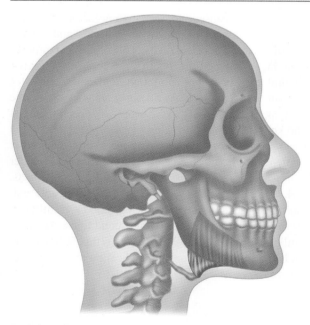

Mylohyoid.

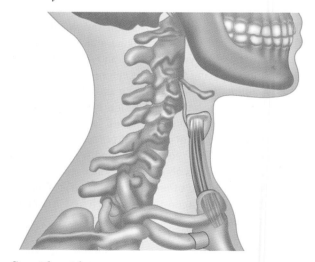

Sternithyroid.

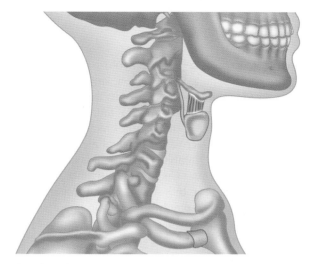

Thyrohyoid.

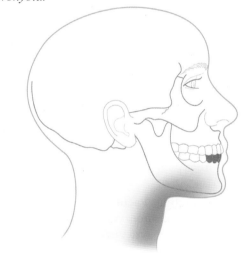

What They Do: Aid in positioning the hyoid bone.

Kinetic Comments: All of these muscles affect the hyoid bone as either hyoid or infrahyoid muscles. The hyoid bone is a floating bone. Muscles attaching above and below the bone support it and direct its integration during respiration, vocalization, chewing, and swallowing. In the neck, stiffness is provided by the infra- and suprahyoids and the SCM during activities such as sit-ups. If the tongue is not placed in its physiological resting position (behind the front teeth on the roof of the mouth), the hyoid muscles cannot contract to create the level of stiffness required through the fascia to offer cervical joint support. The SCM will contract even more to make up the stiffness deficit. This will result in a short SCM, head-forward posture, rounded shoulders, and additional full-body kinetic chain implications.

TrP Comments: If active TrPs occur only on one side, there is a tendency to avoid turning the head to that side because it will aggravate swallowing problems or other symptoms. These TrPs can increase air swallowing (Sato and Nakashima 2009), and that can be significant for patients on CPAP and may even interrupt sleep. These

TrPs may be related to vocal tremor (Finnegan et al. 2003).

Notable Perpetuating Factors: Head-forward posture, whiplash, and upper respiratory infection or irritation such as from allergies. Sleeping or sitting for long periods with the neck tilted to one side and the shoulder hiked up can initiate or perpetuate these TrPs. Head-forward posture places the mandible in a position that puts the masseter under undue stress. Antagonist muscles such as the geniohyoid, omohyoid, and digastric can all become spastic because of poor technique used while overtraining the abdominal muscles. This in turn may inhibit the masseter, with resulting TrP formation to provide stiffness within the muscle. Changes in associated suboccipital muscles lead to changes in the balance of the head and face muscles. Change in the positioning of the temporomandibular joint will also affect the position of the cervical spine. Correct alignment of the TMJ requires treatment of the masseter and pterygoids at the local level, with attention to core efficiency at the global level.

Hints for Control (Patients): Intermittent cold compress, gentle finger pressure (it takes skill to get into specific muscles), stretch and spray, and myofascial release may be helpful. Correct poor posture. At rest and during exercise, keep the tongue in its physiological resting position.

Hints for Control (Care Providers): Injection of the oblique lateral cricoarytenoid muscles can ease the symptoms of a strained/strangled-sounding voice (Young and Blitzer 2007). TrPs in the stylohyoid muscle can entrap the external carotid artery and auricular artery, thus decreasing the flow of blood to the brain, even without calcifications or the presence of Eagle syndrome (Loch and Fehrmann 1990), causing confusing carotid test results.

Stretch: A nice way to maintain appropriate ROM for the anterior neck muscles is simply moving through all the ranges gently, but do not "circle the head." Avoid static stretching and do not hold your neck in hyperextension (the older you are, the more important this becomes!), such as when you bend your neck back to look up at the top of a tall building. This can reduce both blood supply and blood pressure, placing you at risk of falling. Falling, however, is not the problem: the problem is the sudden stop when you hit the ground.

Note: Although physiotherapy has been found helpful for voice disorders (Rubin, Blake, and Matheieson 2007), and hypertonicity in these muscles has been associated with vocal quality (Kooijman et al. 2005), many vocal practitioners are unaware of TrPs that can shorten or weaken these muscles. We encourage collaboration between vocal researchers and TrP therapists.

Omohyoid
Greek *omos* means "shoulder"; *huoeides*, "shaped like the Greek letter upsilon."

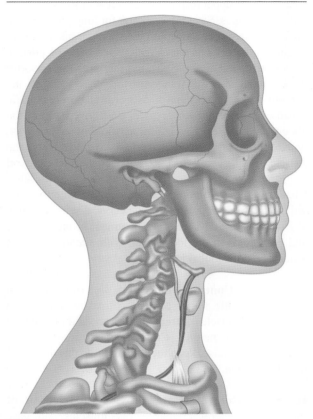

Right omohyoid.

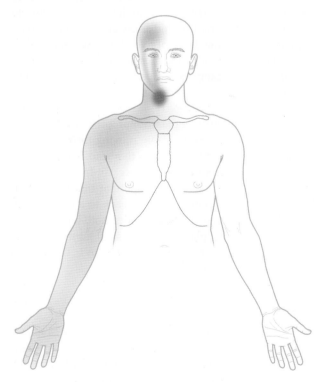

Right omohyoid referral pattern.

What It Does: Depresses the hyoid bone after it has been raised during swallowing.

Kinetics Comments: The omohyoid is a long muscle with two bellies, united by a tendon, and is an important link in the kinetic chain. Because of its fascial investment it picks up the lungs to allow for full lung expansion and deep breathing. A short, tight omohyoid can form a constricting band across the brachial plexus, elevating the first rib. A tight, inhibited omohyoid is also a source of kinetic problems. Contracture of the omohyoid muscle can inhibit a full stretch of the trapezius and scalene muscles. The omohyoid plays an important role in moving food from the mouth into the gastrointestinal system and avoiding it being sent it into the respiratory system.

TrP Comments: Muscle weakness, burning, and/or tingling may accompany aching pain and cause diagnostic confusion. These TrPs may result in a sore throat, difficulty swallowing, and/or constriction of the neck area. TrPs in the omohyoid may cause choking as if "food is going down the wrong pipe." Even swallowing saliva may initiate this sensation. TrPs in this muscle are very common in patients with CMP, and may contribute to excess air from CPAP pressure going into the stomach. Omohyoid TrPs may be disabling and must not be taken lightly (Rask 1984).

Notable Perpetuating Factors: Intense or repeated muscle overload, such as from vomiting, severe coughing, or GERD. Check for systemic illness or nutritional insufficiency.

Hints for Control: *Surgery must not be the first line of treatment for elevated first rib.* That rib is bound to the omohyoid by a deep cervical fascial sling. The omohyoid stands out prominently when the head is tilted to the opposite side. Check for postural problems. TrP finger-point pressure release may help, and may be easier to do during exhalation, but the muscle is long and must be fully treated. TrPs may respond to cold compresses. If these TrPs are active, eat mindfully and slowly, chewing thoroughly. Avoid drinking cold liquids quickly, especially at the beginning of a meal. All perpetuating factors must be thoroughly brought under control.

Stretch: Sit upright with your right arm hanging directly down along the side of your body, and point your right fingers towards the floor. Isolate the movement so that only the right arm moves and your body remains still. Gently bring the left ear towards the left shoulder until you feel a mild stretch and immediately return to the starting position and repeat on the other side, changing both the side of the arm and the side of the ear and shoulder.

Digastric
Latin *digastricus* means "having two (muscle) bellies."

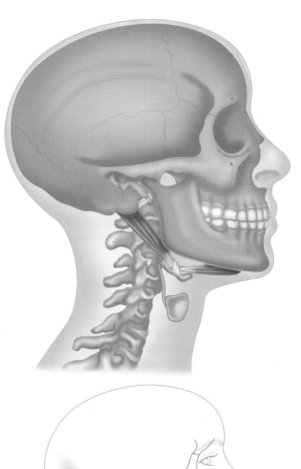

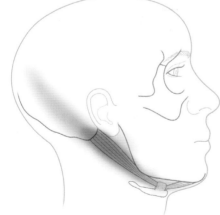

Left posterior digastric TrP referral pattern.

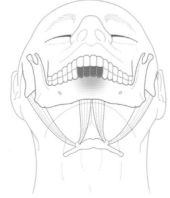

Anterior digastric TrP referral pattern.

What It Does: Raises the hyoid bone; depresses and retracts the mandible.

Kinetics Comments: Digastric TrPs may perpetuate SCM TrPs. The digastric is another muscle that affects the position of the hyoid bone. Every bone in your body has some unique aspect, but the hyoid bone itself is unique: it is the only bone in the human body that does not directly attach in any manner to any other bone. The hyoid bone is located not far below your jawbone (mandible) and literally "hangs," as it is suspended in the neck by the styloid process (a protrusion of bone just behind your ears and part of the temporal bone), as well as by the stylohyoid muscle and ligaments. This horseshoe-shaped bone is responsible for providing the necessary support for the tongue and serves as an attachment point for a number of muscles that move the tongue. The bone can be felt using a pincer grip with your thumb and second finger just below the jaw. When muscles are not playing their part in the team effort required to ensure this bone is in place, the result can be a wide range of sensations. A "lump in the throat" feeling and difficulty drinking or swallowing are generally reported. In our clinical experience a misplaced hyoid bone can lead to head rotation, head tilting, and misalignment of the jawbone—and TrPs!

TrP Comments: The anterior digastric refers pain to the front bottom teeth and to the tissues below them. The referral area may include the middle of the bottom lip and the tongue. Posterior digastric TrPs refer in a curving band from under the jaw line to the back of the head, with the most severe pain in the neck at the base of the jaw beneath the ear; they may refer pain into the ear. There may be a sensation of a lump in the throat. These TrPs can be involved in speech difficulties due to their effect on the hyoid bone. TrPs in this muscle may also cause the feeling of food "going down the wrong pipe," and may lead to choking on saliva. These TrPs often cause swallowing difficulties. TrP contraction nodules may be mistaken for swollen glands. If the SCMs are also involved, this can cause diagnostic confusion.

Notable Perpetuating Factors: Paradoxical breathing (especially mouth breathing), head-forward posture, teeth clenching and grinding, and poor bite. Posterior digastric TrPs may be initiated and perpetuated by Eagle syndrome. Digastric TrPs may be initiated and perpetuated by chronic overload, such as from playing a wind instrument or maintaining a fixed position holding a violin or telephone in place, or by sudden overload, such as whiplash.

Hints for Control (Patients): Pain from the anterior TrPs may be temporarily eased by rubbing the gum and adjacent mouth area with a topical numbing agent; this allows for less painful massage of the area. Intermittent cold may relieve the pain from the posterior section.

Hints for Control (Care Providers): Having carried out a full-body kinetic chain assessment, offer therapeutic intervention at the level of the head/neck, upper torso, and pelvis, and then the lower limbs. Many times the body needs a little push towards "homeostasis" and it can then begin to heal. Clinical experience indicates a superior-to-inferior and medial-to-lateral development pattern in many cases, and this is a preferred sequence in treatment as well.

Self-treatment: Try gentle self-massage of this area, sitting at a table with your elbows on the table to help support your arms. Gently work the area with your fingers, starting under the chin and working back. Massage both sides, even if only one side hurts. Go gently. The area close to the ear may be very tight and may take a while to loosen up to touch. It is a good way to practice self-palpation. Moist heat may help for the tightness, and ice stroking may help for the pain. When we use the word "stretch," we are referring to an effort made to return a shortened muscle fiber or group of fibers, along with the associated fascia, to a more normal length. In this case, opening and closing the mouth through normal range is a really nice finish to a treatment.

Longus Colli
Latin *longus* means "long"; *colli*, "of the neck."

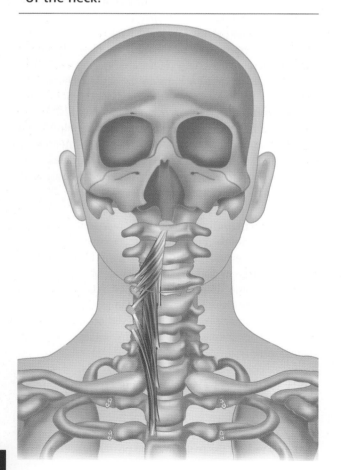

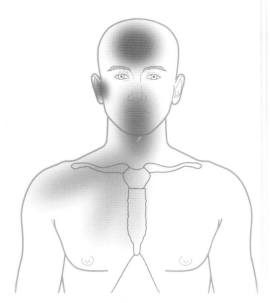

What It Does: Flexes the neck. The lowest section may aid sideways bending and lateral rotation.

Kinetics Comments: This muscle attaches to multiple areas of the spine, adding to its networking skills. A tight and spastic longus colli, together with resulting accommodation by scalenes and other muscles, leads to a stiff neck and head-forward posture, and even to tightness in the psoas and down the leg to the foot. TrPs in the psoas can in turn perpetuate TrPs in the longus colli.

TrP Comments: Referral pain varies in patterns as shown in the figures, and may continue to the eye. These TrPs may be accompanied by a dry mouth, a persistent tickle in the throat, a feeling of a lump in the throat when swallowing, tongue pain, a sore throat, and/or tightness in the chest. Whiplash is frequently an instigator of these TrPs. Check this muscle when the SCM has TrPs.

Notable Perpetuating Factors: Head-forward posture, sudden jerks to the neck (that can occur when falling, near falling, or being pulled by an unruly large dog on a leash), pelvic torsion, and sustained twisting of neck. Lying-down reading with the head tilted to one side, lying on the sofa reading with the neck tilted upward, and other postural nightmares are perpetuating factors.

Hints for Control: Correct any perpetuating factors. Tend to the areas around the muscle up and down the kinetic chain.

Stretch: Most people who feel tightness in these muscles want to stretch them. You may be only "stretching the symptoms." A dynamic stretch can feel good while you are performing the stretch, but if it does not resolve the tension, you need to consider the muscles and tissues further along the kinetic chain. We advise avoiding static stretching of these muscles. Instead, lie on your back on the floor, with a folded towel under your neck for support. Bend your knees and keep your feet flat on the floor. Rotate your head to one side and go as far as feels comfortable. Then drop your ear on that side to the shoulder below, feeling a nice stretch. Return to the starting position and repeat to the other side. Remember to breathe normally and avoid pain.

Longus Capitis
Latin *longus* means "long"; *capitis*, "of the head."

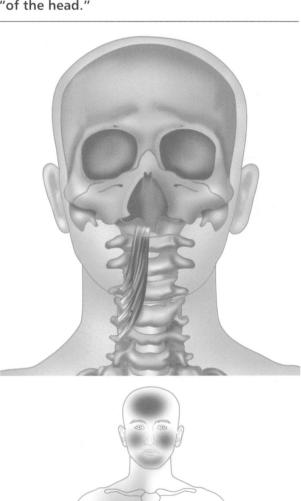

What It Does: Flexes the head on the neck and flexes the superior cervical spine, usually against resistance. This muscle is part of the mechanism that helps to equalize air and sound pressure between the oral and nasal cavities.

Kinetics Comments: This muscle slows down (i.e. decelerates) neck extension, and is frequently part of whiplash trauma. Tightness here may be secondary to spasm in the lower stabilizers, especially the psoas.

TrP Comments: Head and facial pain, including referral to the ear and eye, and pain down the neck, chest, and part of the arm. "Sinus" pain may be reported, as well as significant pain to the front of the neck, with difficulty swallowing and the sensation of a lump in throat. Some of these symptoms are logical when you investigate the research (Yamawaki, Nishimura, and Suzuki 1996).

Notable Perpetuating Factors: Any sustained or chronic movement, trauma, or environmental stressor (such as drafts or other irritants) can be an initiating or perpetuating factor.

Hints for Control: This muscle may be involved when whiplash symptoms persist after other muscles have been treated. It responds to FSM (as do all TrPs), and to stretch and spray. Cold compresses may help. Avoid treating sinus infections with antibiotics unless there is evidence of bacterial infection. If bacteria are present, they should be tested for their susceptibility to specific antibiotics.

Stretch: The longus capitis is another muscle that is difficult to stretch without the aid of a professional. That said, allowing your head to drop back as far as feels comfortable and then bringing your chin to your chest will take this muscle through its ROM. If you feel dizzy when performing the neck extension part of the stretch, seek professional advice before continuing.

Rectus Capitis Anterior and Lateralis

Latin *rectus* means "straight"; *capitis*, "of the head"; *anterior*, "before"; *lateralis*, "relating to the side."

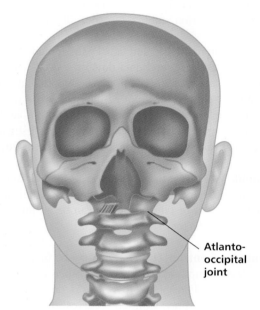

Rectus capitis anterior.

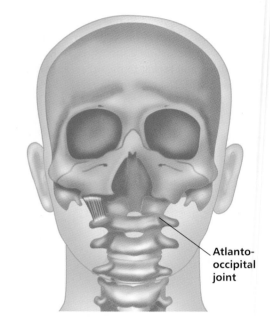

Rectus capitis lateralis.

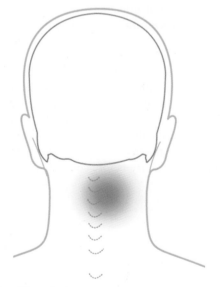

Rectus capitis anterior.

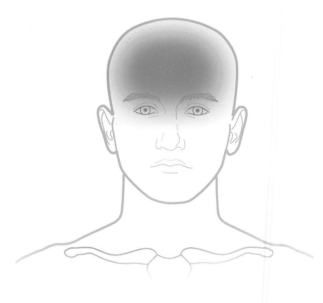

Rectus capitis lateralis.

What They Do: The anterior muscle stabilizes the atlanto-occipital joint during movement, and flexes the head. The lateralis muscle stabilizes the atlanto-occipital joint during movement, and flexes the head to the side.

Kinetics Comments: The average weight of a head is ten pounds, or similar to a bowling ball. The coordinated work of many muscles all the way down the kinetic chain is required to keep it balanced and stable on the top of the spine. When these muscles are shortened, tight, inflexible, and inhibited and lack coordination, dysfunction results. One type of dysfunction relates to proprioception, as signals in the neck tell your brain where you are in space in relation to your surroundings, as well as where your head is in relation to the rest of your body. Although the SCM is well known for proprioceptor dysfunction, many neck muscles are likewise involved, and these are no exception. The tendency to be "accident-prone" or clumsy may have as its root proprioceptor dysfunction. Muscle timing may be off, resulting in missed connections that cause you to plan the day to allow time for frequent cleanup. (Clue: do you buy paper towels by the case?) It may be difficult to keep a sense of humor as you bounce off doorjambs and furniture corners. The question isn't if your glass is half full or half empty, but whether or not you were able to get any liquid in the glass at all. Once you understand *why* this is happening, you can focus on the neck muscles, especially that SCM, with the basic understanding that the primary TrP that started the kinetic compensation could be anywhere in the body—even the foot.

TrP Comments: These TrPs can refer pain to the back of the neck and/or diffuse pain deep into the brain. This can feel like a migraine originating inside the brain and encompassing the whole of the brain, or it can intensify a migraine. Any posterior neck muscle can contribute to or cause what is called "tension headache." The muscle may be tense because of TrPs. Stress is one, but only one, potential initiating factor of this "tension." Emotional stress can always be a contributing factor, but one must consider physical stressors as well. Light sensitivity, sensitivity to touch in the head and neck regions, and loss of ability to focus attention are common, and nerve and/or blood vessel entrapment may be due to these TrPs, but all these symptoms may be blamed on FM.

Notable Perpetuating Factors: Whiplash, cold drafts on a chilled muscle, poor posture, infections, and other physical stressors, including emotional stressors, are common perpetuating factors.

Hints for Control: Ice stroking, correction of perpetuating factors, stimuli reduction for sensitivities, and manual therapy may be useful. A folded hand towel pinned as a gentle soft neck brace may help support the head.

Stretch: Gently bring your chin closer to your chest until you feel a mild stretch in the back of your neck. Return to the starting position and rest a moment. Slowly turn your head slightly to the right and repeat. Rest a moment. Then slowly turn your head slightly to the left and repeat.

Rectus Capitis Posterior Major and Minor

Latin *rectus* means "straight"; *capitis*, "of the head."

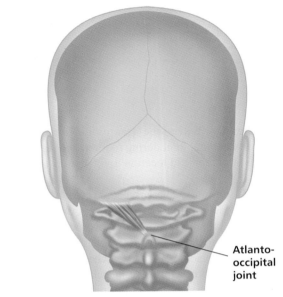

Rectus capitis posterior major.

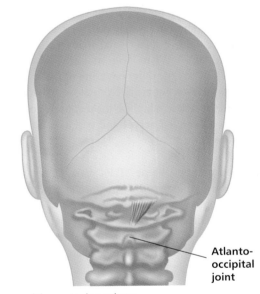

Rectus capitis posterior minor.

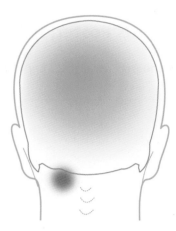

What They Do: Extend the head on the neck, stabilize the atlanto-occipital joint during motion, and send spatial information of the head location to the brain.

Kinetics Comments: There is a connective tissue bridge between the deep part of these muscles and transverse fibers of the atlanto-occipital membrane that extends anatomically into the perivascular vertebral artery tissues. This may explain some of the headache intensity that can be caused by tightness in these muscles, as it can affect the dura (the outer covering of the spinal cord and brain) and the flow of cerebrospinal fluid. These muscles attach directly to the dura mater of both the spinal cord and the brain, fulfilling an important functional role. When these muscles shorten (as they do), their associated fascia pulls on the dura, causing what many patients describe as "brain pain." When you move your head, these muscles "pull" on the outer covering of the spinal cord to ensure that it does not crinkle or get stuck between bony structures. In severe whiplash these muscles can separate from their associated nerves and will eventually atrophy (waste away).

TrP Comments: These TrPs can cause myogenic headache, migraine, and/or postural imbalance. Visual and neurological symptoms may join the headaches and neck pain, including dizziness and/or petit mal seizure-like symptoms. The pain from these TrPs can worsen as soon as the head hits the pillow, affecting the quality of sleep.

Notable Perpetuating Factors: Be attentive to head movements in bed. Raising the unsupported head while lying on the back initiates and perpetuates TrPs, as can articular dysfunction high on the vertebral column, sustained muscle overload (such as during bird watching), and chilling of the muscle. Any suboccipital muscle can be stressed by frequent movements of the head to compensate for bifocals, or by incorrect eye correction. Poor posture, including head-forward posture and reading at the kitchen table with the chin propped on the hands, begs TrPs to form. Muscle atrophy in the rectus capitis minor can occur if the TrPs persist.

Hints for Control: If you have these TrPs, turtleneck shirts are your best friend and may even need to be worn to bed. Unfortunately, if these TrPs are present, you may be unable to tolerate the pressure of turtlenecks, so you need to find another way to keep your neck warm and protected from drafts. Treat with gentle muscle lengthening and light finger pressure. These TrPs can be disabling and frightening. They can be treated, but treatment should be prompt.

Stretch: Gently bring your chin closer to your chest until you feel a mild stretch in the back of your neck. Then return to the starting position. Repeat during the day, but avoid speed, as this may lead to dizziness. We recommend regular manual therapy including fascial release.

Scalenes
Greek *skalenos* means "uneven."

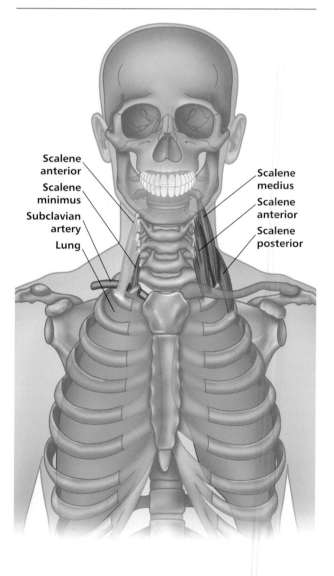

Scalene anterior
Scalene minimus
Subclavian artery
Lung
Scalene medius
Scalene anterior
Scalene posterior

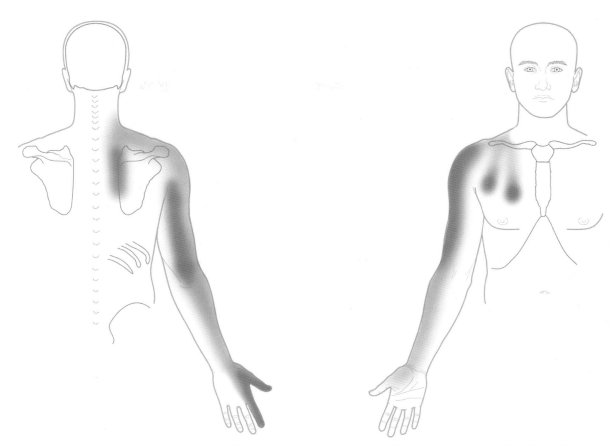

Combined referral pattern for scalenes medius, anterior, and posterior, which, together, are called the scalene major.

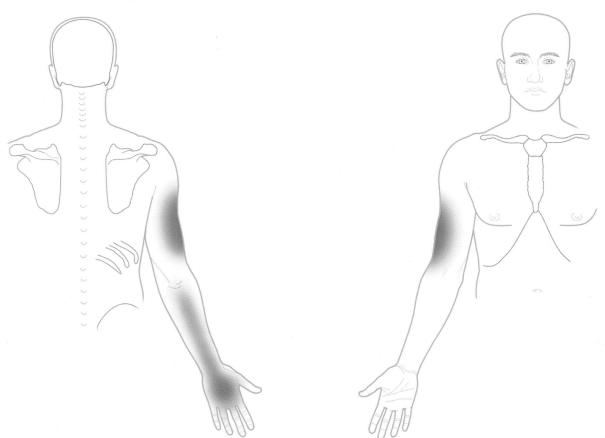

Combined referral pattern for scalene minimus.

What They Do: The three scalene groups on each side (anterior, medial, and posterior) are attached so that they can work together to flex the neck to their own side, with limited rotation on the other side. Anterior and medial scalenes stabilize the first rib during breathing and assist in rib elevation. Posterior scalenes help stabilize, with the scalene minimus, and/or elevate the second ribs during breathing.

Kinetics Comments: The subclavian and brachial plexus are surrounded by the scalenes, and opportunity for nerve or blood/lymph vessel entrapment abounds. If the scalenes are shortened and tight, check the SCM, upper trapezius, and splenius capitis, as they are all part of the same functional unit. Also check the pectoralis major and minor, the long head of the triceps brachii, the deltoid, and all of the arm muscles. The omohyoid may also be involved by forming a constricting band across the brachial plexus, inhibiting the full stretch of the scalenes and trapezius. Medial scalene TrPs may be causing entrapment of nerve fibers, producing symptoms of carpal tunnel syndrome (CTS) and thoracic outlet syndrome (TOS).

TrP Comments: In our opinions, lack of TrP awareness results in much unnecessary surgery. If you hear descriptions such as "carpal tunnel syndrome," "thoracic outlet syndrome," "raised first rib," or "scalene syndrome," surgery should be the last thing on your mind. Scalene TrPs cause a wide variety of symptoms and have a large referral pattern that can be severe enough to disrupt sleep. They can cause median nerve entrapment, with tingling or numbness in the thumb and first finger, and/or blood vessel or lymph entrapment that may lead to puffiness on the back of the hand and stiffness of the hand. Rings may feel tight, often most noticeably in the morning. These TrPs can cause myogenic headache, angina-like pain and chest tightness, and/or persistent pain in any part or all of the referral area, with weakness in the hand or arm that results in loss of grip strength and unexpectedly dropping objects. Pain and other symptoms may vary from day to day or hour to hour, causing diagnostic confusion. If symptoms become worse when turning the head to the extent of the ROM towards the side of the pain (assuming you only have TrPs on one side) and dropping the chin towards the collarbone, scalene TrPs are the culprits. They can also be the source of the phantom limb pain of an amputated arm.

Notable Perpetuating Factors: Poor posture, paradoxical breathing, cool drafts, poor body mechanics in lifting or pulling heavy objects, heavy backpacks, heavy breasts, chronic breathing conditions such as asthma or chronic obstructive pulmonary disease (COPD), respiratory infections, chronic cough, and inappropriate lighting. Lying down on a sofa with the neck propped at an angle while reading or watching television invites these TrPs to settle in, as does lifting your head from the lying position without supporting it. If you're owned by a cat who sleeps on your shoulder, you've got a furpetuating factor. (This requires prompt negotiations with the cat union for substitute nightly feline accommodations so that the cat is not a literal pain in the neck.) To compensate for short upper arms, use an appropriate elbow rest in the car or when sitting and reading. Use a speakerphone if possible. One of the authors (Starlanyl) has seen these TrPs in an equestrian after a long ride on an unruly horse, a long-distance swimmer after a cold day in the water, and a dog walker after a huge, untrained dog yanked him about. Playing some musical instruments such as the violin can perpetuate these TrPs, as can any tilt of the shoulder girdle axis (lower limb inequality when standing, small hemipelvis when seated). Any gait dysfunction can also initiate or perpetuate these TrPs.

Hints for Control (Patients): Have the reading light overhead, not at the side. Learn how to roll over in bed and how to get up from lying on the sofa. Be mindful of your posture at all times (yes, you *can* learn to modify sleep postures), and keep those shoulders from creeping up to the ears by periodically checking and adjusting shoulder position. Prevention is better than treatment. These TrPs can occur as a delayed reaction after a neck trauma or after an infection. If there is trauma, even a fall or sudden neck jerk, take preventative measures with gentle manual therapy and moist heat on the scalene area for 15 minutes before bed. If needed, a folded kitchen towel can be pinned to form a soft collar to help support these muscles. Avoid rigid neck braces. Keep the neck warm and out of chill drafts. Scarves and turtleneck sweaters are your friends. Correct paradoxical breathing and postural stressors, and ensure that eye correction is appropriate. Professional guidance may be helpful for fingertip therapy, as many nerves and blood vessels are in this area. When symptoms are worse after sleeping, check sleeping postures, pillows, and the bed. Avoid using extra pillows, and make sure that your pillow fits the curvature of your neck: neck curvature may change with therapy, and one size does not fit all. If necessary, raise the head of the bed 3–4" (about 7.5–10 cm). Some patients need to sleep in a reclining chair.

Hints for Control (Care Providers): Craniosacral and myofascial release and other manual therapy methods may be helpful. Chiropractic adjustment may help temporarily but must avoid manual thrust techniques if there is a possibility of nerve entrapment. Any adjustment *must* be coupled with TrP soft tissue work and control of the perpetuating factors. TrPs in the medial scalene may entrap the long thoracic nerve. An apparent elevation of the first rib, concurrent with T1 articular dysfunction, may be due to rotation of the vertebra caused by TrPs in the longissimus capitis. There may be C4-C5-C6 radiculopathy or facet pathology as well as scalene entrapment. This neuropathy enhances development of forearm TrPs that refer to the wrist. Check the omohyoid for possible TrPs, as that referral pattern, including tingling, may mimic the scalenes.

Stretch: Sit up straight and place your hands behind your lower back. Grasp the wrist of one arm with the hand of the other as you stretch the grasping hand's side. Move your shoulders downward gently while bending your neck back and to the side. Gently rock your head forward and back, teasing out any restrictions. Return to the start and repeat on the other side. Breathe normally as you stretch. Don't overdo—this stretch can have a profound effect on the vestibular system, which plays a vital role in your sense of spatial orientation and sense of balance. You may feel a little dizzy during or after this dynamic stretch, so do take appropriate care. If you feel an area of particular tension, try breathing into that area and hold the breath for just three seconds. Then gently release. *This stretch is unfortunately not suitable for individuals who are post-coronary operative. Seek medical advice before any physical therapy routine.*

Sternocleidomastoid
Greek *sternon* means "chest"; *kleis*, "clavicle" or "key."
Latin *mastoides* means "breast-shaped" (from Greek *mastos*, meaning "breast").

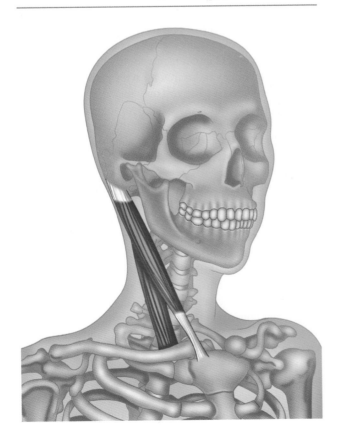

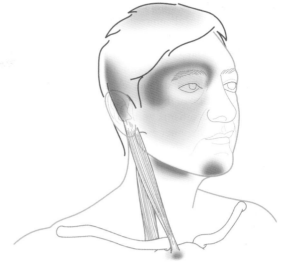

Sternal division.

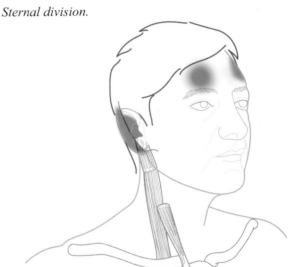

Clavicular division.

What It Does: This muscle is often referred to as the SCM rather than the SternoCleidoMastoid (guess why). It's connected to the mastoid area, but soon divides into two bellies: one with a lower portion connecting to the upper part of the breastbone (sternum), and the other connecting to the clavicle (collarbone). The SCMs pull the head forward when they both contract, raising the collarbone and ribs, thus facilitating inward breath. If only one of the SCMs is contracted by TrPs, the head is tilted to that side because it hurts to keep the head up and straight. This can result in TrPs in the opposite SCM as it tries to compensate. Some additional tension is needed, and, rather than a muscle spasm (which requires a nerve input and lots of energy), muscles often choose to form TrPs (which require little or no energy and no nerve input).

Kinetics Comments: The SCMs and scalenes are often overloaded if the shoulder or pelvic axis is uneven, or if something happens to cause stiffness or relative shortness on one side of the body. Overload occurs because the brain is hard-wired to keep the eyes level, no matter what. An individual's ability to balance is part of what we call "the righting reflex." In all animals there are three systems used to sense change in position: (1) the vestibular (inner ear); (2) the visual (eyes); and (3) the somatosensory (soma = body, sensory = sensations). The vestibular system is located in the inner ear and senses change in motion and position of the head. Righting reflexes involve complicated mechanisms and processes associated with the structures of the inner ear. The visual system provides information to the brain on the body's position in relation to the external world. The somatosensory system is responsible for conveying sensory information from the skin, muscles, and joints to the brain. All three systems are used in combination to help the body balance itself. If muscles are contracted due to TrPs, the resulting head-forward posture becomes a perpetuating factor for gait irregularities, muscle imbalances, and tissue changes that include satellite TrPs, especially along the kinetic chain.

TrP Comments: TrPs in this muscle cause extensive and often misdiagnosed symptoms, and are often blamed on FM. TrPs in each of the two sections produce very different symptoms. An attachment TrP towards the lower end of the sternal division refers pain down over the upper portion of the sternum. Pressing on this TrP may cause a dry cough. Other SCM TrPs refer pain upward. Non-pain symptoms may cause considerable diagnostic confusion. It is possible to have sternal SCM symptoms without clavicular SCM symptoms. TrP nodules and tenderness may be mistaken for glandular swelling. TrPs are not exclusively related to pain; they are also associated with changes in sensations, and this is demonstrated well by SCM TrPs.

Sternal Division: TrPs in this area may cause symptoms similar to trigeminal neuralgia. True trigeminal neuralgia is not accompanied by sternal pain, but when TrPs mimic this condition there often is sternal pain. TrPs do not cause facial grimace such as found in trigeminal neuralgia. Look at the whole picture and history. TrPs in the upper area of this segment refer pain behind but not close to the ear, and to the top of the head like a skullcap, with scalp tenderness. The touch of a hairbrush can initiate the intense soreness, and headbands and hats may be intolerable. At mid level, these TrPs refer pain across the cheek on the same side, often in finger-like projections. Pain is also felt in the jaw, over the ridge above the eye, and deep inside the eye. TrPs along the *inner* margin at mid level refer pain to the throat and back of the tongue during swallowing, causing a sore throat. Pain may also be referred to a small round area at the tip of the chin. Non-pain symptoms include teary eyes, and visual disturbances when confronted by a series of contrasting parallel lines such as an escalator and even some fabric patterns. Even conveyor belts, such as luggage returns in airports, may provoke severe dizziness and/or disorientation. The patterns of light and shadow that fall on the road after the leaves have fallen can cause a petit-mal-like fugue state, irritability, disorientation, or confusion. Possible symptoms include eye reddening and nose running. The eyelid (or eyelids) may droop, which may be due to increased motor unit excitability and spasm of the orbicularis oculi. Pupil size and response, however, is normal. It may be impossible for the patient to raise the upper eyelid. There may be blurring of vision, dimming of perceived light, crackling in the ear, or rare unilateral deafness. Just as with pain, the nonpain symptoms can be amplified by FM. The combination of cognitive disruptions can be overwhelming and devastating.

Clavicular Division: The upper part of this division usually sends pain deep into the ear and the area behind the ear. TrPs in the middle refer pain to the forehead and may extend pain across the forehead, even if the TrPs are only active on one side. These TrPs may refer poorly localized pain to the cheek and molar teeth. Other symptoms include dizziness (e.g. postural) and imbalance. Temporary loss of balance may follow a quick turning of the head, such as when one is turning into traffic. This loss of balance can lead to falls and may also occur after sustained tilting of the head to one side. These motions can lead to vertigo, with the environment seeming to spin around, or even to blackouts (Simons, Travell, and Simons 1999, p. 310). Dizziness episodes can last for seconds or hours. Loss of balance and disorientation can occur separately from postural dizziness. Sudden falls may occur during bending or stooping. Functional veering to one side can occur when walking with both eyes open. This can lead observers to suspect alcohol or drug-related problems. Postural responses are exaggerated: when you look up, you can pitch over backward; if you look down, you can fall forward. Gardening, cleaning out the kitty litter, and birdwatching can be fraught with peril. While lying down in bed or on a sofa, you may feel as if you are tilted and have to put your foot on the floor to gain a feeling of stability. These alterations of sensation may be amplified if FM is part of the picture, but understanding the source may help.

TrPs in this muscle can also cause a disturbed perception of the weight of objects held in the hand. Some of this may be due to proprioceptive neck mechanisms. Electrical discharges from these TrPs disturb the central processing of proprioceptive information from arm muscles as well as affecting vestibular function related to neck muscles. This means that patients fling objects about because they are unable to gauge how much they weigh, and consequently use an inappropriate amount of force to lift them. Suddenly you are surrounded by flying saucers, and cups too! It can be confusing and frustrating. Active TrPs here may also contribute to seasickness or motion sickness, and may cause nausea (vomiting is rare) and anorexia that leads to poor diet. Again, FM can amplify these symptoms. Keep in mind that these TrPs are treatable.

Autonomic nervous system symptoms associated with these TrPs include localized sweating, vasoconstriction with blanching and cooling, or redness. This can seem strange when it occurs on one side of the face, and diagnostically misleading when occurring on both sides. One of the authors (Starlanyl) believes that some SCM TrPs may be able to partially entrap the carotid artery, and baroreceptors in the area may also be affected. We encourage research on this subject.

Notable Perpetuating Factors: Paradoxical breathing, and persistent or severe acute muscle overload (including from excessive head-forward posture or from prolonged sitting with the head turned to the side). Nearsightedness may be a perpetuating factor for head-forward posture. Mechanical stress can include protracted neck extension from painting the ceiling, bird watching, whiplash, or poor sleep posture, including the use of two pillows to prop the head. Intubation during surgery can activate these TrPs, as can head-rolling exercises. Don't ever tilt the head back and roll it from side to side. The SCMs can be stressed by whatever restricts upper limb movement and requires awkward compensation, such as structural asymmetry. Perpetuating factors include anything that produces a severe deviation from the normal pattern of gait, such as limping, even because of shoes that are too tight. TrPs can be activated by TrPs in the pectoralis major, which consequently pulls down and forward on the clavicular head of the SCM. Be attentive to your environment. If you have an acute cough and you get an SCM-pattern headache with each cough, the SCM TrPs are calling out to you. Walking a large and unruly dog or riding a headstrong horse may yank on the SCMs. With SCM TrPs, tennis matches are nearly impossible to watch. Pressure from a tight collar or necktie may also aggravate these TrPs, as may leakage of cerebrospinal fluid after a spinal tap or myelogram, or any chronic infection in the sinuses or teeth. SCM TrPs are perpetuated by swimming the crawl stroke.

Hints for Control (Patients): When you try on clothing, turn your head to the side, because that increases the diameter of your neck. Make sure your clothes give you room to breathe. Don't use your shoulder to hold a telephone against your head. Rounded shoulders and head-forward posture are often clues that these TrPs are present. Learn to roll over in bed without lifting your head from the pillow. Any posture or activity that activates a TrP may perpetuate it. If only one side of the SCM has active TrPs, sleeping on the side of the TrPs, with the pillow properly adjusted, may help. Make sure that your neck is supported and that your face is not bearing any weight. Don't sleep on your stomach. When the SCM muscles are hyperirritable, the muscles must be supported without immobilization. A pinned folded kitchen towel used as a neck support may become a useful companion.

Hints for Control (Care Providers): In cases of dizziness and disequilibrium, the patient can't walk in a straight line towards a point in the room where his or her gaze is fixed without veering to the side of the active TrPs in the clavicular division (if active TrPs are one sided). Patients have neither Romberg's sign nor nystagmus. Vestibular dysfunction is a common coexisting condition, especially if FM is also present. Imbalance due to SCMs may mimic ataxia. Proprioceptive concomitants mostly involve spatial disorientation and may be misdiagnosed as neurological. Some may be caused by referred pain areas encompassing the locus of the fifth cranial nerve. SCM TrPs in areas of the muscle supplied by upper cervical and spinal accessory cranial nerves may cause dizziness, photophobia, unsteadiness, falling, and even anorexia.

Treat the short muscle first. Normal neural function of the inhibited muscle should be restored once the opposing muscle is rid of its TrPs. Place the previously inhibited muscle under a stretch and gently tap it to stimulate muscle spindle activity and restore normal tone. If SCM TrPs are contributing to throat pain, hold the SCM tightly and ask the patient to swallow. If the throat pain disappears, TrPs are involved. Patients may have decreased hearing due to TrP-induced reflex disturbance of the tensor tympani muscle tension on the same side. When the spinal accessory nerve (cranial nerve XI) penetrates the SCM on its way to the trapezius, myogenic torticollis due to contracture of the SCM can cause paresis of the same-side trapezius muscle. To palpate, laterally flex the neck to that side and turn the head to the opposite side. Pincer palpation works well with parts of this muscle. If TrPs are active on one side of the SCM and history indicates that they have been active before, check the other side for latent TrPs, and check the scalenes as well. When SCM TrPs are active, always check for TrPs in the longus colli. If using stretch and spray therapy, the patient must not hold the rewarming heating pad. The patient's arms must be at her or his sides for TrP release to proceed. Use a strap to secure the heating pad.

The SCM TrPs may react to injection and manual therapy with more extreme head pain and much more local soreness than many other TrPs. TrP releases must always be done in both sides of the SCM, although injection of both sides at the same time is inadvisable due to temporary symptom increase immediately after injection. Manual release of one side might result in reactive cramping of the other side, enhancing pain and dizziness. Patients with active TrPs on both sides of the SCM may require a driver and help with home care after therapy, even if only one side is treated; they should be sent home with a written guide to post-treatment care and warning of possible proprioceptor and autonomic changes. Treatment of the SCM may accidentally activate platysma TrPs, causing a prickling pain response. A comfortable collar formed with a soft kitchen towel, folded in half and pinned lightly around the neck, may offer enough support for passengers on the homeward trip and when these TrPs are active. There must be room for easy head rotation. Dramamine may be useful for nausea but does not help the dizziness.

Stretch: Be very careful not to rotate the head while you stretch this muscle. The stretch can be performed while you lie on your back. Slowly bring your left ear down to the left shoulder and rest a moment there. Then return to the center and rest a moment there. Next bring the right ear down to the right shoulder. Rest a moment there, and then return to center. The resting is as important as the stretch. This stretch avoids harming the back of the neck, and also avoids contributing to the head-forward position.

Obliquus Capitis Inferior
Latin *obliquus* means "inclined"; *capitis*, "of the head"; *inferior*, "lower."

It is the larger of two neck oblique muscles but "inferior" because it lies below the "superior" muscle.

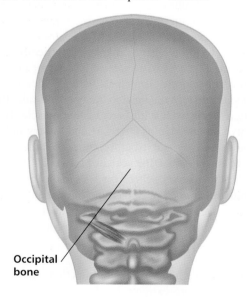

Occipital bone

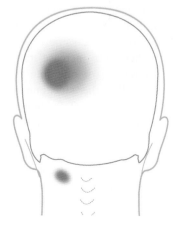

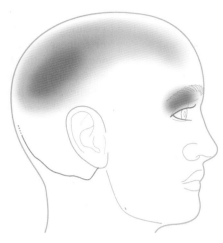

What It Does: Rotates the first vertebra in the neck and rotates the head. Despite its name, it does not attach directly to the head, but to the first cervical vertebra (C1).

Kinetics Comments: This deep suboccipital muscle can entrap the greater occipital nerve. Like the other suboccipital muscles, it is rich in proprioceptors. Sustained shortening of this muscle, such as that caused by TrPs, can result in difficulty in maintaining standing balance. (These difficulties may be compounded by vestibular dysfunction and eye inequality. They are not exclusive.) Therapists who work on the occipital muscles know their importance in and contribution to spine health and sacral distortion.

TrP Comments: When TrPs occur in the suboccipital muscles, extension and rotation of the head can enhance entrapment of the vertebral arteries. This can occur when a driver looks over the shoulder while backing up the car, resulting in instant headache, dizziness, and loss of control.

Notable Perpetuating Factors: Lasting or frequent emotional stressors; physical stressors such as head-forward posture, sudden cooling, and drafts; and poor posture habits.

Hints for Control: Be attentive to the link between postural changes and symptom onset. If dizziness or other symptoms are enhanced when backing up the car, use mirrors as an aid in these maneuvers, and avoid parallel parking. Ice compresses may relieve some pain. Cool water above the eyes and on the lids may temporarily relieve some tension and pain there.

Stretch: This muscle and its associated muscles (rectus capitis posterior minor and major, obliquus capitis superior) are intrinsically linked to eye movement. A secret to changing the level of tone within the muscle lies in the eyes. Bring your chin towards your chest, looking up with your eyes until your chin has gone down as far as it can. Once you reach that point, look down towards the floor. As you look down, bring your chin closer to your chest if you can. Magic! Do not be surprised if you feel a fall in tension all the way down the spine. If you feel strain in your eyes, check the eye muscles for TrPs. If movement of the head into extension is contraindicated for you, try changing the tone of this muscle through eye movement. Place two or three fingers gently into the tissue on either side of your neck, just one fingernail-width out from the spinous process directly beneath the occipital bone. Roll your eyes up and down and side to side, and note when you feel the tone reduce in the muscle. This is known as "reciprocal inhibition," and can be held for up to ten seconds. Breathe normally. We give thanks to Dr. Karel Lewit for all the work he has done on the connection between eye movement and muscle tension.

Obliquus Capitis Superior
Latin *obliquus* means "inclined"; *capitis*, "of the head"; *superior*, "higher."

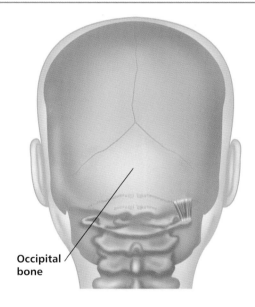

Occipital bone

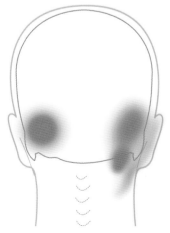

What It Does: Extends and flexes the neck to the side.

Kinetics Comments: This small occipital muscle is loaded with proprioceptors and charged with keeping the head in as efficient a position atop the vertebral column as possible. Our hypothesis is that these small suboccipital muscles have more to do with fascial bracing and proprioception than with producing movement.

TrP Comments: These TrPs refer dull, deep pain, including into the ear, and can cause a deep itch in the ear. It can be very painful to lie with the back of the head on a pillow, and there is the temptation to angle the pillow, resting your side weight on the side of your face. That position can set up TrPs elsewhere. TrPs in the obliquus capitis superior can be associated with dizziness and a variety of proprioceptor dysfunctions that may be mistaken for neurological problems. Look for the pattern of TrPs, referral pain, and other symptoms.

Notable Perpetuating Factors: Jerky, unexpected head movement, postures such as lying on the back on a sofa with the head propped upward at a steep angle, pressure of a helmet, CPAP or other straps.

Hints for Control: Craniosacral work and other manual therapy can relieve the tension on these muscles. Ice or cool compresses may provide temporary relief, but extra care is needed when applying any cold or ice compress to the suboccipital area.

Stretch: See Obliquus Capitis Inferior.

9 Muscles of the Trunk

Introduction

The trunk is the physical center of the body, encompassing the heart, lungs, gastrointestinal system, and other organs, as well as the tissues that support them, and much of the spinal column. The fascia affects it all. Many trunk TrPs are responsible for enigmatic symptoms often labeled as "functional" (medspeak for "we don't know the cause") and usually interpreted as "imaginary." Nothing could be further from the truth. Did you know that frequent voiding or defecation may be an attempt to relieve pressure and pain in the pelvic area (Doggweiler-Wiygul 2004)? Sitting with the weight on one side and putting a leg under the pelvic area to ease this pressure will stress the front thigh muscles and the foot and ankle area. TrPs can "spread" that way too. What you don't know can hurt you.

For example, it was once believed that distention in the gut caused by air or fluids caused sensations of bloating and swelling only. The gut couldn't feel pain, right? Wrong! We know better now. In central sensitization states such as FM, migraine and IBS, distention of the gut often causes *pain*. TrPs can also cause or contribute to cardiac arrhythmia, impotence, IBS, prostate symptoms, diarrhea, vomiting, food intolerance, pain with intercourse, colic, urinary urgency or incontinence, dysmenorrhea, gastroesophageal reflux, burping, and an assortment of other symptoms often considered "visceral," meaning originating in the organs. TrPs can even cause seemingly unrelated symptoms such as anorexia. TrPs in the rectus abdominis (and to a lesser extent other low abdominal muscles) can even cause (or be caused by) a lax, distended abdomen with excessive gas. When the TrPs are causing the symptoms, successful treatment of the TrPs and control of the perpetuating factors resolves the symptoms. If the symptoms come back, there is at least one perpetuating factor.

Regional Kinetics: In this segment you will meet the first of the **core muscles**. The core includes the abdominal muscles, erector spinae, multifidi, psoas, gluteals, and hamstrings, and the deep connective tissues that attach to the pelvis and help protect the spine. Vertebra are grouped into segments, and muscles attached to those segments are often referred to as belonging to those segments. For example, posterior cervical muscles are associated with the cervical spine.

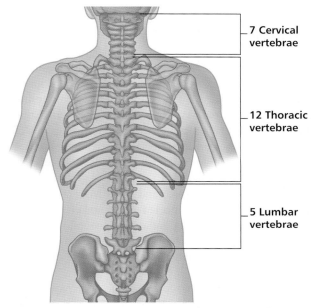

7 Cervical vertebrae

12 Thoracic vertebrae

5 Lumbar vertebrae

The vertebral column is separated into three divisions for anatomical convenience. Muscles attached to these areas often interact with spinal dysfunction in the same segment, and disfunctions of one segment eventually usually affect the others following the kinetic chains.

Many people fall into the trap of training superficial muscles while neglecting training that involves both superficial and deep muscles working together. This muscular coordination is important. The function of the peripheral muscles is greatly dependent on the stability and strength of the core. Weakness in the core musculature requires the rest of the body to compensate, overworking other muscles and often initiating one or more TrP cascades. Using the body in a healthy and efficient manner requires the integrated relationship of local muscles as links within any kinetic chain. We can combine existing research to show this. People with chronic low back pain have problems adjusting their postural movements (Jacobs, Henry, and Nagle 2009); their trunk is stiffer and their proprioception is altered (Brumagne et al. 2008). Trunk and hip stiffness increases the possibility of falling (Gruneberg et al. 2004). This research, in combination, has implications for people with TrPs, even though TrPs are never mentioned. Chronic low back pain itself influences breathing patterns (Smith, Coppieters, and Hodges 2005), which can perpetuate other TrPs that cause low back pain. The cycle must be interrupted, and knowing TrPs, we can do that.

Regional TrP Comments: The trunk is the most likely segment of the body to be affected by organ/TrP interactions. Somatovisceral interactions occur when TrPs cause or contribute to organ symptoms and disease. TrPs cause nerve, blood vessel, and lymph entrapment. For instance, TrPs can entrap a nerve and cause symptoms typical of renal colic (Eken, Durmaz, and Erol 2009). Entrapped nerves can also cause burning pain, itching, redness, and/or numbness between the thoracic spine and the shoulder blade (Williams et al. 2010); although this condition, called notalgia paresthetica, is often considered dermatological or psychological, some cases have been successfully treated with botulinum toxin, surgical release of fascial entrapment, or osteopathic manipulation. Logic indicates that TrPs may be significantly involved in at least some of these cases. Not only can TrPs cause symptoms mimicking diseases of the gall bladder, gastrointestinal system, genitourinary system, cardiac system, and spine, but they can also interact with true organ illnesses as well. Viscerosomatic interactions occur when visceral illness forms a reciprocating relationship with TrPs. Ulcers, gall bladder disease, esophageal reflux, IBS, gastrointestinal infections, cardiac disease, and other visceral illnesses can activate TrPs in the affected region and elsewhere. So TrPs can influence organs, and organs can influence TrPs. Together they can create a mutual grievance network, with symptoms worsening until successful intervention occurs.

The abdominal area is separated into four parts called quadrants. Some abdominal TrP referral patterns cross quadrants, referring across the midline, or on a diagonal, or to the back. They're not as consistent in their patterns from patient to patient as most other TrPs. TrPs in the back can be as complicated as in the abdominals. Paraspinal TrPs can refer pain to the upper buttock, kidney area, groin, and scrotum, or cause retraction of the testicle. Assessment and control of TrPs has implications for preventing some cases of scoliosis, bulging discs, and DDD. Treating TrPs first can avoid some surgeries and may prevent "failed surgical back." Failed surgical back is the description (not diagnosis) given when a patient has had back surgery but the symptoms remain. Research indicates that less than 1% of all cases of chronic low back pain require orthopedic, neurosurgical, or neurological attention (Rosomoff and Rosomoff 1999). Chronic low back pain is a description, not a diagnosis. One must search for the cause of the pain.

We've seen too many patients who've had multiple back surgeries. First one disc degenerates or bulges and there is an operation. Nothing is done to treat the TrPs, so the stress on the vertebrae remains. Then the disc above or below (or both) begins to compensate. Eventually, there are more surgeries, which are often unnecessary. There is a significant association between bulging discs in specific cervical (neck) disc areas and specific active TrPs, as noted by Hsueh et al. (1998). These researchers found that levator scapulae and latissimus dorsi TrPs are associated with C3–C4 disc bulges; splenius capitis, deltoid, levator scapulae, rhomboid minor, and latissimus dorsi TrPs are associated with C4–C5 disc bulges; splenius capitis, deltoid, levator scapulae, latissimus dorsi, and rhomboid minor TrPs are associated with C5–C6 bulges; and latissimus dorsi and rhomboid minor TrPs are associated with C6–C7 disc lesions. One of the authors (Starlanyl) believes that TrPs and disc and/or facet pathology interact along the spine. The tight muscles, contractured by TrPs, pull the vertebrae slightly out of position, creating problems for associated tissues and the bony spine. Osteoarthritis of the spine and, often, disc and facet pathologies may follow. When pain and dysfunction begin to appear, one should identify and treat the TrPs and control the perpetuating factors before disc degeneration and osteoarthritis occurs. Karel Lewit, in *Manipulative Therapy: Musculoskeletal Medicine* (2010), wrote that early neck spinal involvement may first present as migraine, and the first sign of lumbar spinal involvement in women may be menstrual pain. At that point, nothing shows on imaging, but if TrPs are found and perpetuating factors brought under control, much future misery may be prevented.

Regional CMP Comments: In the trunk, CMP may interact with multiple coexisting conditions such as congestive obstructive pulmonary disease, degenerative disc disease, and GERD. TrPs can mimic organ conditions, but there is always the risk that the TrPs are being perpetuated by organ conditions. When in doubt, check it out. The following patient scenario has been simplified for teaching purposes, as have all scenarios in this book. It is unusual for patients to have untreated TrPs that fail to spread to other regions. In this example, a 51-year-old male nurse was frequently called upon to lift heavy patients. Even with good body mechanics, he has had chronic low and mid back pain for the last five years. Recently he had episodic pain behind the eyes, with a headache in a hatband pattern, but his eye doctor said his eyes were fine. Although he'd been coping with chronic low back pain, he was increasingly fatigued: he would come home after work and collapse, sometimes being unable to fix dinner. Two weeks ago he played golf in a tournament and was unable to finish due to severe back pain; he had to be driven off the course. Imaging showed L4–L5 minimal disc degeneration.

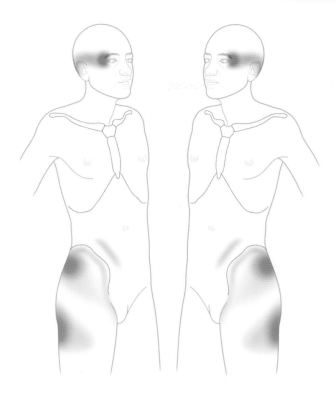

Patient lateral views.

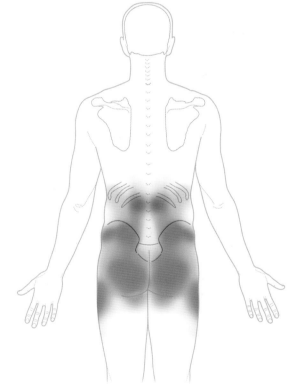

Patient posterior view.

Examination showed bilateral TrPs in the splenius cervicis, erector spinae, low back multifidi, and deep and superficial quadratus lumborum. The TrPs were treated with electrical stimulation, stretch and spray, and strain-counterstrain. Resistant TrPs were treated with local injection. He was given a stretch routine to perform several times during his night shift, and warm-up exercises to be done before golf. He was taught tennis-ball compression, and prescribed a small microstimulation unit and instructed in its use. The back pain eased considerably, and, with successful treatment of the quadratus TrPs, any abnormal fatigue went away. A five-year follow-up has revealed that the disc degeneration is still there, but it has not increased.

Regional Perpetuating Factors: These include interactive conditions—especially anything affecting, for example, respiratory, circulatory, gastrointestinal, and other organ systems—as well as surgery and other traumas, and their aftermath such as scars and adhesions. The spine, shoulder, and pelvic girdle interact with trunk TrPs. A leaky gut (permeable bowel) can be a major factor in multiple metabolic conditions, so healing the gut is a priority. Work on the sources of the problems. All this interaction has a positive side: when you begin to control one perpetuating factor, it will often help control others.

Regional Hints for Control (Patients): Once you start working with a tennis ball, you may find that you have TrPs everywhere. Consider this. You had them before you found them. Now, you know what they are and where they are. You've spent your life accumulating them. Now, you can start to treat them. Keep hope and faith. Help your care providers discover the perpetuating factors and bring them under control. Don't be surprised if new TrPs appear as others are treated. Don't be discouraged and don't be overwhelmed. Give yourself time, and give your care providers time too.

Regional Hints for Control (Care Providers): Any myofascial therapy for the low back should start with bilateral release of the hamstrings. Consider the way the muscles work together (or don't). Remember to check deep stabilizing ligaments and tendons for TrPs. When there are multiple perpetuating factors and coexisting conditions, it is easy to get discouraged. We guarantee that this process is tougher for the patient. Don't get frustrated. Patients and care providers must work together with myofascial therapy. An educated patient is your best resource.

Posterior Cervical Muscles
(semispinalis capitis, semispinalis cervicis, longissimus capitis)
Latin *semi* means "half"; *spinalis*, "relating to the spine"; *capitis*, "of the head"; *cervicis*, "of the neck"; *longissimus*, "longest."

The term "cervix" can be confusing for those outside the field of medicine. It does mean "neck," but an anatomical structure such as a uterus also has a "neck," and thus, a cervix. The cervical mutlifidi and rotators will be addressed in their own sections.

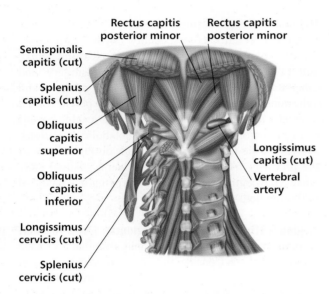

Posterior cervical anatomy.

Posterior Cervical TrP Referral Patterns

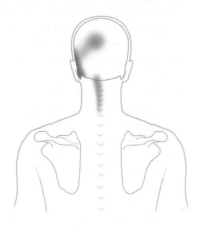

Longissimus capitis. This referral pattern may include deep periorbital "behind-the-eye" pain.

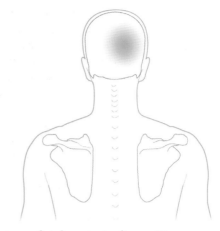

Middle superficial semispinalis capitis.

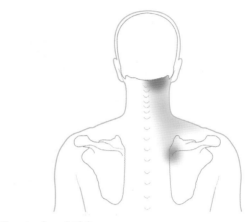

Cervical multifidi.

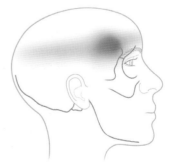

Upper semispinalis capitis.

What They Do: The semispinalis capitis is the main muscular component for head extension; it also assists head rotation. The longissimus capitis is a **core muscle** that extends and rotates the head, helps maintain healthy postural anatomical placement of the erect upper spine, and maintains upper back spinal curvature. The semispinalis cervicis extends the erect upper spine and assists in its rotation. The semispinalis muscles allow us to look upward, and to turn our head around to look behind us. We suspect that the suppleness of these muscles and their attachments can affect the tightness and position of the dural tube and thus the CNS.

Kinetics Comments: Humans lack the ability to rotate their heads totally like owls. Tightness in the slender semispinalis muscles can restrict head rotation to the point where we need to move our whole body to see what is around us. The longissimus muscles are slender, yet help give our spine the flexibility and movement that we need for supple motion. Together, they provide healthy curvature of the upper spine. These muscles work in conjunction with the multifidi and other spinal support muscles. Be attentive to other tissues in the area: if one is tight, it will affect the others. The links in the kinetic chain seem to be especially closely woven along the spine. Check for TrPs in attachment areas. We suspect that these TrPs can cause sufficient tightness to pull the vertebrae slightly out of alignment, leading to OA and/or degenerative disc disease, and that a "dowager's hump" can not only perpetuate these TrPs but also be caused by them.

TrP Comments: The upper area semispinalis capitis TrPs call out in their hatband-shaped pattern above the level of the eye, with emphatic intensity in the temporal region. It may be painful to lie down with the side of the head on the pillow. TrP tightness in this area can entrap the greater occipital nerve. There may be difficulty wearing hats or headgear such as some CPAP straps. TrPs in the middle regions of the semispinalis capitis and semispinalis cervicis (considering the muscles lengthwise) cause pain and sometimes burning in the back of the head. These TrPs may make it uncomfortable to rest the back of the head on a pillow, or to wear any heavy or constricting headgear that presses on that region. All of these TrPs can contribute to neck pain, stiffness, and restricted ROM. These TrPs affect whatever affects the spine, and can thus interact with the CNS. They require careful and often continued attention when FM coexists. When these TrPs are chronic, this area may be fibrotic; rock hard and tight. Palpation may be difficult. Be patient and persistent. Longissimus capitis TrPs refer pain to the ear and surrounding area and may make it difficult or impossible to wear headbands, eyeglasses, or headphones.

Notable Perpetuating Factors: Whiplash is a common initiator of these TrPs, as is chilling of the neck muscles, chronic extension or flexion through sustained head-forward posture at work or sustained bird watching, inadequate lumbar support, a long neck, ill-fitting and unsupportive sleep pillows, use of multiple pillows under the head, improper eye correction, emotional depression, spinal articular disease or deformity, or degenerative disc disease.

Hints for Control (Patients): A neck support made by pinning a soft hand towel or kitchen towel gently around the neck can provide support without restriction during the day. Stretch and spray or stretch and ice stroking can be effective for immediate easing of some symptoms for those who are not cold intolerant, to be followed by rewarming and manual therapy combined with a daily home self-treatment program. The treatment regimen must include control of perpetuating factors. If no disc disease is present, the use of two tennis balls in a knotted knee sock can be very helpful (see Chapter 14). Avoid head-rolling exercises. Become mindful of how you use your body.

Hints for Control (Care Providers): These TrPs may require chronic care. Work with the patient to uncover perpetuating factors such as bad furniture and posture. Check for associated articular dysfunction; if present, it may be correctable manually using techniques for suboccipital decompression (Simons, Travell, and Simons 1999, p. 445).

Stretch: Sit up erect or stand if you prefer. Allow your chin to drop towards your chest, while at the same time dropping your shoulders by pointing your fingers towards the floor. Alternatively, you can place one hand behind your head and gently assist your head as you drop your chin towards your chest. A gentle rotation left and right can be added when you feel the stretch. Breathe normally, and go slowly.

Erector Spinae

Latin: *erigere* means "to lift up" or "to erect"; *spina*, "spine" or "thorn."

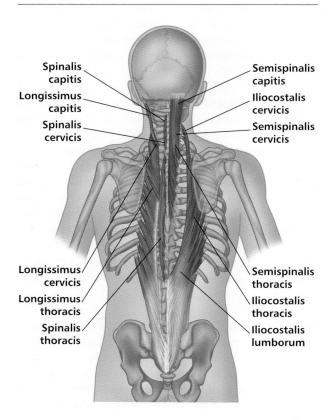

Spinalis capitis
Longissimus capitis
Spinalis cervicis
Semispinalis capitis
Iliocostalis cervicis
Semispinalis cervicis
Longissimus cervicis
Longissimus thoracis
Spinalis thoracis
Semispinalis thoracis
Iliocostalis thoracis
Iliocostalis lumborum

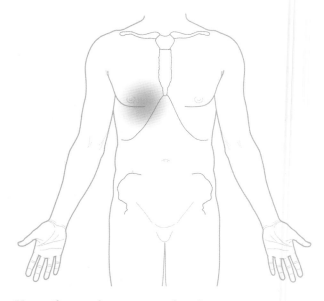

Upper iliocostalis anterior referral pattern.

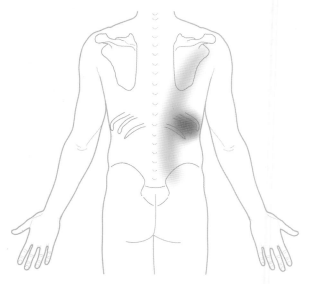

Posterior iliocostalis thoracis referral pattern.

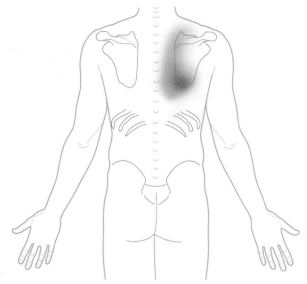

Upper iliocostalis posterior referral pattern.

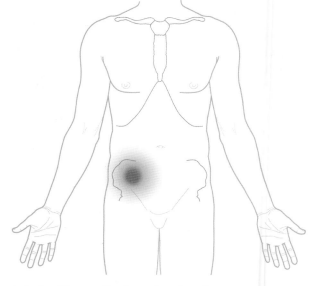

Anterior iliocostalis thoracis referral pattern.

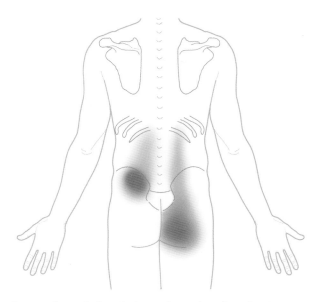

Lower thoracic longissimus thoracis referral pattern.

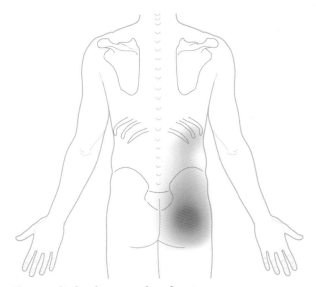

Iliocostalis lumborum referral pattern.

What They Do: This complicated and important group of **core muscles** can be confusing. The muscle names themselves can add to the confusion. Each is made up of small paired muscle fibers and tendons that form vertical columns close to the spine. The pairs vary in thickness. The erector spinae group is composed of muscle chains called iliocostalis, longissimus, spinalis, and multifidi. (The longissimus capitis and multifidi have their own sections.) The semispinalis capitis and longissimus capitis rotate the head and pull it back; the ilicostalis cervicis and longissimus cervicis extend the vertebrae of the neck; the longissimus thoracis, iliocostalis thoracis, and ilicostalis lumborum extend and side-bend the chest spine and help rotate the ribs; and the semispinalis thoracis and longissimus lumborum extend and rotate the spine. Some of these muscles are vertical and others are shorter and diagonal; some lower ones merge into thick tendons.

They all work to stabilize the spine and maintain posture and spinal curvature, and their coordinated work allows us to walk erect. This is the simplified version. Honest.

Kinetics: These long chains of muscles reach from the skull to the base of the spine, also connecting to core ligaments, and some of the columns divide or branch along their length. Tightness in the ilicostalis can affect the position of the lowest rib and the hip, squeezing all the tissues in between. When the abdominal muscles are weak, the erector spinae (their antagonists) are at greater risk of injury.

TrP Comments: These TrPs can cause severe restriction of spine flexibility. They can lead to hip pain, buttock pain, marked change in spinal curvature, sacroiliac pain, deep spinal "bone" pain, and/or low back pain that worsens towards the end of the day. They can cause tailbone pain, retraction of the testicle, or pain down the back and outside of the thigh. Some of these TrPs refer pain to the front of the body, usually at the same level as the TrP. This pain may be mistaken for angina, renal colic, gall bladder pain, or other organ pain. They can even cause deep tenderness and abdominal rigidity that mimics appendicitis (Simons, Travell, and Simons 1999, p. 916). TrPs in the iliocostalis thoracis along the side edge of the spine of the shoulder blade may contribute to cramping of muscles under the breast (of the same side as the TrPs); this cramping is likely to occur as you lean over to tie your shoe or pick something up. Disc and facet problems can interact with the TrPs, causing a worsening symptom spiral. Some spinal nerves travel through the paraspinals, so when the muscles are tight, the nerves may be compressed. This can result in burning or lancing pain, numbness, or other altered sensation across the skin of the back. Check for coexisting conditions, but deal with the TrPs promptly as well. You may have an accumulation of muscle stressors, and then one wrong move—*Ouch*! Suddenly you can't get up out of a chair without help.

Notable Perpetuating Factors: Trauma such as a fall or whiplash (these muscles are in the neck too); using poor body mechanics when lifting (especially while twisting and bending), or even straining during birth labor, a bowel movement, or coughing; chronic or acute muscle overload; structural asymmetry; dehydration; gait irregularities; sleeping on a bed with inadequate support (such as a water bed); immobility; holding awkward postures; repetitive motions such in golf; and unbalanced weight during late stages of pregnancy. Lumbar facet joint and disc problems perpetuate these TrPs, but may respond to non-surgical options.

Hints for Control (Patients): Some people sit at a desk all week and then try to dig a whole garden or play hard at sports all weekend. Weekend athletes overusing tight, unconditioned muscles may think that they've gotten away with it, but then they turn the wrong way or when they wake up the next day, wham!—a whole back column bulges out like a fat rope. Life happens. We may have to deal with a two-foot snowfall that must be shoveled, but we must do it with care, and there will be consequences. Immobility affects these long chains of little muscles. We need to keep them flexible and strong. Tight erector spinae are often paired with weak, overextended abdominal muscles, so the abdominals must be assessed as well. An ergonomic check of the workstation and an examination of sleeping and recreational postures (reading, computer, television, etc.) may be needed, as well as a review of good biomechanics.

Hints for Control (Care Providers): Slow, gradual stretching of tight muscles and connective tissue is important, and may be eased by stretch and spray. The cold is sprayed on for immediate effect to dampen muscle spindle activity, along with the stretch, and followed by rewarming. Electric stimulation, a back knobber and a tennis ball work well on these muscles. Frequent change of position can be helpful. These TrPs may cause difficulty climbing stairs or getting out of a chair, especially if facing directly forward. These tasks are somewhat easier if the patient turns to the diagonal. If the skin is stuck to subcutaneous layers over TrPs, skin rolling may be too painful. On lateral pressure, the skin may ripple like orange peel over the TrPs.

Stretch and Self-treatment: Staying hydrated is an important factor in healthy, supple, pliable tissue. These muscles are not designed to stretch a lot, contrary to popular belief. While sitting on the edge of a chair, give yourself a really big hug by wrapping your arms around you. Ensure your feet and knees are wide apart. Now slowly bend forward, concentrating on moving each vertebral segment before the one below it. Or start at the base of the head and roll your spine forward and down, leaving your arms hanging by your sides. When you have gone as far as feels good, return to an upright position and repeat this dynamic movement. You can also use your breath to help you, by breathing out as you roll forward and "deflate." Then breathe in as you "inflate" and return to the upright starting position.

Splenius Capitis
Greek *splenion* means "bandage" or "patch." Latin *capitis* means "of the head."

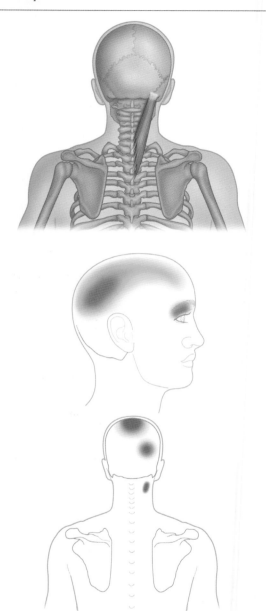

What It Does: Works with the splenius cervicis to extend the neck.

Kinetics Comments: These muscles are part of a complex interweaving of tissues in the neck and surrounding areas that help support the head and allow it to move. Other tissues, including discs and facet joints, are affected and can interact when these muscles are tight and inflexible.

TrP Comments: TrPs in these muscles are often part of myogenic "tension" headache, although splenius capitis TrPs may add an explosive pain to the mix that can stop you in your tracks. Other symptoms may be met with disbelief ("Your *hair* hurts?"). The referral pattern includes the crown of the head, and can be combined with headache, pain in the back of the eye, and blurring of near vision on the same side as the TrP (or on both sides if there are bilateral TrPs). These TrPs can cause numbness and other altered sensations, including an itch that can be terribly distracting and confusing to patients and care providers alike. TrPs in the chest and anterior neck may need to be treated before splenius cervicis TrPs can resolve.

Notable Perpetuating Factors: Whiplash is one type of acute overload of these muscles. Chronic overload can come from peering long hours through a microscope or prolonged working on a jigsaw puzzle. The muscles don't care why; they react to the extreme posture stress of sudden trauma or a prolonged head-forward static posture. Attempts to avoid glare on a computer screen may contribute to these TrPs. If the computer or other workstation is not ergonomically designed, the head may be forced to tilt in a way that stresses this muscle. This may create particular problems for people who are required to periodically change workstations. Any activity that thrusts the head forward repeatedly or continuously may initiate or perpetuate these TrPs, as may body asymmetry of any kind. Neck muscles are especially vulnerable when tired and then exposed to a cold draft. Avoid head-rolling exercises with full rotation.

Hints for Control (Patients): Eliminate perpetuating factors, and pace activities carefully. Be mindful of posture. Minimize excessive twisting and turning of the head and neck. Sleep with the head in a neutral position and not flexed with the chin down to one side or the other. A gentle touch of cool water on the referral area above the eye may relieve the optical symptoms temporarily. A cold compress on the TrP area may help ease the headache.

Hints for Control (Care Providers): These TrPs may cause symptoms that could be mistaken as neurological or psychological. Check for the possibility of interactive cervical spine dysfunction.

Stretch: To stretch this muscle, your neck should be flexed and rotated laterally away from the side you wish to stretch. Keep the shoulder of the involved (or more involved) side stable and down by holding onto a chair seat with the hand on the (more) involved side. Bring your ear closer to your shoulder until you feel a mild stretch. Then return your head to a neutral (face-forward) position and rest a moment. Stretch the other side. Repeat the stretch once or twice on each side, changing the stabilizing hands, and keeping it dynamic.

Splenius Cervicis
Greek *splenion* means "bandage" or "patch."
Latin *cervicis* means "of the neck."

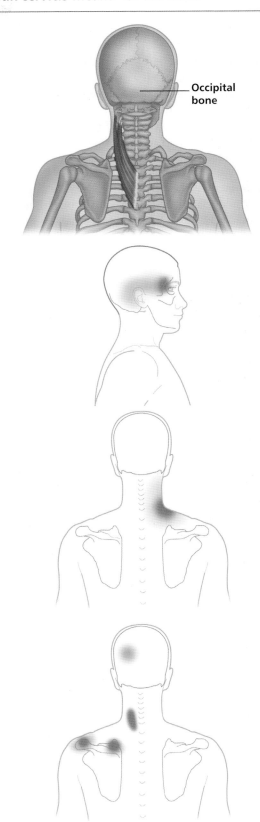

Occipital bone

All or any combination of these referral patterns may occur, depending on the locations of the TrPs.

What It Does: Works with the splenius capitis to achieve neck extension. Slightly rotates the head and bends it to the side; turns the neck to that side. Also helps keep the cervical spine upright.

Kinetics Comments: These muscles are part of a complex interweaving of tissues in the neck and surrounding areas that help support the head and allow it to move in many ways. Other tissues are affected when these muscles are tight and inflexible: discs, facet joints, and other stressed areas interact with these muscles. Tightness of this muscle can cause a domino effect of postural compensations up and down the kinetic chain, and may initiate TrP cascades.

TrP Comments: These TrPs can cause headache inside the skull and behind the eye, as well as pain in the neck and shoulder blade. Some symptoms may be met with disbelief ("What do you mean, your *brain* hurts?"). Restriction of ROM caused by these TrPs can cause neck stiffness. There can be blurring of vision on the same side as the TrPs, and pain referred down to the shoulder girdle and angle of the neck. Numbness in the occipital area is especially common. One patient was told, "If you are numb, you don't have pain. That's good!" (Patients, if this happens to you, get it in writing. Then change care providers *fast*!) Spontaneous numbness is *not* good. TrPs can cause altered sensations that usually follow the referral pattern. So how do you tell your care provider that your brain itches? Bring this book in.

Notable Perpetuating Factors: Whiplash, body asymmetry, and head-forward posture. Acute overload may be caused by excessive weight on an exercise machine or when lifting weights. Chronic overload can come from a workstation (including a kitchen table) requiring a bent-over static neck posture. Neck muscles are especially vulnerable when fatigued and exposed to a cold draft. Avoid head-rolling exercises with back rotation. Body asymmetry may be acquired rather than inherited, such as when one leg is in a cast and the heel of the casted foot is higher than the other, or while using a cane that is too high.

Hints for Control (Patients): Eliminate perpetuating factors and work with your care provider to set up a program of daily stretching, and then do it. Minimize frequent twisting and turning of the head and neck. A soft neck support made from a kitchen towel or hand towel can be useful when these TrPs are active or if you plan riding over bumpy roads. Check sleeping posture as well as working posture—keep the neck in neutral position as much as possible. See if ice or moist heat on this area works better for you.

Hints for Control (Care Providers): TrPs in the chest and anterior neck may need to be treated before these TrPs resolve. Check for interactive cervical dysfunction.

Stretch: Your neck should be flexed and rotated laterally away from the side you wish to stretch. Keep the shoulder of the involved (or most involved) side stable and down by holding onto a chair with the hand on the (most) involved side. Bring your ear closer to your shoulder until you feel a mild stretch. Then return your head to a neutral (face-forward) position and rest a moment. Stretch both sides. Repeat the stretch once or twice on both sides, keeping it dynamic.

Multifidi
Latin *multi* means "many"; *findere*, "to split."

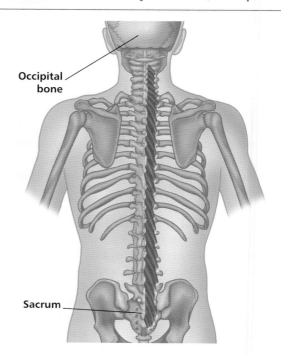

TrPs can be present in more than one multifidi muscle, and the referral pattern(s) depends on the location of the TrPs.

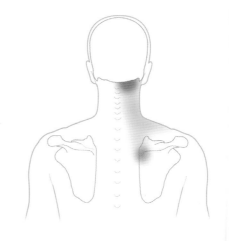

Cervical multifidi.

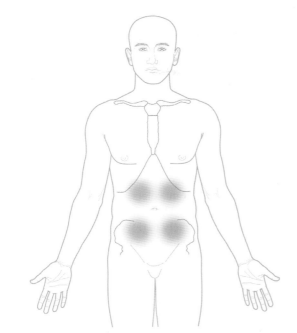

Anterior multifidi referral patterns.

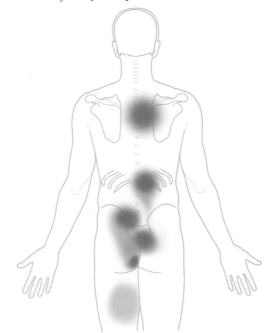

Thoracic and lumbar multifidi referral patterns.

What They Do: Rotate, extend, and flex the spine at all levels. Extend and laterally rotate the pelvis, and help to stabilize the vertebral column. These are **core muscles**.

Kinetics Comments: Multifidi are deep muscles that act as shock absorbers and tension buffers between the spine and the prime movers of the trunk. Their fibers go from the top of the neck to the posterior sacrum. When these muscles shorten, stiffen, and tighten, the shock-absorbent quality is lessened or lost and the neuromuscular integrity of the spine is affected. The multifidi and rotators both work to stabilize the structures of the spine and fine-tune the spatial relationship between the vertebrae.

TrP Comments: Cervical multifidi refer more superficial pain to the occiput and vertebral neck, and sweep pain to the rhomboids. The multifidi TrPs at the thoracic (chest) level cause back and shoulder blade pain patterns. Low back multifidi TrPs at the L1–L5 level can refer pain to the *front* of the body, at the level of the abdomen; they may also perpetuate IBS, no matter what initiates it. There are reports that this front referral may occur at any level, but it has not been documented in the chest and neck. Multifidi TrPs can cause an amazingly relentless, deep low backache that is resistant to treatment. The pain may feel as if it originates in the bone. There may be a distinct palpable or even visible bulge of muscles along the affected area of the spine. When the multifidi of the sacral spine are involved, the base of the spine may appear swollen. Low back pregnancy pain can be caused by multifidi TrPs, as the unbalanced body tries to compensate for the growing child within. At the S1 level, multifidi TrPs refer pain to the tailbone. Lower paraspinal muscles can refer pain to the upper buttock and kidney area, or produce pain in the groin and scrotum. Symptoms may include retraction of the testicle.

Multifidi TrPs can cause marked restriction of spinal ROM, as well as nerve entrapment symptoms, including supersensitivity, numbness, and lessened sensitivity of the skin in the area of the TrP. Other symptoms may occur depending on which nerves are entrapped. If TrPs are allowed to persist, the multifidi involved may atrophy; studies have shown this in chronic low back pain patients (Wallwork et al. 2009). We suspect that multifidi TrPs can cause sufficient tightness to pull vertebrae slightly out of alignment, leading to degenerative disc disease. This poses the question: could myofascial TrPs be a common cause of OA? When TrPs are routinely diagnosed and treated promptly, one of the scourges of aging may be prevented or at least minimized.

Notable Perpetuating Factors: Chronic or acute overload. A sudden bend and twist motion may initiate the pain, often immediately. Whiplash, diving accidents and other sports injuries, and falling on the head or other shock to the spine can initiate multifidi TrPs, as can pushing muscles to work when they are fatigued and/ or chilled. Then all it might take is a sudden bend and twist motion. "I just moved my back the wrong way and it went out" is a frequent comment. Nobody ever says where it went. It may take a while to return. Low back pain in pregnancy may initiate multifidi TrPs. A long second-stage labor can either initiate TrPs or aggravate existing ones.

Hints for Control: Pacing and careful body mechanics, moving mindfully, and using the muscles with respect are all important. Muscles are forgiving, but only to a point. Control perpetuating factors and avoid initiating factors. In pregnancy, a belly support may help. A case of the "good-sport syndrome" stressing multifidi and other paraspinals can be costly beyond imagination.

Stretch: Dynamic stretches such as the one described for the erector spinae will work just fine for the multifidi. A standing stretch for these muscles begins with the feet and knees shoulder width apart. Start at the base of the head and roll forward and down, leaving your arms hanging by your sides. Slowly bend your spine forward, concentrating on moving each vertebral segment before the one below it. When you have gone as far as feels good, slowly return to the starting position, moving vertebra by vertebra. Repeat this dynamic movement once or twice. You can also use your breath to help you during this Stretch: breathe out as you roll forward and "deflate," then breathe in as you "inflate" and return to the upright starting position.

Rotators
Latin *rotare* means "to rotate."

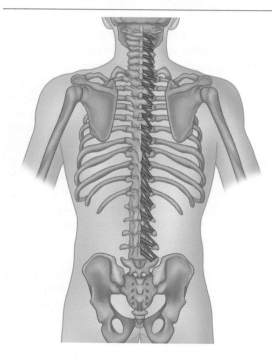

Compare the rotators with the multifidi and note the differences. They both form deep layers of paraspinal muscles. A rotator TrP in a rotator muscle will have the same or similar referral pattern as a multifidi TrP in a muscle in the same location, even though it is in a different layer of muscle.

What They Do: Extend and rotate the vertebrae, primarily in the thoracic region.

Kinetics Comments: The rotators (also called rotatores spinae) are major **core muscles** but act more like ligaments, as they form a bridge from one vertebra to the next in a diagonal pattern. They help to stabilize the

vertebrae, acting as shock absorbers as they lengthen or tighten in response to changes in posture. Thus, they fine-tune the spatial relationship between the vertebrae. They are highly proprioceptive and may play a significant role in controlling upright posture (McGill 2004, p. 325).

TrP Comments: The rotator TrPs are virtually identical to multifidi TrPs as to symptoms. Since the pain feels like it is deep in the bone, it can cause great concern as well as diagnostic confusion. Rotator TrPs often cause pain to the base of the skull, neck, shoulder blade, or low back. The level of the rotator muscle(s) involved is often a clue to the level of the TrPs. Thus, the rotator muscles closest to the head are more likely to refer pain to the base of the skull, and the rotators closest to the lower back will refer pain there. TrPs in these muscles may be affected by, and affect, disc dysfunction, and may also be implicated in OA of the spine. We suspect that rotator TrPs may also be involved in the development of scoliosis. Although some research that implies this connection has been done by van der Pallts, Veldhuizen, and Verkerke (2007), those researchers were unfamiliar with TrPs. It may be possible to prevent many cases of scoliosis by assessing for these TrPs and treating them in infants and young children.

Notable Perpetuating Factors: Chronic or acute overload may initiate these TrPs. A sudden bend and twist motion may initiate the pain, often immediately. Whiplash, diving accidents and other sports injuries, and falling on the head or other shock to the spine can be rotator TrP initiators, as can pushing muscles to work when they are fatigued and/or chilled. During mid to late pregnancy, chronic tension on these muscles and their attachments may cause chronic overload in these muscles and their adjoining attachments, especially if the mother is carrying more than one child or if the baby is large. This problem seems more common in ten-month pregnancies that may occur in some mothers who also have FM.

Hints for Control: See Multifidi. Care should be taken when getting in and out of chairs, and climbing steps. Pointing the body diagonal to the steps rather than facing them while climbing stairs is helpful in reducing stress on these muscles. Likewise, positioning the body so that it is diagonal to the chair when sitting down and rising can avoid unnecessary stress. It just takes a little effort to achieve a slightly altered point of view, and the muscles will thank you for it by not kicking up a fuss. This is especially important during late pregnancy, when the developing baby should be the only one doing the kicking.

Stretch: Sit in a chair and allow your knees to be as wide apart as possible. Slowly drop your torso into full flexion with your arms hanging straight down, and allow a small rotation of your body to one side and then the other. This only requires a slight rotation, and should target all the superficial and deep tissues all along the length of your spine. Try to feel each muscle. Your spine will love you for it. When returning to an upright position, place your hands on the front of your legs to help you rise back up to the starting position—move slowly. Repeat the stretch. Try breathing out on the stretch down and breathing in on the way back up.

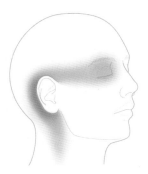

Longissimus Capitis
Latin *longissimus* means "longest"; *capitis*, "of the head."

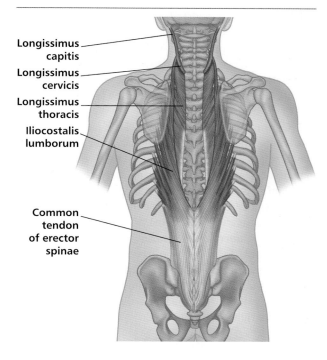

Longissimus capitis

Longissimus cervicis

Longissimus thoracis

Iliocostalis lumborum

Common tendon of erector spinae

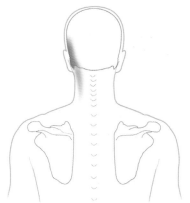

What It Does: The longissimus capitis, along with its paired muscle on the other side of the spine, extends and rotates the head. Healthy longissimus muscles help us keep upright and maintain good spinal posture.

Kinetics Comments: This deep neck muscle belongs to a paired column called the longissimus, which is part of the erector spinae. The longissimus capitis extends from the vertebrae to the skull; the longissimus thoracis connects vertebrae to ribs. In the low back, the longissimus merges with the ilicostalis lumborum.

TrP Comments: TrPs in the longissimus capitis can cause headache, neck pain and stiffness, and decreased ROM. Pain behind the ear can be intense. These TrPs may be associated with numbness and tingling in the scalp. The pain pattern may extend across the neck and behind the eyes. *TrPs in the longissimus capitis may cause rotation of the T1 vertebra, resulting in apparent elevated first rib and eventual articular dysfunction.* Longissimus thoracis TrPs transmit pain downward to the sacroiliac region as well as the buttock. They create a deep, steady ache in the spine, which can quickly spread to the other side as muscles there attempt to compensate for the weaker side. This leads to formation of satellite TrPs. TrPs may also be found in the tendon attachments. A wide variety of conditions may cause similar symptoms, and they may interact with TrPs. Pain referred along the tendon attachments in the longissimus thoracis is suspected by one of the authors (Starlanyl), as is the contribution of these TrPs, to the development of scoliosis in young children. Research is greatly needed.

Notable Perpetuating Factors: Acute overload of the longissimus capitis includes whiplash trauma and falls. Chronic overload perpetuators include poor posture, inappropriate visual correction, overuse of repetitive-motion athletic machines, and inadequate neck support during sleep.

Hints for Control: Keep the spinal muscles supple and long. Mindful moving and control of perpetuating factors is critical. Check your photographs for spinal posture. It may take several trials to find a pillow offering correct neck support for a particular person—one size does not fit all. As neck curvature changes due to treatment and healthier spinal curvature, pillows may need to be adjusted or changed. An adjustable water pillow may help.

Stretch: Sit on the floor with your legs folded. Slowly bend forward, concentrating on moving each vertebral segment before the one below it. Start at the base of the head, dropping your chin towards your chest, and roll forward and down. Leave your arms hanging by your sides. When you have gone as far as feels good, return to an upright position. Repeat this dynamic movement. Use your breath to help you: breathe out as you roll forward and down and "deflate," then breathe in as you "inflate" and return to the upright seated starting position.

External and Internal Intercostals

Latin *inter* means "between"; *costa*, "rib."

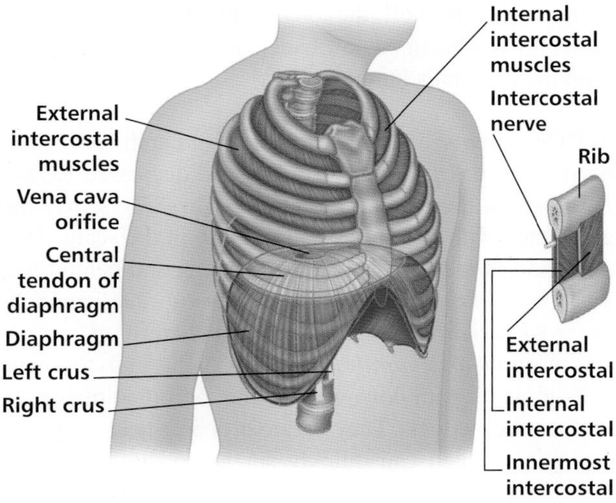
External intercostal muscles
Vena cava orifice
Central tendon of diaphragm
Diaphragm
Left crus
Right crus
Internal intercostal muscles
Intercostal nerve
Rib
External intercostal
Internal intercostal
Innermost intercostal

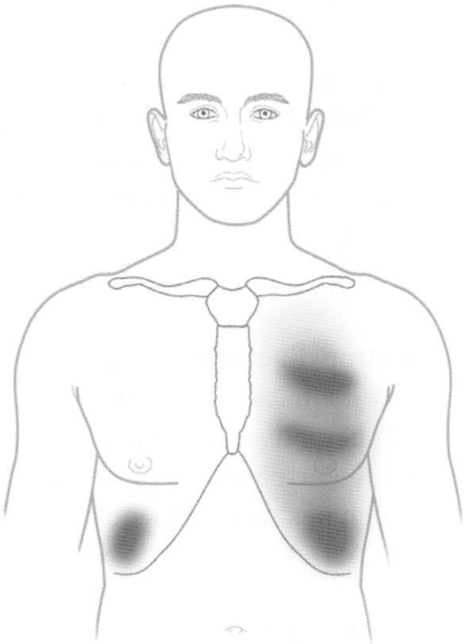

What They Do: Change the dynamics of the ribs, providing about 25% of the total force of breathing, and may help stabilize the chest wall.

Kinetics Comments: The intercostals are three layers of muscles that pass between the ribs. Each external outer layer intercostal attaches to the lower border of one rib, and, on a diagonal line, to the upper border of the rib below. The lowest intercostals merge with the external oblique muscles. The internal intercostals connect each rib from the cartilage to the upper border of the rib below it. There is also a deeper, innermost intercostal layer. The intercostal nerve runs between it and the more superficial internal intercostal, and TrPs in the areas along the nerve can entrap that nerve. The intercostals draw the central tendon of the diaphragm downward during respiration. The health of these muscles can profoundly alter the acid/base balance of the body. Shortening of the intercostals affects the kinetic front chain along the lateral line.

TrP Comments: Intercostal TrPs cause pain locally and restrict the thoracic rotation of the spine. These TrPs may result in a significantly reduced lung volume, which may first become noticeable during exercise, leading to a mistaken diagnosis of exercise-induced asthma. Suddenly, jogging is not an option, because these TrPs can feel as if there is a spear sticking into the ribs when you try to jog. The combination of chest pain and reduced vital capacity can be critical for those who have coexisting breathing impairments such as COPD or emphysema. Any sort of forced respiration such as coughing or sneezing may be extremely painful. A cardiac arrhythmia may result from TrPs in the right-side intercostals.

Depending on their location, intercostal TrPs may interfere with the ability to tolerate a bra. The bra that fits comfortably in the morning may be unbearable an hour later. Women's wardrobe changes may include tops with strategically placed opaque pockets. Anything that puts pressure on these TrPs, including lying on them, may be intolerable. Intercostal TrPs under the right breast in right-handers and left breast in left-handers may cause the muscle to tighten in a visible clump. This may occur during prolonged computer work, or may happen suddenly when you bend over to tie a shoe. Untreated intercostal TrPs can lead to subscapularis TrPs and "frozen shoulder" symptoms. Intercostal TrPs may be described as "painful rib syndrome" (Hughes 1998), "chest wall pain," postherpetic pain (Weiner and Schmader 2006), "abdominal intercostal neuralgia," or mistakenly diagnosed as costochondritis.

Even more posteriorly located intercostal TrPs tend to refer pain towards the front of the chest, and the referral pattern may overlap several ribs. If you locate one TrP, check for others. The presence of these and TrPs in other areas may become apparent when a patient is put on CPAP or other respiratory assistance. The chest cavity is finally expanding to its intended volume, and those muscles are being stretched, perhaps for the first time in a long while. The resulting temporary pain can be frightening unless the reason for it is understood and expected.

Notable Perpetuating Factors: Common perpetuating factors include paradoxical breathing, head-forward posture, diaphragm TrPs, constricting clothing, chronic cough, inhalant allergies, lower respiratory infections, vomiting, coughing, sneezing, leaning over a workstation such as a computer desk, and coexisting chest and abdominal illness. Chest surgery may initiate these TrPs, as may local blunt-force trauma such as a steering wheel impact. These TrPs can crop up following a herpes zoster attack, rib fracture, breast implant surgery, or secondary to tumors.

Hints for Control: These TrPs respond to finger pressure, barrier release, and gentle manipulation of the tissues, but perpetuating factors must be kept under control. The intercostal muscle tension that resembles a spasm may be prevented by attention to posture and other perpetuating factors. Topical carisoprodol 350 mg/ml on the cramped muscle area may help to relax the cramp-like tension. Intercostal TrPs are often accompanied by abdominal TrPs. Whenever these TrPs respond poorly to treatment, look for perpetuating factors. Get them all.

Stretch: Begin in a neutral position, standing with your feet together, and raise both arms over your head with the palms of the hands in contact with each other. Breathe in as you bend to one side, going as far as feels comfortable. Breathe out on the return to neutral. Rest a moment. Repeat this dynamic stretch on the other side. Pay attention to unwanted movement, including the pelvis rising up while stretching. If you have a difficulty with balance, place your feet wider apart to provide a wider base. Remember, movement is life.

Diaphragm

Greek *dia* means "across"; *phragma*, "partition" or "wall."

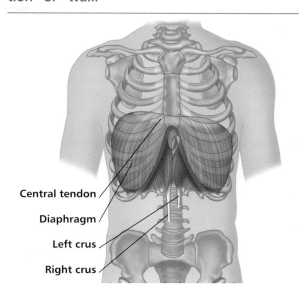

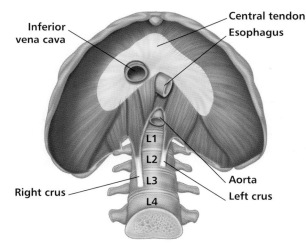

Diaphragm from below.

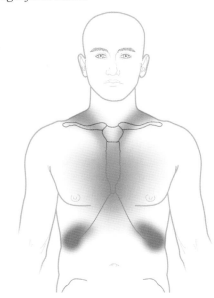

What It Does: The diaphragm is responsible for creating most of the respiratory flow. During quiet breathing, its action produces 70–80% of the force required to inhale.

Kinetics Comments: Among those of us who bother to contemplate it, there is a popular misconception of the thoracic diaphragm as a nearly rectangular flat muscle. Nothing could be further from the truth (unless you are in very big trouble). A relaxed diaphragm is a flexible, dynamic, cloverleaf-shaped convex dome. The right and left halves of this musculotendinous sheet arch and merge to form a large central tendon. When the central tendon pulls down, the lung volume increases and allows full inhalation. As the diaphragm relaxes, air is exhaled. When we breathe more heavily, the abdominal muscles join in to help push the air in and out.

Openings in the diaphragm, called hiatuses, allow structures such as the vena cava, esophagus and aorta to pass through. If the gastroesophageal junction intrudes through an opening, it's called a hiatal hernia. Other veins and arteries pass through the diaphragm. It's also involved in increasing abdominal pressure, which allows expressive acts such as vomiting and defecation; spasms of the diaphragm produce hiccups. The diaphragm affects spinal stiffness through regulating intra-abdominal pressure, and also affects the quality of the voice, influencing singing, whistling, and vocal tone.

Two tendinous structures—the right and left crura (singular: crus)—extend from the lumbar (low back) portion of the diaphragm, attaching it to the spine as the structures merge into the anterior longitudinal ligament. Tightness of the crura affects the anterior longitudinal ligament, which affects the tension of the spine (Shirley et al. 2003). Crural attachment release must be part of any manual release of the dural tube. The diaphragm helps to prevent acid reflux by creating pressure on the esophagus, and the right crus itself is actually part of the lower esophageal sphincter system. Injuries to the neck at C3, C4, and C5 can change the tonic state of the diaphragm, as the phrenic nerve controls diaphragmatic tension.

TrP Comments: Pain can be referred in two distinct patterns: TrPs in the central tendon of the diaphragm refer to the same-side upper border of the shoulder near the angle of the neck, and TrPs in the peripheral areas of the diaphragm refer pain to the region of the rib (costal) margin and can cause a "stitch in the side" pain. Diaphragm TrPs can cause or contribute to chest pain, shortness of breath, and low back pain, and can also cause an odd fluttery feeling in the belly. These TrPs activate when nervousness or anxiety tightens the area, and are called "butterflies in the stomach," because that's what they feel like. These TrP "butterflies" can also cause hiccups. Leaning forward and inhaling can aggravate diaphragm TrP symptoms.

Remember that TrPs are areas of oxygen depravation, and the amount of oxygen in the body depends on many things, including the working of the diaphragm. If the diaphragm is rigid with TrPs, there will be shortness of breath and chronic oxygen depravation. In times of chronic stress or acute severe stress, these TrPs are butterflies with fangs. Along with the pain, episodic diaphragm spasms may occur, resulting in inability to get a deep breath. Patients may fear that death is approaching, adding to tension and feelings of desperation. Both patient and care provider must know about these TrPs to prevent this state or to regain control. Research indicates there is a proprioceptive side to these TrPs which has not yet been clarified (Pickering and Jones 2002). This may include nausea, dizziness, and cardiac symptoms such as arrhythmia. It may explain why some patients with active TrPs in the diaphragm experience a pounding heartbeat when they have a bowel movement. It is our hope that these research avenues will be explored.

Notable Perpetuating Factors: These TrPs can be initiated by laparoscopic surgery, especially if there are other TrPs in the area and/or if the patient already has FM. Other initiating and perpetuating factors include paradoxical breathing, persistent coughing, retching or vomiting, head-forward and slumped-over posture, shallow breathing, and/or hiatal hernia. These TrPs can cause interactive symptoms: for example, TrPs causing shortness of breath may lead to the muscle tightening, which causes more shortness of breath, resulting in more TrPs.

Hints for Control: Manual working of the costal portion of the diaphragm attachment may be accomplished by having the patient seated on a table and leaning into the manual worker, with the patient's arms resting on the worker's shoulders. This position often allows access to much of the diaphragm. Alternatively, the patient may sit in a chair and lean over, with the manual worker behind them, hands under the patient's rib cage. Check for attachment TrPs, especially if there has been protracted coughing or retching, and don't forget to check the crura. Crural tightness can spread TrPs in back muscles adjacent to their attachments. The presence of these and other nearby TrPs may become apparent when a patient is put on CPAP or other respiratory assistance. Those muscles are being stretched, perhaps for the first time in a very long while. The resulting pain could be frightening unless the reason for it is understood and expected.

Stretch: Healthy abdominal breathing and deep belly laughs are good exercise for the diaphragm. One of the authors (Sharkey) has had the privilege of working for many years with leading bodywork expert Leon Chaitow. Dr. Chaitow always highlighted the importance of breath in our work—breath for the therapist and the patient. We tend to think that the diaphragm is out of reach, and perhaps therefore out of out influence, to stretch it. A lovely way to give this muscle a safe dynamic stretch is to sit down on a chair and take your feet shoulder width apart. Place the palms of your hands on top of your knees and allow your back to bend into a mild flexion. Purse your lips and forcefully breathe out fully. This may cause you to cough or feel a little dizzy at the beginning, but you will become accustomed to it in no time. Two or three cycles of forced expiration through pursed lips should be sufficient.

Internal Abdominal Oblique
Latin *internus* means "internal"; abdomen, "stomach"; *obliquus*, "slanting."

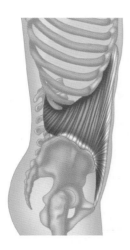

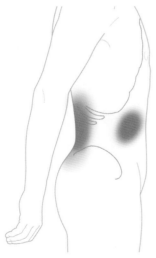

Abdominal oblique TrPs can vary considerably in pain patterns from patient to patient.

What It Does: This **core muscle** supports the wall of the abdomen, helps to raise abdominal pressure, assists in forced respiration, and helps the muscles on either side to move the upper trunk away from the midline. It works with the external abdominal oblique and rectus abdominis to produce trunk flexion. The lower fibers of this muscle combine, forming an aponeurosis (flat tendon) that blends into the lower transversus abdominis,

merging into the conjoint tendon attaching to the pubis. The conjoint tendon itself supports the posterior wall of the inguinal canal.

Kinetics Comments: The abdominal obliques are part of a network of muscles that contain the major body organs and connecting tissues. They help support and protect these organs, and work to provide increased intra-abdominal pressure when needed for deep breathing, defecation, and other "force" work, including birthing labor. Abdominal muscle problems and chronic low back pain would go hand in hand, if they had hands.

TrP Comments: Abdominal TrPs are less consistent from patient to patient than other TrPs, although the approximate location of some TrPs can be suggested by the symptoms. For example, heartburn may indicate TrPs in the upper external oblique, whereas diarrhea indicates TrPs in the lower obliques. Abdominal TrPs are tricky: TrPs on the right side can refer pain only to the right or left abdomen, to *both* sides of the abdomen, and/or up into the chest. They can send pain diagonally as well as straight, and can even cause back pain. These TrPs can cause abdominal swelling, bloating, gas, and burning as well as or instead of referral pain. They can also cause projectile vomiting, burping, groin pain, genital pain, dysmenorrhea, diarrhea, food intolerance (Simons, Travell, and Simons 1999, p. 958), or indigestion.

These TrPs can cause urinary retention problems. They are common in children, causing bed wetting, and in those of us much older, causing the same. You may feel as if you have to "go" all the time. They can cause urinary spasms or inability to empty the bladder. Readers, check with your health care professional. Look for TrPs before you head for medication or surgery. Note that the muscle extends around the back; some of the TrPs, especially the ones that cause burping, may therefore be found in the posterior segment. Check the whole muscle and its attachments for TrPs.

Notable Perpetuating Factors: Abdominal surgery, strain such as birthing labor, trauma, sustained or repetitive twisting of the torso, sustained or severe coughing, paradoxical respiration, poor posture, body asymmetry, prolonged or severe vomiting or other exertion that can over exercise these muscles, stress, infection, or infestation.

Hints for Control: Care must be taken in treating any abdominal pain—it is important to be aware of somatovisceral and viscerosomatic possibilities. TrPs can mimic many complaints, but they can also be hiding visceral pathology. When in doubt, check it out.

Stretch: The abdominal muscles must be exercised together. Healthy function depends on each of the muscles in this area working in concert with the others. Isolated stretches defeat the purpose of integrated function and can change a healthy pelvic tilt, initiating kinetic stress up and down the kinetic line. Place some pillows under the most involved side as you lie on that side on a bed or the floor. Keep your legs straight out, or bend them slightly at the knees. Raise the arm on the least involved side above your head, and allow that arm to gently fall behind your ear, stretching that side. Once you feel the stretch, return to the start and repeat. Then turn and stretch the other side. The pillows under your midsection provide an added arc to the side being stretched.

External Abdominal Oblique

Latin *externus* means "external"; abdomen, "stomach"; *obliquus*, "slanting."

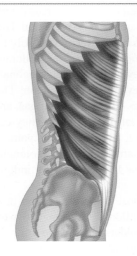

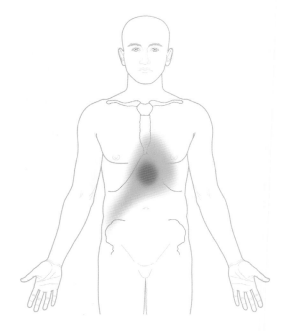

External abdominal oblique. Abdominal oblique TrP referral pattern can vary considerably from patient to patient.

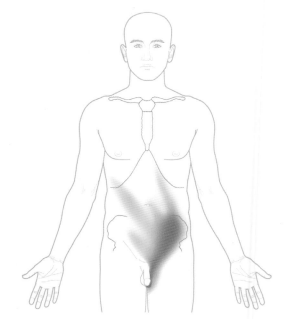

Lateral lower abdominal wall.

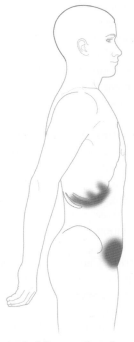

External abdominal oblique referral pattern.

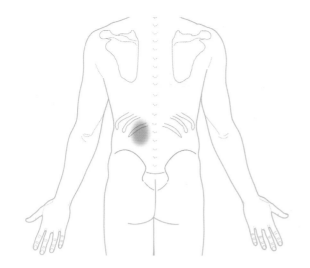

Belch button, posterior lower abdominal wall.

What It Does: This multitalented core muscle supports the wall of the abdomen, helps to raise abdominal pressure, assists in forced respiration, and helps the muscles on either side to move the upper trunk away from the midline. It also works with the external abdominal oblique and rectus abdominis to produce trunk flexion.

Kinetics Comments: The upper fibers of this muscle attach to the lower ribs. The lower fibers blend into an aponeurosis (flat tendon) that goes on to form the inguinal ligament, which in turn attaches to the tensor fasciae latae.

TrP Comments: External oblique TrPs can mimic gall bladder pain and hiatal hernia, or produce a deep stomachache. The abdominal pain can be severe, although non-pain symptoms of these TrPs often cause more misery than the pain and include nausea, heartburn, IBS, diarrhea, colic, dysmenorrhea, bladder pain and urinary dysfunction, and groin and/or genital pain. TrPs in the lower oblique can intensify during menstrual periods. Remember that abdominal TrPs can cause a variety of referral pain patterns. TrPs on the posterior edge of the muscles can cause or contribute to back pain, belching, or vomiting, and TrPs along the ribs may be misdiagnosed as costochondritis. External oblique TrPs under the breast can contribute to a bulging spasm in that area. TrPs in the rib area of the external oblique may cause symptoms similar to an appendix attack, and TrPs in the right upper lateral border can be mistaken for a gall bladder attack. Before you attack the gall bladder or appendix in retaliation, be kind to your body. Check for TrPs.

Notable Perpetuating Factors: Paradoxical breathing, body asymmetry, infections or infestations, over exercising the muscles with job-related activities, flat twisting sit-ups or abdominal exercise machines, toxins, coexisting visceral illness, total body fatigue, emotional stress, trauma, scar tissue, straining due to constipation, and chilly drafts are common initiating or perpetuating factors. Upper frontal external oblique TrPs can be perpetuated by reflux.

Hints for Control: Care must be taken in treating any abdominal pain—it is important to be aware of somatovisceral and viscerosomatic possibilities. TrPs can mimic many complaints, but they can also be hiding visceral pathology. The pain may be temporarily relieved by TrP treatment because there are TrPs *and* an organ disease perpetuating them. For example, TrPs can mimic gall bladder disease, but gall bladder disease may be perpetuating TrPs. You may need to attack that gall bladder after all. When in doubt, check it out.

Stretch: Open and closed kinetic chain movements are important for exercising the external obliques. The muscles need to be both contracted and stretched, with relaxation in between. T'ai chi chuan is good for this, as is swimming the crawl stroke. If your balance is good, you can mimic swimming motions carefully while leaning through a doorway. If your balance isn't good, t'ai chi chuan helps balance too. Laughter, especially deep belly laughs, stretches these muscles. The yoga cobra stretch helps these muscles, but don't hold that stretch. Follow it with the yoga child pose, which moves the muscles in the opposite direction.

A wonderful stretch starts as you lie on your back. Move both arms above your head and to one side. Now add to the stretch: bend your legs at the knees, and drop both of your legs to the opposite side. This will create a lovely rotation of your torso and give a dynamic stretch to the targeted muscles and associated fascia all the way up and down the kinetic chain. Return to the starting position and repeat to the other side. Move slowly, and breathe naturally.

Transversus Abdominis
Latin *transversus* means "across"; *abdominis*, "of the stomach."

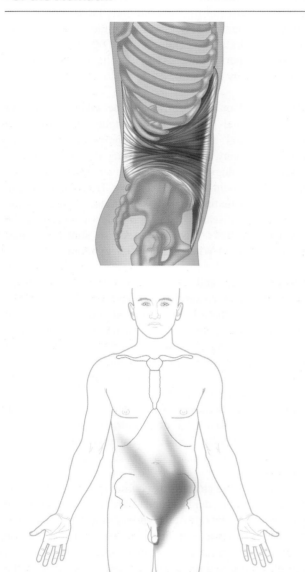

What It Does: This **core muscle** supports other abdominal wall muscles, raises intra-abdominal pressure for forced, "expulsive" actions, and works with obliques to rotate and bend the trunk.

Kinetics: The transversus abdominis (or transversalis muscle) is the deepest abdominal wall muscle. It's called transversus because its fibers are nearly horizontal. It assists with forced expiration, urination, defecation, vomiting, and the final stages of childbirth, as well as helping to produce a strong cough or sneeze. Its effectiveness in raising intra-abdominal pressure depends on the healthy muscle tone of the diaphragm. The broad tendon at the bottom of the transversus joins the internal oblique to form a conjoint tendon.

TrP Comments: This muscle produces somatovisceral symptoms as well as, or instead of, pain in the characteristic patterns. Active TrPs in this muscle can cause heartburn, nausea, vomiting, food intolerance, colic, bloating, diarrhea, groin pain, and/or genital pain. TrPs in the upper regions of this muscle can cause pain at the xiphoid process, sometimes mistaken for cardiac pain. TrPs in the rib attachment areas can cause severe pain on coughing.

Notable Perpetuating Factors: Poor posture, paradoxical breathing, body asymmetry, trauma (including surgery), chronic repetitive motion, total body fatigue, adhesions, overdoing and/or improperly doing repetitive abdominal exercise, cold exposure, straining during defecation, difficult birth labor, infection, infestation, and/or sustained emotional stress.

Hints for Control (Patients): This deep abdominal muscle is more difficult to reach by pressure release methods, although they can be effective, especially with the help of a knobber tool. TrPs in this muscle often mean there are TrPs in other abdominal muscles. Care must be taken in treating any abdominal pain—it is important to be aware of somatovisceral and viscerosomatic possibilities. TrPs can mimic many complaints, but they can also be hiding pathology, and FM can amplify all these symptoms. When in doubt, check it out.

Hints for Control (Care Providers): Palpation for TrPs in this muscle can be difficult. Identification is helped by the transverse nature of the fibers. The spermatic cord may run though its lower border in some men; when it does, entrapment may occur. An infection can activate TrPs, and, when this happens, the symptoms can remain after the infection has gone. That second course of antibiotics, antifungals, or antivirals may not be what is needed. Check for TrPs.

Stretch: Ensure that TrP muscle exercises are aimed at lengthening muscles, not strengthening them. Pelvic tilt and yoga cobra and cat exercises are helpful, as are deep belly laughs.

Rectus Abdominis and Pyramidalis

Latin *rectus* means "straight"; *abdominis*, "of the stomach."
Greek *puramis* means "cone-shaped."

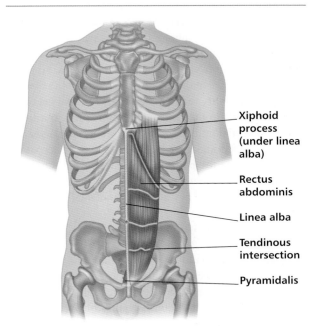

Xiphoid process (under linea alba)

Rectus abdominis

Linea alba

Tendinous intersection

Pyramidalis

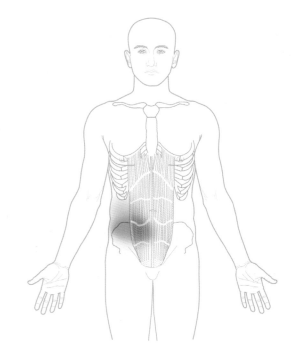

Right lateral rectus abdominis, McBurney's point.

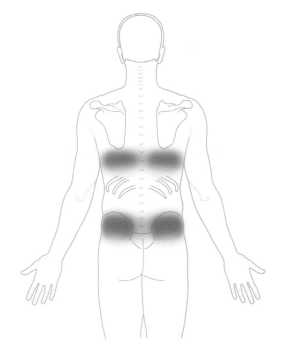

Rectus abdominis.

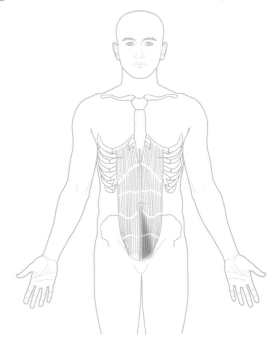

Pyramidalis.

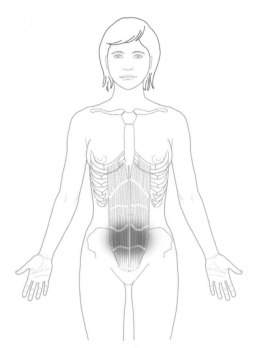

Middle lower rectus abdominis.

What They Do: The rectus abdominis flexes the lower thoracic and lumbar spine. The pyramidalis is a small **core muscle** that creates tension in the linea alba, helping to stabilize it during flexion of the abdominal muscles.

Kinetics Comments: The rectus muscles are **core muscles**. They are enclosed in fibrous sheaths, forming the "abdominal six-pack" look that body builders crave, although there are more than six divisions. Each division is separated from the others by a tendon. The linea alba is a fibrous white band running down the midline between the two rectus abdominis muscles, providing attachment for the transverse and oblique abdominal muscles. It stretches during the late stages of pregnancy to accommodate the further separation of the two rectus abdominis muscles. The pyramidalis is found (if it has been lost) inside the rectus sheath in front of the rectus muscle. It isn't present in everyone, so may not be found at all.

TrP Comments: TrPs in the rectus abdominis can cause non-pain symptoms, but they also refer pain in horizontal bands across the back, although a TrP in the vicinity of the McBurney's point causes one-sided horizontal pain across the belly. If the back pain is confined to one side, it is usually not due to rectus abdominis TrPs. Look for the TrPs in this muscle at the same level as the pain bands in the back. *As TrPs can* occur anywhere in the muscle, so the referred bands can occur at any level. The figure gives *examples only.*

Symptoms from TrPs in the rectus abdominis often give clues as to their location. TrPs in the upper rectus abdominis may cause pain between low-level ribs,

vomiting, colic and excess gas in infants, indigestion, pain similar to heart pain, a feeling of stomach fullness, and/or anorexia. Those beneath the navel level can cause dysmenorrhea; diarrhea; premenstrual pain; pelvic pain; moderate to severe cramping; pain similar to gall bladder or kidney disease; pain similar to appendicitis, prostatitis, cystitis, or diverticulosis; colic; burping; and/or pain to the penis or vulva. A TrP located in the pyramidalis in the area immediately above the pubis can cause spasm of the detrusor urinae and urinary sphincter muscles. The detrusor is the muscle that helps expel urine, so these TrPs can affect the ability to urinate or empty the bladder fully, and the ability to hold that urine until you get to the bathroom. TrPs in the rectus abdominis (and to a lesser extent other abdominals) can cause (and be caused by) a lax, distended abdomen with excess gas. The patient may not be able to "pull in the stomach." All too often, abdominal strengthening exercises are then prescribed for this belly bulge. They are contraindicated for TrPs.

These TrPs can have life-altering effects, and must be taken seriously. Multiple TrPs and FM may be a destructive combination. Premenstrual and menstrual pain due to pressure of extra fluid at those times of the month can lead to many days lost at school or work every month, and to a much-reduced quality of life. In severe cases, the effects of one menstrual period may extend to the next. They can join with psoas and other TrPs to send throbbing pain down the back and the thigh. The rectus abdominis muscle or its sheath may entrap an anterior branch of the spinal nerve, producing sharp pelvic pain. Care must always be taken in treating any abdominal pain—it is important to be aware of the possibility of somatovisceral and viscerosomatic possibilities. TrPs can mimic many complaints, but they can also be hiding visceral pathology. When in doubt, the possibility of underlying disease must be investigated.

Notable Perpetuating Factors: Abdominal surgery, including laparoscopy and Cesarean section, and acute muscle overload, such as from lifting heavy objects or from trauma, can initiate these TrPs. Poor posture, paradoxical breathing, body asymmetry, anterior pelvic tilt, cold exposure, constricting clothing, infections or infestations, sit-ups and crunches (or machines that create the same motions), and other chronic overload such as from repetitive motions during work or repetitive sports (e.g. golfing) can perpetuate them. Emotional tension or water retention can add to the symptoms of these TrPs, and cause TrP activation themselves.

Hints for Control: Patients can learn the barrier release method for these TrPs. Surgical TrPs can be prevented by injecting the area around the incision with local anesthetic before the cut is made in each layer. Ice may relieve symptoms temporarily, but it must be applied on the TrPs themselves. The temptation is to put the ice where it hurts rather than the source. Remember that there may be multiple TrPs, and all must be treated. If the psoas is involved, tilting the knee out at an angle sideways with the ice at the groin can provide temporary relief as well as confirming psoas involvement. In cases of colic, cramping, and excess gas, check for periumbilical TrPs.

Menstrual cramps may be eased by ice packs or moist heat over the pubis, but remember there are other TrP sources of menstrual pain, so move the ice pack around—and include the low back—until you find the source(s). Between menstrual periods, the pubic area may be worked lying on a tennis ball on a rug, but be very gentle—TrPs hurt! The good news is that this helps confirm their presence. Menstrual pain-causing TrPs can cause extreme tenderness, and are most easily worked with pressure release between periods. Gently separating the stuck tissue of the rectus abdominis manually is extremely helpful treatment, but no fun to experience, and may cause TrP activation in itself. Manual work on this muscle may require extra medication before and after, and may cause delayed pain reaction, especially if FM is part of the picture. Patients need to understand this and know that it doesn't mean things are getting worse. When these TrPs roar, check the skin of the abdomen for TrPs as well. Take into consideration the possibility of FM amplification, and be cautions in adding medications to control these symptoms. Work on the cause.

Stretch: Laughter is good medicine for these TrPs, even though they are no laughing matter. This muscle and its associates can be stretched in a dynamic fashion sitting, standing, or lying down. The use of a stability ball may add to the enjoyment and variety of this stretch, but may not be appropriate for those with balance problems. Check with your therapist or doctor, and have a spotter nearby the first time you try this stretch. Lie on the ball, making sure that your back is well supported and your feet are hip-distance apart. The ball should be inflated to a height that ensures that your knees and hips are in line with each other, and your knees are bent at a right angle. Hold a light object, such as a small ball, in your hands. Starting with your hands resting on your belly button, raise your arms up and over your head. Reach with your arms while making sure that your feet keep you stable. Reach as far as feels good and return to the start. This stretch can also be performed sitting or standing. Too many people try to avoid arching their back, but slightly arching as you stretch is in fact a good thing. Remember, speed is the enemy, so listen to your body and avoid bouncing or jerky movements. Breathe in while taking your arms over your head, and breathe out on returning to the starting position.

Psoas Major and Minor
Greek *psoa* means "loin muscle."
Latin *major* means "larger"; *minor*, "smaller."

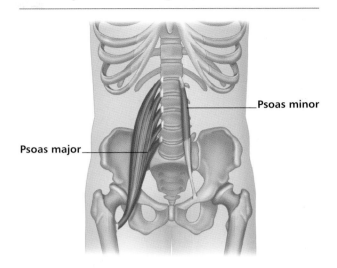

Psoas minor

Psoas major

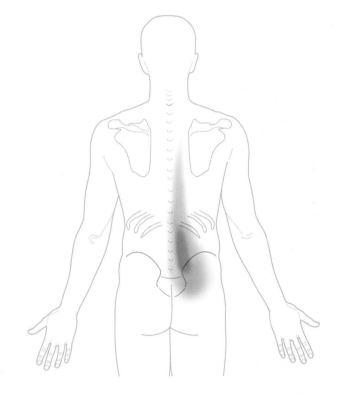

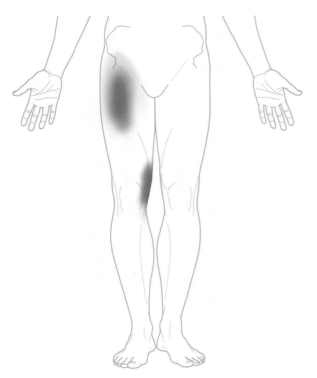

What They Do: The psoas major flexes and medially rotates the hip. It helps us to sit and walk upright, and, through its attachments, *it may significantly affect the stability of the spine and the tightness of the pelvic floor.* The psoas minor is a weak trunk flexor. These are **core muscles**.

Kinetics Comments: These deep muscles form a link from the trunk to the lower body. The psoas major and minor are often grouped with the iliacus and referred to as the iliopsoas, although the psoas minor is missing in about half of all human beings, who are left with a fascial band rather than a muscle. A short, tight psoas causes inhibition of the gluteal muscles, often initiating a TrP cascade down the kinetic chain. Imbalances in other core musculature cause the psoas muscles to compensate, leading to additional tension and tightness. It is important to learn to move mindfully and with care in respect of stress placed on this muscle—it can be unforgiving. These muscles attach to the lumbar spine and play an important role in the position of the lumbar vertebrae and the pelvis.

TrP Comments: Psoas TrPs love company and are frequently associated with other TrPs in the region. You won't love their company, as they can produce extreme pain, especially when they exist in a group with iliacus, quadratus lumborum, and gluteus minimus TrPs. Psoas TrP pain, known for its distinct vertical spinal component, is usually worse during weight-bearing activities, and may ease somewhat in intensity when weight is taken off the muscle. Along with the back and anterior thigh pain, the referral area may include a tight, painful zone on the same side of the navel as the TrP. Psoas TrPs can also refer pain and weakness to the inner knee area. With these TrPs, it may be difficult or impossible to get up from a deep chair. If the TrPs are severe, walking may be impossible, and crawling may be the only endurable way to move. These TrPs can worsen during menstruation. The front component may worsen with constipation, especially if a ball of feces presses against the iliocaecal valve. Massage of the valve may help the passing of the feces and relieve some pain. Psoas pain may mimic appendicitis, and this pain can be severe, resulting in a sharp jab during movement while lifting a heavy object. That lifted object may be dropped due to the sudden intensity of the pain, and/or the patient may fall to the ground in agony. Possible entrapments include the femoral, ilioinguinal, iliohypogastric, obturator, genitofemoral, and lateral femoral cutaneous nerves. Check the lateral and medial border of the muscle for entrapments, which can cause sharp pain, and paresthesia or decreased sensation of the groin, genitals, and/or upper thigh. These TrPs are common contributors to vulvodynia.

The stooped "psoatic gait," walking bent over with a pronounced hyperlordosis of the pelvic spine, is far too common in older people and can reduce height by several centimeters (an inch or more), with the space between the top of the hipbone and the bottom of the ribs (and everything therein) compressed. When this situation is due to TrPs, it can often be corrected. Psoas TrPs are often the cause of failed low back surgery. There may have been a surgical problem in addition to the TrPs, or there may have just been the TrPs. TrP assessment and treatment is necessary *before* surgery is even contemplated.

Notable Perpetuating Factors: Muscle overload that perpetuates psoas TrPs often comes from impaired circulation due to immobility of hip flexors. If you sleep curled up in a fetal position or with hips otherwise flexed, you may not be able to stand up straight when you get out of bed due to these TrPs. It may be difficult to stand up after a long meeting. Common perpetuating factors are: repetitive kicking, jogging, or running; lumbar disc pathology; poor posture; scoliosis; lumbar fusion; chronic constipation; sacroiliac dysfunction; pregnancy; gait irregularities; structural asymmetry; and sit-ups (or machines that copy this motion). Seated abdominal curls, with or without machines, are perpetuating factors and we recommend avoiding these exercises. Psoas TrPs are usually satellites of other TrPs, but can be initiated by prolonged sitting with the knees flexed, or sleeping in a fetal position.

Hints for Control: On long drives, cruise control provides an opportunity for the driver to shift position, and frequent stretching stops are helpful. During airplane trips, stretch: get up and move around the cabin. Any sustained immobility must be avoided. It is possible to change a habitual sleeping position, but this requires commitment and an understanding of TrP perpetuation. Before lying on the back, place a small pillow under the knees to help ease tension on these muscles, unless you have TrPs there too. Moist heat over the entire front length of the muscle may ease the pain. Kneeling on hands and knees may also be helpful for temporarily relieving tension on the muscle. Tilting the knee out at an angle sideways, with the ice or moist heat at the groin, may provide temporary relief. Check both sides for TrPs; as healing occurs, the pain may shift from side to side as latent TrPs are activated. It is to be expected—don't worry.

Care Provider Note: When psoas pain occurs, be alert to the possibility of hemorrhage in these muscles, especially if the patient is on anti-coagulant therapy. Psoas hemorrhage may occur spontaneously or from even relatively minor trauma.

Stretch: We recommend a dynamic stretch using a stability ball to aid balance. As you become more proficient, you can reduce air in the ball or stretch without the ball. Sit on the ball or balance beside the ball with a split stance while keeping upright, as shown in the diagram.

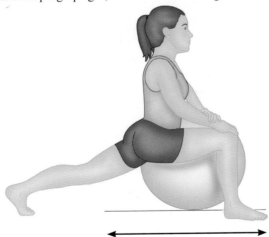

Psoas stretch.

Keep your head lifted and suspended. Imagine you have a cord tied to the top of your head and someone is pulling it up. Your lead leg should bend at the knee, keeping your knee and heel in line. You're "up on your toes" on the back leg. Keeping the knee straight, you will feel the stretch in the front of the hip. Use the ball to rock back and forth with control, avoiding speed and jerky movement. Repeat several times and change sides.

Iliacus
Latin *ilia* means "the flanks."

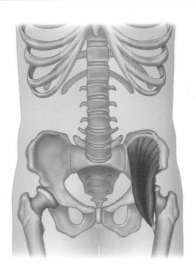

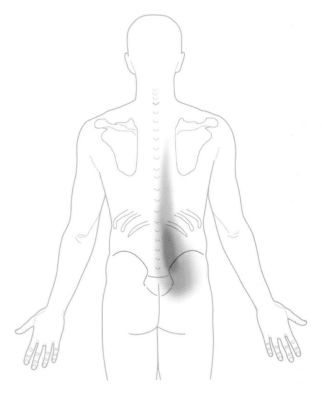

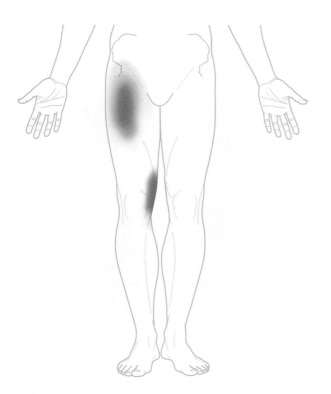

What It Does: Flexes and stabilizes the hip.

Kinetics Comments: These **core muscles** line the pelvic wall, and blend with and join the psoas major as the iliopsoas. The iliacus works with the psoas to bring us to a sitting position when we are lying down, and assists in pulling the leg up as we walk. It helps to connect the thighbone to the hip. It is also connected to the anterior inferior iliac spine. This muscle, along with the psoas major, is rich in muscle spindles and thus prone to shortening when stressed. Tightness on the iliacus pulls on its connections, including the spine, and lower spine pathology can affect the iliacus.

TrP Comments: See Psoas.

Notable Perpetuating Factors: Anything that stresses the connections of the iliacus—such as the psoas, thighbone, spine, or deep ligaments—stresses the iliacus itself. Repetitive kicking, jogging, running, lumbar disc pathology, poor posture, scoliosis, lumbar fusion, constipation, sacroiliac dysfunction, pregnancy, gait irregularities, structural asymmetry, sit-ups (or machines that copy this motion), and muscle imbalances are common perpetuating factors.

Hints for Control: Much of the iliacus—a deep muscle lining the hipbone—is difficult to access manually. Freeing those structures attached to the iliacus can help relieve tension indirectly. As always, control of perpetuating factors is the key to controlling TrPs.

Stretch: This stretch can be achieved sitting, but standing is preferred. Place the foot of the uninvolved (or less involved) side behind the other leg: in other words, cross your legs at the ankle. Now reach the hand of the involved side up towards the ceiling, and bend sideways to the uninvolved (or less involved) side. While you are side-bending, you can reach towards the floor with the fingers of the other hand. This will intensify the stretch, so do take it slowly and avoid speed. Do not bounce the stretch. Avoid holding your breath: breathe in and out comfortably. Return slowly to the start, and then stretch the involved (or most involved) side.

Quadratus Lumborum
Latin *quadratus* means "squared-off"; *lumbus*, "loin."

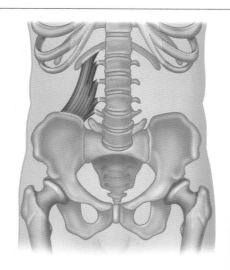

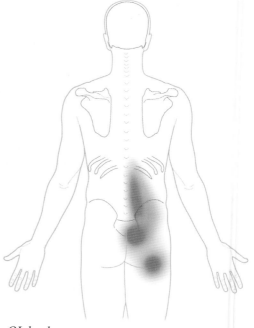

Deep QL back.

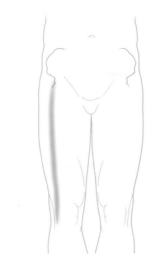

QL lightning bolt.

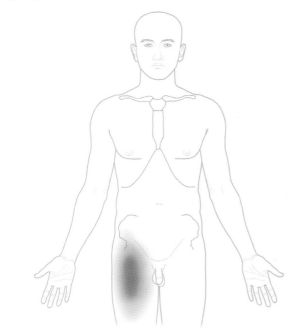

QL thigh.

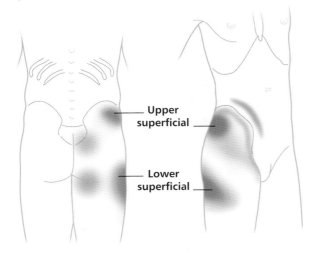

— Upper superficial

— Lower superficial

Superficial QL.

What It Does: The quadratus lumborum (nicknamed QL) flexes the trunk laterally on the same side. It stabilizes the twelfth rib during a deep inward breath, keeping the upper roots of the diaphragm steady. It also keeps the pelvis from dropping on the non-weight-bearing side when you stand on one leg. Both sides of the QL act together to extend and stabilize the lower vertebrae. The QL works with the diaphragm, helping to stabilize the lower spine.

Kinetics Comments: The health of this **core muscle** can determine tolerance for standing and sitting. These muscles are attached to the twelfth rib, the L1–L4 lumbar vertebrae, and the hipbone. When the QL is tighter on one side than on the other, the kinetic chain attempts to compensate. The pelvis rotates anteriorly on the most affected side. The adductors on the other side shorten to level the hips and better stabilize the thighbone in the hip socket. The thigh on that side can be drawn up into the hip, giving the impression of that leg being shorter than the other one. Too often, a heel lift is then recommended, which worsens the problem, as the leg is only functionally, not anatomically, shorter. Tightness in the QL on one side may cause functional scoliosis; in addition, the stress on the pelvis can lead to subluxation, or partial dislocation, of the cartilage joint in the pubis (the pubic symphysis) and/or the sacroiliac. *These muscles are key players involved in low back pain, yet often overlooked.*

TrP Comments: One cannot overstate the intensity of QL TrP pain—it can be overwhelming. FM will amplify its intensity. Even when these TrPs are relatively mild, climbing stairs can be painful. As TrPs persist, the pain may not cease during rest, and can worsen on standing. You may have to stand with your hands pressing in and downward on your hips to relieve some of the pain. This action bypasses the lumbar spine and takes some of the pressure off the QL. Lying down with a small pillow under the upper part of the muscle may give some relief. These are temporary measures, as these TrPs mean business and must be treated promptly. You may need to use hands and arms to lift yourself out of a chair or roll onto your side. Bending forward may be out of the question; walking may be impossible. You may not be able to stand at all, and even need to crawl to get to the bathroom. Referral pain may include the sacroiliac region, groin area and genitals.

QL TrPs can cause a feeling of heaviness in the thighs, cramping in the calves, and a burning sensation in the hands and feet. When these TrPs are active and you attempt to engage the QL, it may feel as if you have a knife in your back. Lightning-bolt pain may jolt down the front of the thigh, from the hip to the outside of the kneecap. That pain feels electrical in nature, and patients will go to great lengths to avoid coughing or sneezing or any other action that might initiate it. They may fall to the ground when this pain occurs—it is so devastating. Hip joint pain caused by these TrPs is often mistaken for trochanteric bursitis, and can wake you up when you move during sleep, especially if you try to roll over. The trochanter area (where the thighbone fits into the hip socket) is too tender to allow any pressure on it. These TrPs cause significant additional energy expenditure that increases general fatigue.

Notable Perpetuating Factors: Trauma, stooping and twisting, lifting and twisting motions, body asymmetry (including short upper arms), poor posture, weak abdominal muscles, scoliosis, abdominal area infections, aortic aneurysm, lower spinal pathology, constant heavy sneezing or coughing, any motion that shortens one side of the QL (such as often holding a child or other weight on the same side), walking or running on a tilted surface, shoveling snow, frequent getting-up from a lying-down position, or holding an awkward position. Sports that stress one side repeatedly, such as golf, are major QL TrP activators. If you pull on pants while standing and lose your balance, or stand and lean over a workstation, you're asking for these TrPs. Sleeping position can profoundly affect this muscle.

Hints for Control (Patients): You can learn to treat this muscle manually by lying on the least affected side and working the other one, with the top leg placed behind the bottom one, working down the ropy bands and lumps of TrPs with the fingers. You can open the QL area to palpation and treatment by placing a small pillow underneath the opposite side. The QL is easier to identify during deep inhalation. Posterior QL areas can also be worked using tennis-ball pressure. Check the gluteal muscles for TrPs as well. All perpetuating factors must be brought under control. Yes, this may mean golf must wait for a while, and please, don't try to substitute bowling or other activity that also stresses the same side. Get someone else to walk that unruly dog, and arrange dog obedience training. These TrPs are unforgiving. If you need to climb stairs, do so with the feet pointed at a diagonal to the stairs (at a 45-degree angle) to help stabilize the body. A lumbosacral support may be helpful in acute cases, but attention must be given to remedying the TrPs. Carefully strengthen weak abdominals once those muscles are free of TrPs.

When QL TrPs occur bilaterally, it is not unusual for pain to switch from one side to the other as therapy resolves some TrPs and muscles try to compensate. Work and stretch both sides. Ensure that your bed provides proper support, and evaluate common postures and furniture. Be mindful of body mechanics and movement. A pillow beneath the legs when sleeping on the side, or under the knees when sleeping on the back, may help relieve some pressure on this muscle.

Hints for Control (Care Providers): When patients are bedridden with low back pain, look first for QL TrPs. If low backache won't go away in spite of treatment of other muscles, check the QL. If one hip is hiked and one leg appears short, check for pelvic rotation and compensation. If the unequal leg length is functional, adding a lift to the "shorter" leg will add another perpetuating factor. Once QL TrPs are present, a difference of only 1/10" (about 3 mm) may be sufficient to perpetuate them. Investigate why the leg is short: this may require weight-bearing imaging. Correct pelvic rotation and check for unequal hemipelvis. When these TrPs occur in younger patients, they may cause functional scoliosis and change growth patterns. It is critical to identify and treat these TrPs as soon as possible. The sacroiliac and pubic symphysis may sublux as the bones are pulled out of alignment by contracted muscles. Attempts to compensate for this may lead to TrPs in all four quadrants of the body. The history will often reveal the onset of the first TrP cascades. QL TrPs are often the cause of "failed surgical back." They may be mistaken for disc pain, or called lumbago. They may cause pudendal neuralgia. They rarely occur alone: when QL TrPs are active, check for TrPs in the erector spinae, multifidi, gluteal muscles, piriformis, iliocostalis, abdominal obliques, rectus abdominis, latissimus dorsi, iliopsoas, and deep pelvic stabilizing ligaments. The pain that QL TrPs and their friends can cause is unrelenting and all consuming, and may include a feeling of impending doom that may be mistaken as psychological. The QL may be most easily worked manually by lying on the least affected side with a thin pillow between the knees, and the upper knee behind the back of the lower knee. When the patient is standing and there are TrPs on only one side of the QL, there is a pelvic tilt downward on the opposite side. When there are bilateral QL TrPs, the space between the lower ribs and the top of the iliac crest is often substantially shortened.

Stretch: Stretching the QL requires control: ensure you do not overstretch. This stretch can be performed sitting or standing. Sitting upright, let your arms hang down by your sides and let your fingers drop towards the floor slowly. Then bend to one side. Control your movement and go slowly, bending as far as feels comfortable, then return to the starting position. If you are seated, keep your buttocks firmly on the chair. Repeat on the opposite side. To advance this stretch, reach the arm of the side to be stretched over your head and up, while bending slowly to the other side until the stretch is felt. Return to the starting position, and repeat on the opposite side.

Pelvic Floor

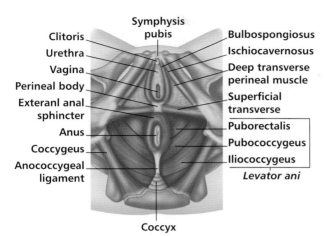

Third layer perineum (female).

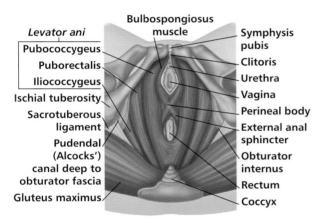

Second layer perineum (female).

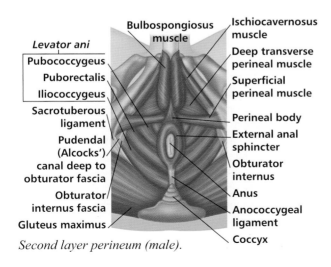

Second layer perineum (male).

The pelvic floor is part of the **core muscles**. It's formed by muscles and many other structures, and they can all develop TrPs. Far too many people are unaware of the multitude and diversity of symptoms generated by TrPs in this complex area. Interior pelvic floor TrPs aren't typical TrP contraction nodules: most are longitudinal bands. Symptoms generated by TrPs in this area are usually misdiagnosed. We tend to hold tension in the pelvic floor—that tension becomes part of life, and we become unaware that we are holding these muscles up and tight. For example, when we stand, the buttocks tend to be held tight with the anus clenched. Pelvic structures are not designed to be kept under extra chronic tension. The first step towards healing is becoming aware of this tension so that we can begin to let it go.

Symptoms from pelvic floor TrPs are referred to using a wide variety of terms, including: chronic abacterial prostatitis, chronic pelvic pain, coccygodynia, erectile dysfunction, levator spasm, levator ani syndrome, pudendal neuralgia, proctodynia, tight pelvic floor, prostatodynia, tension myalgia, urgency-frequency syndrome, and vulvodynia. These labels are descriptions: they don't identify the symptom cause, and that's what needs treatment. Neurotransmitters control pelvic activity, and much neurotransmitter research has been done in the fields of fibromyalgia and mental health. Healthy pelvic function requires healthy muscle tension. Myofascial TrPs are the most common cause of pain in the pelvic floor, and they can greatly affect quality of life (Itza et al. 2010). They cause symptoms that are indistinguishable from a variety of organ diseases; they may occur in conjunction with those diseases and can perpetuate their symptoms long after those illnesses have been treated. Many of these symptoms are associated with fibromyalgia, but FM *amplifies* the symptoms, whatever the cause. To treat them, and to begin healing, one must identify the cause. These symptoms are often, but not always, *caused* by TrPs.

Pelvic floor tissues with TrPs don't work in coordination with each other or with tissues in surrounding areas. It is uncommon for seniors to have a flexible pelvic floor, and that lack of suppleness can cause extreme dysfunction. Disruptions to normal healthy pelvic function may be obvious, such as an infection or trauma, or they may occur subtly and without notice over time. They are cumulative. When pelvic symptoms occur, check for possible pathologies, such as an ovarian cyst, prostate infection, or malignancy. That being said, TrPs can be the sole cause of interstitial cystitis, chronic pelvic pain, and many voiding dysfunctions (Doggweiler-Wiygul and Wiygul 2002). Muscle weakness in a tight pelvic floor is usually due to TrPs, not muscle fatigue (Fitzgerald and Kotarinos 2003a). Attempts at strengthening TrP-laden muscles are counterproductive. Fortunately, much can be done to eliminate or significantly reduce symptoms, often without surgery (Fitzgerald and Kotarinos 2003b). Some conditions linked with the aging process may be preventable as well. For example, studies have shown that, as they age, women with urinary stress incontinence recruit the pelvic floor muscles to compensate for weakness in the urethral sphincter or fascia (Madill and McLean 2010). This may be true in men as well.

Regional Kinetics: The pelvic floor provides a foundation and protection for the pelvic organs, controls continence of the bowels and bladder, and includes the mechanisms for sexual and reproductive functions. A healthy, flexible pelvic floor contributes to postural and even respiratory function (Hodges, Sapsford, and Pengel 2007). It helps to support a growing fetus, aids in stabilizing the pelvis and the spine, and contributes to sexual arousal. When the pelvic floor muscles are tight and weak, all these functions and more are affected. Even though nerves in the S2–S4 vertebrae control central bladder function, the process of urination is basically a learned behavior. When TrPs lurk in the pelvic floor, it may hurt to sit for any length of time. Laughing, coughing, sneezing, lifting, or bending forward may cause stress incontinence. In women, urine may dribble sideways or run down the leg, especially at the end of urination. Men may experience premature ejaculation or post-urinary dribbling. For men and women, muscles may get so tight it can be difficult to urinate or defecate smoothly unless you are blowing your nose or otherwise increasing abdominal pressure. Sexual sensation and desire may diminish.

Regional TrP Comments: We ask our readers who are patients (we hope you are all patient readers) to understand that care of these TrPs often requires professional help, so much of this segment requires medical language. The figures will help. *Many pelvic floor TrPs refer pain to the area in between the buttocks*, but not all do that in all patients. Individual muscle TrPs cause specific symptoms that give clues to their location. There is a complete book dedicated to these TrPs—*A Headache in the Pelvis* by Wise and Anderson (2008). Some TrPs cause painful intercourse in women (dyspareunia), particularly during entry, pain in the external female genitalia (vulvodynia), and aching between the anus and the genitalia (the perineum). Some TrPs cause or contribute to erectile dysfunction or "chronic prostatitis." TrPs in the back half of the pelvic floor cause diffuse, hard-to-locate pain; with these TrPs, you may need to shift sitting position frequently, and getting up after prolonged sitting may cause obvious pain and require extra effort. Some of these TrPs can contribute to vulvar or anal itching and burning. It is not known at this time if TrPs are involved in blood vessel and lymph entrapment contributing to pelvic floor congestion, but it's suspected. Pudendal nerve entrapment can be a contributor to pain here, and generally occurs between the sacrotuberous and sacrospinous ligaments or inside Alcock's canal. The dorsal nerve of the penis or clitoris can be entrapped close to the pubic bone (Sedy 2008), but this generally causes numbness rather than pain.

There are two common uses of the term interstitial cystitis (IC). It may be used to mean any combination of pain in the pubis and perineum pain with urinary burning and urgency. Others restrict IC to describing a condition with an unknown cause that includes fragile bladder wall, mucosal irritation, micro hemorrhage in the bladder, and ulceration. TrPs can contribute in both situations, but can be the sole cause of the first. That may begin with frequent urination to relieve pressure and pain caused by area TrPs, developing a frequent voiding habit (Doggweiler-Wiygul 2004). Frequency of defecation may likewise occur in attempts to relieve pressure on the rectum and surrounding muscles. The patient may develop a tendency to sit on one side and put a leg under the pelvic area to relieve pressure there. This posture is an avoidable perpetuating factor that stresses the front thigh and can initiate a TrP cascade.

Regional Scar TrPs: TrPs in scar tissue produced by any pelvic or abdominal surgery are common, especially in the vaginal cuff following hysterectomy. They can cause pain that feels like ovarian pain, menstrual cramps, or bladder spasms; they can also cause lightning-like jolts of pain. The amount of pain does not reflect the size of the scar. Some scars are hidden, as when an appendix or ovaries are removed during hysterectomy. The chance of developing surgical scar TrPs is lessened if the surgeon injects the incision area with topical anesthetic immediately before the incision. Also common in this area are non-myofascial TrPs in fat layers under the skin, in the fat pads overlying the sacroiliac region, and in fatty tumors called lipomas.

Regional CMP Comments: This will be discussed by means of an example. A 42-year-old teacher with a history of pelvic pain had been on birth control pills since age 16 to decrease the symptoms, which kept developing. Her menstrual flow had always been membranous, containing clots. It was a struggle for her to get through school because of the symptoms, which started a week before her period and lasted for some time after. Pain radiating down her thighs, including the pelvic and abdominal regions, was eventually coupled with IBS. She had multiple laparoscopies with negative results. After a complete hysterectomy at age 35, she stopped birth control medication briefly. The monthly pain was gone, but abdominal cramping and other IBS symptoms remained, along with episodic back and leg pain. She resumed hormones and they seemed to help with the pain. She had married at age 28. In the last five years, chronic pelvic pain and vulvodynia caused increasing loss of interest in sexual relations. She had urinary urgency and frequency as well. She got restorative sleep and ate organic, well-balanced meals. She had been going to a psychologist and psychiatrist for over a decade and was on very heavy medication for depression. She said she was depressed because she felt helpless to control the pain. She could not sit for any length of time, and needed to get up and move several times during the history. Her psychologist had told her that she didn't love her husband and may have had early sexual abuse with suppressed memories, which she denied. Her husband was supportive and they had an otherwise happy relationship. She mentioned that, with all the anti-depressant medications, she couldn't be other than happy, but the chronic pain was still unendurable. Healing began as soon as she recognized her own TrP pain patterns.

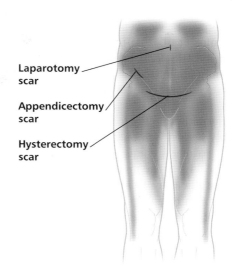

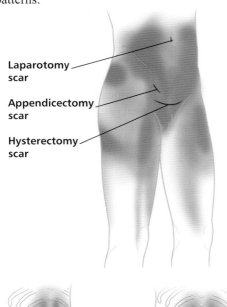

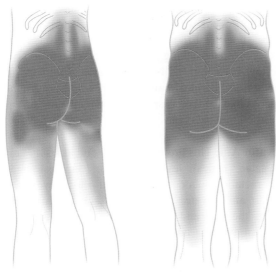

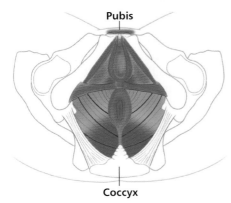

Patient pain patterns.

Examination revealed active TrPs in all abdominal obliques (referring downward only) and multiple scars, and in the rectus abdominis, pyramidalis, quadratus lumborum, perineum, adductor magnus, levator ani, sphincter ani, ischiocavernosus and bulbospongiosus, piriformis, and gluteus medius and maximus. Latent TrPs were found in several other abdominal, paraspinal, gluteal, and thigh muscles. Perpetuating factors included a tight pelvic floor, paradoxical breathing, head-forward posture, stress, short stature, proportionally short lower legs, and IBS. After TrP treatment and temporary worsening of symptoms due to TrP activation, she dispensed with the antidepressants with the blessing of her newly educated psychiatrist. She temporarily required extra pain medication, including topicals, to help her get through internal manual therapy and the start of a home exercise program, t'ai chi classes, and stretches. Her symptoms significantly diminished within a few weeks.

Membranous dysmenorrhea, often associated with high progesterone levels, is a perpetuating factor of pelvic floor pain. Estrogen replacement therapy can be helpful in decreasing central sensitization and visceral sensitivity (Sanoja and Cevero 2010). The history indicated that there had been membranous flow and that hormone therapy was helpful. Blood testing was done to find the levels of each estrogen component, and a topical was compounded for her. After she'd been on the replacement therapy for several weeks, subsequent testing showed the levels to be those of an intact female. The patient found footrests for use at home and in the classroom so that she could elevate her feet to avoid compressing the hamstring area. The IBS improved significantly with TrP therapy, rectal lidocaine, simethicone, and control of perpetuating factors. The patient required mental counseling to help her grieve for the lost years of her life, although she switched psychologists. Uneducated care providers can be major perpetuating factors. Chronic pelvic pain and IBS often occur in the same patients (Rodriguez et al.

2009); abnormal pelvic floor function occurs in IBS patients (Suttor et al. 2010). In patients with chronic pelvic pain and IBS, 72% had their symptoms relieved or significantly minimized for 12 months after just two osteopathic treatments (Riot et al. 2004).

Regional Perpetuating Factors: Common perpetuating factors apply here. When one is focusing on a specific region with so many unique and daunting symptoms, it is easy to forget that thyroid or insulin resistance, nutritional insufficiency, slumped posture, or a chair that does not fit might be a perpetuating factor. The habit of holding pelvic floor muscles tight can be very old: it can start during toilet training, or can develop if you do not have sufficient time to urinate or defecate, and therefore start forcing the pelvic floor muscles with some extra abdominal pressure to speed things up. It can happen during school if insufficient bathroom time is allowed between classes. Acute muscle overload stressing the pelvic floor can occur during sports (such as gymnastics), dance, and trauma (including childbirth or pelvic surgery), or may result from sustained compression due to carrying a heavy baby (or babies) low during pregnancy. Anything that can interfere with blood circulation, even constrictive clothing, can perpetuate these TrPs, as can prolonged bicycling, motorcycling, horseback riding, sitting at a computer, and chronic hemorrhoids. Other perpetuating factors include chronic pelvic inflammatory conditions (such as endometriosis), IC, and chronic infection (viral, bacterial, or fungal), as well as adhesions, scars, and disc or joint pathology (including the sacroiliac joint and pubic symphysis). Lax ligaments and tendons can perpetuate TrPs. Tightness in the dural tube and pelvic torsion can cause the coccyx to be pulled in towards the pelvis. This can cause compression of the area in both sexes, but is very treatable. Perpetuating factors include straining such as with constipation. The straining itself can be due to a feeling of fullness in the rectum caused by TrPs. Physical abuse, especially sexual abuse, may initiate and perpetuate TrPs; because of the abuse factor, all symptoms may be considered psychological, so specific TrP therapy may be delayed or omitted. Pelvic floor tightness should optimally be assessed before pregnancy, and certainly before delivery, and TrPs treated promptly, as there will be less chance of sphincter laceration or pudendal nerve compression and damage. Pelvic floor TrPs require patience and time to unravel.

Specific Muscle Referral Patterns

Perineum: The perineum is a common location for TrPs (Jarrell 2003a). One common TrP site is just distal to the hymen on the perineal body; this TrP can be treated with 1 to 2 cc of 1% Xylocaine injected into the perineal body (Jarrell 2003b).

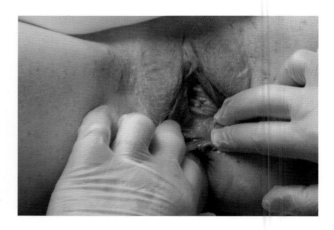

Location of a common perineal trigger point just distal to the hymen. Photo supplied by John Jarrell MD.

This TrP area can be sufficiently painful to prevent sexual intercourse. Perineal pain can also be due to nerve entrapment of the inferior cluneal nerve, referring burning pain to the lateral anal margin, scrotum or labia majora, medial buttock, and upper thigh (Darnis et al. 2008).

In males and females, perineal TrPs refer pain at the site of palpation and in the rectum. Perpetuating and initiating factors include prolonged compression from sitting, vaginal birth, sports injuries, and repetitive sprinting, kicking or twisting. In about a third of vaginal deliveries, a surgical incision in the perineum is made to prevent irregular tearing. TrPs in scars from this incision, or from tears that occur without it, can cause sharp pain. TrPs in the superficial transverse perineal muscle may cause poorly localized aching pain that may seem to come from the low back, hip, tailbone, anal area, and/or posterior pelvic floor. Perineal pain from TrPs in the surrounding mucosa may be temporarily eased with the use of topical anesthetics or relaxants.

Levator Ani: This group of muscles includes the levator prostatae (males), levator vaginae (females), and the puborectalis, pubococcygeus, and iliococcygeus. The levator ani elevates and supports the pelvic floor and assists the anal and urethral sphincters to help control bowel movement and urination. TrPs in the levator ani group cause poorly localized aching pain that seems to come from the low back, hip, tailbone (coccyx), anal area, and/or posterior pelvic floor, as well as pain in the sacrococcygeal region. Coccyx pain may be called "levator ani syndrome." The puborectalis anterior superior in men refers pain to the tip and/or shaft of the penis, to the bladder, and/or to the urethra, with a sensation of pressure and fullness in the prostate. The puborectalis anterior inferior in men refers pain and pressure to the perineum, the base of the penis, and the prostate. Of all pelvic muscles, this section of the levator ani is the one most commonly afflicted by significant TrPs. TrPs in the puborectalis fibers behind the rectum respond to transvaginal or transgluteal TrP injection (Kotarinos 2010). The levator prostatae refers pain and pressure to the base of the penis, the prostate, the bladder and/or the pelvis, with urinary frequency and/or urgency. The iliococcygeus refers lateral pain to the pelvic wall, perineum and anal sphincter, anterior levators, and prostate, and can cause a sense of prostate fullness. The anterior inferior levator ani in women refers pain to the vagina, bladder, urethra, clitoris, and mons pubis, and causes bladder and urethral discomfort and urgency. In both sexes, the pubococcygeus muscle contracts during orgasm, which can be extremely painful if this muscle has TrPs. Contraction of this muscle also helps empty the urethra at the end of urination. When it is contractured by TrPs there may be urinary incontinence, stress incontinence, and/or premature ejaculation; it can also cause the testicles to be held up close, heating them and lowering active sperm count. Kegel exercises are used by men and women to strengthen this muscle, but if the levator ani has TrPs, the exercises may make TrPs and their symptoms worse.

Sphincter Ani: The external band of circular muscle around the anus is a voluntary muscle, but may not always be under total voluntary control, as anyone who has had diarrhea well knows. TrPs here are the most common source of perineal pain, which gets worse when you lie on your back. They make sitting uncomfortable. Often, but not always, the pain is also aggravated by defecation. These TrPs refer pain to the back of the pelvic floor and vagina, and may cause poorly localized aching pain that feels as if it comes from the low back, hip, tailbone, perineum, anal area, and/or posterior pelvic floor. It may cause painful bowel movements, rectal burning, itching, pressure, or pain. The sphincter ani is in a state of constant contraction that is increased by straining, speaking, coughing, laughing, or weightlifting, all of which aggravate these TrPs.

Ischiocavernosus: In males, these TrPs refer pain to the perineum and adjacent urogenital structures, especially the base of the penis beneath the scrotum, and can be involved with erectile and ejaculatory dysfunction and post-urination dribble. Likewise, in females, these TrPs refer pain to the perineum and adjacent urogenital structures. They can cause dyspareunia (particularly during entry) and aching pain in the perineum. Kegel exercises tone this muscle, but, if TrPs exist, these strengthening exercises will make things worse until the TrPs are resolved.

Bulbospongiosus: In females, these TrPs contribute to dyspareunia (particularly during entry), aching pain in the perineum, and vaginal pain. In males, they refer pain to the area behind the scrotum and/or the base of the penis, and cause discomfort when sitting upright. They refer pain to the perineum and adjacent urogenital

structures, and may contribute to erectile and ejaculatory dysfunction and post-urination dribble. TrPs in men and women occur at the junction of the bulbocavernosus and the superficial transverse perineal muscle; this refers, in both sexes, to the urethra as a sense of urethral urgency, or, in men, to the opening at the tip of the penis as a sharp stabbing sensation (Kotarinos 2010).

Coccygeus: If we had a tail, this is the muscle that would wag it; TrPs here cause pain to the sacrococcygeal region. Coccyx pain arises mainly in the agitator caudae and coccygeus muscles. Whether called coccydynia, coccyx pain, or tailbone pain, it is certainly a pain in the … tail. These TrPs may occur after a fall on the buttocks, especially if the base of the spine is impacted. No matter how well padded, the coccyx is not a good place to land—there can be a shock to the whole CNS, with reflex contraction of the dura. Coccygeus TrPs refer pain to the tailbone, hip, and back, and the coccyx may be tender to the touch. They can cause anal pain, pain to the gluteus maximus, pain before or after a bowel movement, or the sensation of a full bowel, and are often responsible for low back pain late in a pregnancy. An immobile or jammed coccyx is a major perpetuating factor in pelvic pain: it must be mobilized.

Rectal TrPs: To our knowledge, rectal TrPs have thus far not been described. Unlike vaginal TrPs with palpable taut bands, these are small areas of thinned rectal mucosa, sometimes within an inch or two of the anal opening, and are extremely sensitive. They may feel close to the mucosal surface, but referral pain can be deep inside the gut. They begin relatively flat, but, as the mucosal lining of the rectum becomes thinner, they form what feels like contraction nodules. Gastroenterologists have confirmed areas of irritated mucosal thinness at the point of pain. All five patients in whom these TrPs were noted had multiple pelvic TrPs and IBS. When the rectal TrPs worsened, the pelvic floor tightened as well. These TrPs refer pain to the perineum and anal sphincter as well as the gut, and may be related to urinary urgency. They can cause or contribute to allodynia in the bowel, which can be due to constriction of the small blood vessels (Kotarinos 2010). This TrP pain can be eased temporarily with the application of topical lidocaine. Verne et al. (2003) found that using topical anesthetic (lidocaine) rectally decreased visceral and cutaneous hyperalgesia of IBS, and concluded that this was due to CNS blockade, but perhaps area TrPs could have been involved.

Vaginal TrPs: These TrPs refer pain to the lower abdomen and uterine cervical area; this pain may be called bladder spasms, dysmenorrhea, or cramps. TrPs in the vaginal wall about 2.5 to 3.8 cm inward from the vaginal opening can refer pain and tenderness to the lower abdomen (Simons, Travell, and Simons 1999, p. 956). These vaginal TrP bands can be felt during a pelvic exam, and may crisscross the entire vagina. A pelvic exam may activate these and TrPs in other areas, and cramping and other pain may occur for a week or so after. This can be minimized by the use of muscle relaxants before the exam, and the use of topical anesthetic (lidocaine) or relaxant (carisoprodol or diazepam) during the exam. Vaginal wall TrPs may contribute to vulvodynia and perineal pain. TrPs in the vaginal cuff post-hysterectomy region are common, and can be prevented by injecting the incision area with a local anesthetic before surgery.

CNS hypersensitivity is part of vaginismus, a spasm of the pelvic floor muscles that can cause the opening of the vagina to be so tight that sexual penetration is impossible. Even using a tampon or speculum insertion for a pelvic exam may be unendurable. TrPs and fibromyalgia may be perpetuating this condition, but more research is needed. Muscles outside the pelvic floor can impact on this region: rectus abdominis and other abdominal wall muscles, adductors, gluteus (minimus, medius, and maximus), iliacus, piriformis, psoas, and quadratus lumborum can refer pain to the pelvis. Often overlooked are TrPs in the upper adductor magnus that can cause diffuse, hard-to-locate pain throughout the pelvic area. They can also cause perineal, rectal, vaginal, bladder, deep groin, or pubic bone pain; sharp lances of pain shooting up inside the pelvis; pain only during intercourse; or the sensation of a foreign body in the rectum. TrPs in the obturator internus can cause pudendal nerve entrapment. They can refer pain to the external female genitalia (vulvodynia), and around the anus and tailbone, and can cause a full sensation in the rectum. They are associated with urinary hesitancy, frequency, burning, urgency, constipation, and/or painful bowel movements. The pectineus refers pain and sensations to the groin; the quadratus lumborum or lateral abdominal oblique can refer pain to the exterior female genitalia and vagina; the gluteus medius can refer pain to the vagina; and the gluteus minimus can cause pain deep in the vagina. The key to diagnosis and treatment of these TrPs is familiarity with the complete referral patterns, patience, and gentleness, and the awareness that healing is possible.

Regional Hints for Control: Once underlying pathology has been eliminated and the symptoms are known to be caused by TrPs, they can often be significantly relieved by manual methods, even if they are severe and have been present for some time. Research has shown that:

- myofascial therapy has been very successful in dealing with chronic pelvic pain, chronic prostatitis, and IC/painful bladder syndromes (Fitzgerald et al. 2009);

- pelvic floor pain and associated symptoms can be managed by connective tissue manipulation, TrP release, neural mobilization, lengthening short pelvic floor muscles, and correction of structural/biomechanical deformities impacting the pelvic floor (Fitzgerald and Kotarinos, 2003b);

- urinary incontinence can often be significantly alleviated or minimized by retraining the pelvic floor muscles and deep abdominals, and coordinating with deep belly breathing (Hung et al. 2010);

- IC and urinary frequency and urgency can be effectively treated by specific manual pelvic floor therapy (Weiss 2001);

- sexual dysfunction in men with chronic pelvic pain and/or chronic prostatitis—including decreased libido, ejaculatory pain, erectile dysfunction, and ejaculatory dysfunction—was significantly helped by TrP release and paradoxical relaxation training (Anderson et al. 2006);

- pelvic floor exercises and manometric biofeedback are as effective as Viagra for erectile dysfunction (Dorey et al. 2004);

- TrP release and paradoxical relaxation technique is associated with "significant improvement in pelvic pain, urinary symptoms, libido, ejaculatory pain, and erectile and ejaculatory dysfunction" (Anderson et al. 2006).

Pelvic floor TrPs respond to moist heat, massage for reachable areas, stretch, ultrasound, pulsed galvanic stimulation, and posture correction. Control of perpetuating factors is crucial. FSM can be used to treat the area safely. A Botox injection into the bulbospongiosus and ischiocavernosus has been proposed as a treatment for lifelong premature ejaculation, pelvic floor spasm, and chronic pelvic pain for men and women. We suggest that manual TrP release and other noninvasive TrP therapies should be tried first. Treatment of other muscles referring to the pelvic floor can be useful. Muscles as far away as the infraspinatus and supraspinatus can reproduce pelvic referral symptoms (Doggweiler 2010). Check for any TrPs in muscles along a kinetic chain that could impact the pelvic area. Prolotherapy for hyperlax connective tissue should be used only with great care, ensuring that hyperlaxity is not caused by torsion due to TrPs.

Internal manual work on TrPs can be exceedingly helpful, but it may be difficult to find a practitioner who is experienced. Some clinics specialize in pelvic floor work, while others have nurses, physical therapists, or technicians who are specialists in this field. If you cannot find anyone who can do this work, study the Wise and Anderson book mentioned earlier in this segment. Use their diagrams to help locate your internal TrPs with the pelvic floor massage tool available at Current Medical

Technologies, Inc www.cmtmedical.com may enable you to treat the TrPs. Go slowly, carefully, and safely. Treating these TrPs can cause TrP cascades, but bring eventual symptom relief. You may need the help of small amounts of topical lidocaine to do this. Men may need to find urologists who know TrPs, and some pelvic floor clinics take male patients. Myofascial TrPs in the pelvic floor may not have the typical palpable nodules, but the taut bands extending over the muscle bellies are often prominent in those areas that are reachable (Jarrell 2004). If necessary, such as with cases of vaginismus, start internal work gently with a cotton swab. Oral diazepam tablets of 5 or 10 mg can be used intravaginally, or compounded creams of 20–40 mg/ml baclofen, 20 mg/ml amitriptyline, or 300 mg/ml gabapentin can help, with use tailored to the patient (Doggweiler 2010). Topical carisoprodol 350 mg/ml in a transdermal gel base can relax the vaginal and rectal tissues. Vaginal diazepam suppositories may be useful (Rogalski et al. 2010). Topical lidocaine 5% ointment can facilitate manual internal TrP work that would otherwise be unendurable. Internal stripping massage of TrPs can be excruciatingly painful—use lidocaine or another internally safe topical anesthetic or muscle relaxant. An oral muscle relaxant and extra pain medication may allow work to be done that otherwise could not be done, with less pain afterward. An internal pelvic myofascial TrP wand has been developed that may be extremely useful (Anderson et al. 2011).

The first time any new type of therapy is tried, start slowly and gently, for a brief time, to see what the reaction is. There may be delayed cramping and other aftereffects. Keep the pain level low during such work—in the best of all worlds use the 1–10 VAS pain scale. In reality, it's not unusual for the patient to be at level 7 or above before treatment. Inducing or increasing central sensitization must be avoided. The ability to tolerate this work depends on many variables—the patient, TrP sensitivity, presence of central sensitization, etc. The patient must have a sense of safety, and treatment must allow sufficient time for care and sensitivity; nothing can be rushed. Hold each TrP for the amount of time it takes to release, with the patient breathing deeply with intention "into" the pressure. The TrP and the muscle need time to release. It's taken a long time for the tension to build up: it can take time to let go. There may be one release after another, and they may come with emotional releases as well. Patients, please avoid using topical anesthetics if you are planning sexual intercourse immediately after. Yes, patients have tried this—but never, to this author's (Starlanyl's) knowledge, more than once.

When the vaginal cuff is injected with local anesthetic, abdominal TrPs may release. Dense fibrous tissue and post-hysterectomy fibrous nodules may also contain TrPs that respond to TrP injection as well (Jarrell 2003a). The use of TrP injections during labor, even when epidural analgesia has been administered, can be of great preventative benefit (Tsen and Camann 1997). Scar TrPs will respond to local anesthetic injection; again, such scars may be prevented with use of injected (not topical) local anesthetic.

Patients can learn to recognize tension and contraction of muscles in the pelvic floor. It's easier on the body if the pelvis is tilted backward for defecation, and tilted forward for urination (Carriere 2002). Chairs are not friendly, no matter how well designed. The body was not designed to sit in them. Squat when you can, and stretch those pelvic muscles. T'ai chi is a wonderful exercise for awareness of muscle activity, and greatly recommended. Any exercise must be done with the goal of lengthening muscles, and there are books written just on stretches for the pelvic floor. TrPs *must* be resolved before the pelvic floor can be strengthened.

Stretches such as the pelvic tilt, cobra, squat, knee pulls, and lunge can be advantageous. There are many exercises to help develop an awareness of the individual muscles in the pelvic floor. Once you become aware of these muscles, you can learn to appreciate the amount of tension that is being held there. For example, start flat on your back in a comfortable position, breathing slowly. Allow awareness to come into the pelvic area. Raise and bend one knee very, very slowly, engaging just one muscle at a time. Slowly bring that knee to your chest. This should take several minutes. Then, just as slowly, bring it down, one muscle releasing at a time. Rest a few minutes, and then go through the same process with the other knee. Another useful exercise is to clench the buttocks and anal opening tightly and hold this for a count of three, and then let the muscles go. The release should be very noticeable. Don't do repetitions, but do it once several times during the day. Readers who are patients—find a bodyworker who knows TrPs, and learn more exercises that work for you. The focus should first be on returning the normal muscle tone, and then on treating the inhibited muscles to increase their tone.

Be very careful in (care givers) assigning or (patients) allowing internal therapy. Most physical therapists, especially, who do this work are taught to strengthen, strengthen, and then strengthen some more when they find a weak muscle. They may not understand trigger points, and that muscle weakness is caused by the TrPs due to reciprocal inhibition. You cannot strengthen a muscle that has a TrP. They need to know this. Be careful choosing internal pelvic workers and make sure that they understand TrPs, and understand that strengthening exercises are counterproductive and may set off one or more trigger point cascades. It is hoped that this book will help educate internal workers to become the care providers their patients need and deserve.

10 Muscles of the Shoulder, Arm, and Hand

Introduction

A simple thing such as getting your food on to a fork and bringing it to your mouth is an exercise in coordination. We take it for granted, unless something goes wrong and food intended for the mouth becomes abruptly reclassified as an item in the ready-to-wear category. When tissues fail to work together, TrPs are often the cause of, or at the least a contributor to, the failure of kinetic integrity.

Regional Kinetics: The body was designed to move as it carries out various tasks. Jobs and hobbies that keep us in one position lead to trouble. We may fail to notice if our reach gets shorter and our ROM decreases. Suddenly, we're in a box—a box of tight myofascia and contractured muscles. In the past, if we were fortunate, by the time this happened we were told it was old age. Now, if we are exceedingly fortunate, we are familiar with myofascial medicine and so are our health care providers. Much of this degeneration can be prevented; even TrPs that have been present for decades can often be reversed, if perpetuating factors can be controlled.

Regional TrP Comments: True "frozen shoulder" is adhesive capsulitis: the capsule surrounding the bone is frozen into place. That label may be given to TrPs that restrict motion in the shoulder region. Even true frozen shoulder may have a hefty TrP component that, when treated, can resolve the problem because the shoulder capsule got "stuck" to immobile shoulder muscles. TrPs could have developed in the tissue of the joint area.

Rotator cuff problems often begin when the muscles that comprise the cuff (supraspinatus, infraspinatus, teres minor, and subscapularis) develop TrPs. Prompt treatment of these TrPs may prevent further damage if all perpetuating factors are brought under control, including inappropriate exercise. We frequently expect far too much from these muscles. In the gym, people train or exercise them in a seated position; this breaks the kinetic line and dissociates the shoulder joint from the lower limbs. The forces needed to move the shoulder in an appropriate and effective manner are generated in the lower limbs and translated by the fascia through the torso to the shoulder. Small rotator cuff muscles allow movements to be fine-tuned. Strong force is generated some distance away in the kinetic chain. For example, if we have tight

psoas muscles, they can cause inhibition in the gluteus maximus. These lower body dysfunctions cause tensions along the chain, setting up the conditions for rotator cuff tears. To enable rotator cuff muscle function, first release the spastic psoas and fire up the gluteus maximus.

Thoracic outlet syndrome (TOS) describes brachial plexus nerve and subclavian artery compression, often by TrPs in the attached muscles in the region of the first rib and the collarbone. TrPs in the scalene, pectoralis minor, and subclavius muscles can produce true TOS. There is also something called "pseudo TOS," which is common in stroke patients, and involves TrPs in the pectoralis major, latissimus dorsi, teres major, and subscapularis muscles.

Carpal tunnel syndrome (CTS) is another often-misunderstood condition; it's caused by median nerve entrapment. Numbness and tingling of the thumb, next few fingers, and palm, pain to the elbow, pain in the hand, loss of fine motor control, grip failure, and muscle weakness are often assumed to result from entrapment of the nerve where it enters the hand—an area called the carpal tunnel. Myofascia can entrap the median nerve at any point along its length. Rather than cutting tissues around the nerve, manual treatment of TrPs to free the nerve can relieve those symptoms without the need for surgery or steroids. Control of the perpetuating factors can often prevent recurrence. Research indicates that manual myofascial release plus a stretching and exercise program for the patient can be more effective than surgery (Sucher 1993).

Regional CMP Comments: Someday, patients with "coracoid pressure syndrome" will be routinely checked for TrPs compressing the brachial plexus. The round-shouldered posture will be corrected; TrPs in the pectoralis minor, sternal portion of the pectoralis major and lower trapezius will be treated; and the latissimus dorsi will be checked to see if it is causing depression of the humerus. That is currently not the typical scenario. Time for a change.

Example: A 37-year-old violinist had been experiencing recent trouble with fine motor control in his left hand, and was in danger of being unable to perform. He denied a history of chronic pain, although he admitted periodically dropping his music case during recent travel. He had attributed this to nerves, as he was on his first visit by invitation to play overseas. He had pulled heavy luggage with his left hand—the one used to hold his violin. History revealed a forward fall off a ladder, with his left hand outstretched, six months prior. A possible rotator cuff injury was mentioned. He had treated the injury with ice, worn his arm in a sling for a while, taken aspirin, and minimized shoulder movement. Having worked steadily for the past two months, he was preparing for a big concert, spending increasing hours at practice. He admitted to wearing a wrist brace when he played, as the muscle was "weak." When questioned, he described intermittent feeling of pins and needles in the back of his hand. When this occurred, he would wear the sling again, further restricting movement.

Examination revealed restricted ROM in the neck, left shoulder, left arm, and hand. His posture was head-forward with a tilt to the left. Latent TrPs on the left side included levator scapulae, infraspinatus, subscapularis, teres minor, latissimus dorsi, forearm flexors, adductor pollicis, adductor pollicis longus, and extensor carpi radialis brevis. A manual therapy program was instituted, including a home program with stretching, tennis-ball, and back-knobber work. His violin grip was adjusted, and he was told to avoid the arm sling. After he was taught a basic barrier release technique, work pacing, and how to avoid stressing the arm, his function eventually returned.

Regional Perpetuating Factors: TrPs in the forearm can not only enlarge TrP referral patterns elsewhere, but also contribute to central sensitization (Fernandez-Carnero et al. 2007); prompt TrP identification and treatment could prevent those from developing. Look for connections. For example, patients with coronary illness often develop shoulder TrPs, as the area is held in tension; such disability is assumed to be part of the primary condition. If coexisting TrPs are identified and treated, some function may be restored and symptoms and medications minimized.

Regional Hints for Control: Often multiple TrPs exist, which can be difficult to separate at first. Find the ones you can single out: treat them and control the perpetuating factors. Look to the kinetic chains. As other TrPs make themselves known, treat them too, and don't be discouraged—it's part of the healing process.

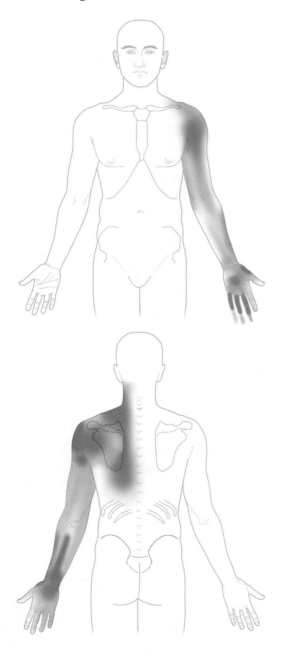

Trapezius
Greek *trapezoides* means "table-shaped."

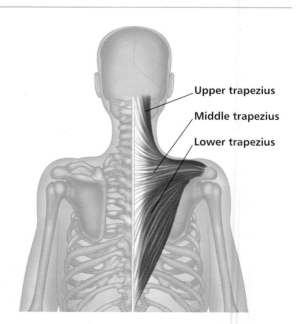

Upper trapezius

Middle trapezius

Lower trapezius

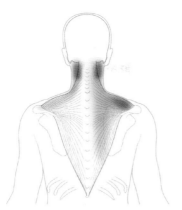

The referral pattern on the left of this figure is from TrPs found in the left most horizontal upper trapezius muscle fibers. The pattern on the right side is usually from TrPs found in the right lower trapezius, between the shoulder blade and the spine, fairly close to the shoulder blade.

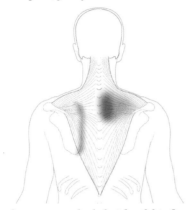

The referral pattern on the left side of this figure is usually from TrPs found in the left side, in the upper top corner attachment of the muscle covering the shoulder blade. The pattern on the right side of this figure is usually from TrPs found to the inside of the worst pain (deepest red) in the middle horizontal fibers of the middle trapezius.

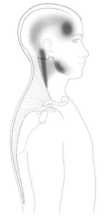

The referral pattern may be entire or in part, and usually results from TrPs in the most vertical upper trapezius fibers, occurring along the side of the neck between the collarbone attachment and the occipital attachment.

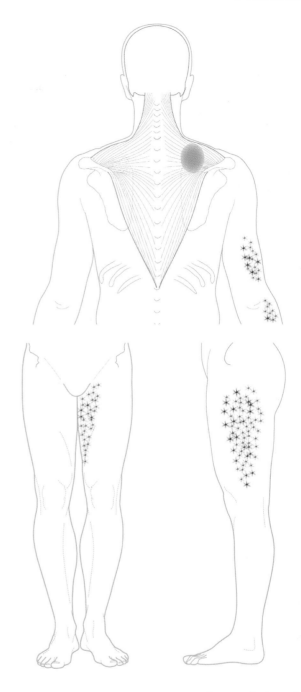

These figures represent patterns of gooseflesh rather than pain, and vary with individuals. The TrPs producing them are often found in an oval trigger area above the upper inside edge of the shoulder blade triangle. Another area of TrPs can occur at the outer attachment area of the upper trapezius. TrPs in this area cause local pain.

What It Does: Stabilizes the shoulder blade as the foundation for the upper quarter and for arm movement. It elevates, retracts, and laterally rotates the shoulder blade. The upper trapezius elevates the shoulder girdle. Both sides work together to extend the neck, but if only one side contracts, the upper portion flexes the head to the side. The middle portion retracts the shoulder blade, and the lower portion pulls the shoulder down.

The upper and lower portions work together to rotate the shoulder blade. This is a simplified description of a complex muscle that can act differently depending on many variables; for example, if the shoulder blade is fixed, the trapezius extends and laterally flexes the neck. The trapezius attaches to the thoracic vertebrae, and we are sure that tensional force through the fascia affects vertebrae in ways that have not as yet been described in medical texts.

Kinetics Comments: The trapezius is a large, flat, superficial sheet covering a lot of territory, with many attachments and varied referral patterns. The upper, middle, and lower sections of the right and left trapezius have their own jobs and personalities. The upper area, attaching to the base of the skull and to the collarbone, is the one most often affected by emotional stress. The trapezius makes it possible for you to shrug your shoulders, but when it's fatigued or weakened, it's difficult to hold your arms above your head for any length of time. This muscle often compensates in rotator cuff injuries. Tension in the trapezius adds to tension in the multifidi, and that can lead to pinched spinal nerves. Tightness in the upper and lower trapezius and serratus anterior is related to shoulder-joint stiffness.

TrP Comments: Upper trapezius TrPs are frequent sources of myogenic and cervicogenic headaches. Bilateral TrPs can result in a migraine encompassing both sides of the head, while TrPs on one side of the head can cause either a one-sided migraine or a bilateral migraine. One-sided migraines, however, will generally have a one-sided TrP component. The TrPs refer pain in a characteristic hook shape on the side of the head; the temple, jaw, and neck pain can be very sharp, and may include the lower molars. Upper trapezius TrPs can contribute to shoulder and neck pain in FM patients (Ge et al. 2009). Although trapezius TrPs may not restrict active rotation of the head and neck to the side opposite the TrP (if there is only one side involved), they can cause that rotation to be painful. Side-bending to the uninvolved side, if there is one, may be moderately restricted. Trapezius TrPs may restrict shoulder ROM. These TrPs can cause sensitivity or intolerance to the weight of clothing, especially that of a heavy coat. Occasionally, pain is referred to the angle of the jaw, or even to the outer ear. Nausea, visual disturbances, and imbalance can be part of the trapezius TrP symptoms (Teachey 2004). TrPs in the horizontal part of the upper trapezius tend to cause neck pain beneath the occiput, without a headache unless there is a contribution from other TrPs or FM. TrPs often lurk between the shoulder blade and the spine, where the trapezius fibers travel in a downward direction, and can be hidden if the tissues in the area are swollen. They can be responsible for satellite TrPs in the upper back and neck, and are often overlooked until more obvious perpetuating factors have been eliminated.

Middle trapezius TrPs can cause burning pain that seems to be skin deep but can penetrate deeper. TrPs in this region can cause dizziness and loss of balance, and may be misdiagnosed as disc pain, neuralgia, bursitis, or arthritis. TrPs in the mid-trapezius shoulder attachment region can cause aching pain in the top of the shoulder. Superficial middle trapezius TrPs above the interior top (superior) corner of the shoulder blade can cause goosebumps in a characteristic pattern that is an objective sign that may be accompanied by a disagreeable shivery sensation.

Notable Perpetuating Factors: These TrPs may be initiated by repetitive or continuous physical or emotional stressors, including sustained shoulder elevation such as when painting a ceiling, hanging blinds, or folding sheets. They can be perpetuated by head-forward posture; holding a telephone without elbow support; acute trauma as in whiplash from the side; and compression from a tight bra strap, heavy purse, bag, or coat. Avoid using a desk or keyboard that is too high, or working or reading on the lap with elbows unsupported. A walking stick or cane that is too tall for the patient can initiate and maintain these TrPs. A properly fitted cane or stick should cause the elbow to bend by 30–40 degrees with the stick or cane alongside the foot and with the shoulders level.

For patients with heavy breasts that contribute to symptoms, reduction mammaplasty can significantly reduce disability, muscle weakness, and pain in the middle and lower trapezius and in the rhomboids (Chao et al. 2002). Long telephone calls can activate these TrPs. Playing the violin, or otherwise a prolonged rotation of the head to one side, perpetuates trapezius TrPs. Check for body asymmetry, short upper arms, and pillows that don't provide adequate support or fit the curvature of the neck. Any job requiring a static position is a breeding ground for TrPs. Continuous trapezius muscle activity of anything over eight minutes can be associated with a risk of neck pain (Ostensvik, Veiersted, and Nilsen 2009). Typing text messages is a relatively new perpetuating factor that stresses the upper trapezius, abductor pollicis brevis, and opponens pollicis. Emotional stress, such as tension or grief, can cause the "weight of the world" to settle on the upper trapezius and crush it with emotional pressure.

Hints for Control (Patients): Correct any round-shouldered posture and excessive head-forward position. Find a pillow that supports and fits the curvature of the neck. Develop an ergonomic work place that allows for varied motions and significant changes of position and movement. Trading one set of repetitive motions for another will not be successful. Check the scalene muscles, levator scapulae, and SCM for TrPs.

Hints for Control (Care Providers): "Trapezius myalgia" is simply a term meaning pain in the trapezius: the cause of the pain must be found. A patient with these

TrPs may be misdiagnosed with cervical radiculopathy or atypical facial neuralgia. Trapezius TrPs can be secondary to cervical facet or vertebral lesions, or these lesions may be perpetuating factors. Attend to whatever can be treated with the least invasive therapies possible. Ultrasound may be helpful. Spine manipulation affecting the C3–C4 segment can relieve pressure/pain sensitivity of TrPs in the upper trapezius (Ruiz-Saez et al. 2007). Patients who have undergone breast removal require TrP assessment of back and chest soft tissues, including the trapezius; TrPs could be causing weakness and loss of function (Shamley et al. 2007). TrPs in the upper trapezius secondary to cervical radiculopathy may be resolved by C4–C5 facet joint injections (Tsai et al. 2009). Some therapies may activate latent TrPs and the patient may need a driver to take them home afterwards, as temporary dizziness or disorientation may result. This reaction may be delayed and occur the day after therapy or even later. Any new therapy must proceed cautiously.

Stretch: Most of us will experience tense short upper trapezius muscles at some time or another. What do most of us do when we feel that tension in our shoulders and neck? We statically stretch, which may compound the problem by creating a contraction in the target tissues. Instead, move your shoulders up and down and back and forth in a flowing movement. Once this feels good, you can add to this stretch by moving your head side to side or forward and back.

Rhomboids
Greek *rhomboeides* means "parallelogram-shaped with oblique angles" (the only sides that are equal in this shape are the opposite ends).

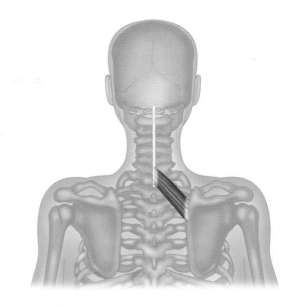

Rhomboid minor.

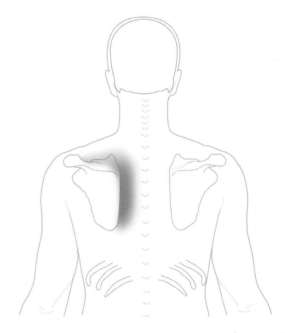

TrPs in the rhomboid major and minor and associated attachments have similar referral patterns.

What They Do: Attach shoulder blades to the spine, and help stabilize them; work with other muscles to move shoulder blades towards midline, and elevate and inwardly rotate them as the arms move.

Kinetics Comments: Rhomboid flexibility affects positioning and movement of the shoulder blade, which affects positioning and movement of the serratus anterior. This, in turn, affects the external obliques, and so on, setting up the development of a TrP cascade. Working with the trapezius, the rhomboids shrug the shoulders, and must be assessed when the trapezius is tight. The rhomboids work the middle trapezius to pull the shoulder blades towards each other, and work with the levator scapulae to elevate the shoulder blades.

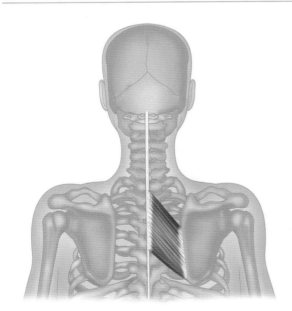

Rhomboid major.

TrP Comments: These TrPs cause pain that persists at rest. Crackling and popping during shoulder blade movement are often cries from the rhomboid letting you know they have TrPs. Pain from these TrPs can become obvious when you reach forward or stretch down to reach for something. If there are rhomboid TrPs, check for pectoralis TrPs. When the rhomboids have TrPs, they don't work well with other muscles, but you can bet those muscles probably have TrPs too.

Notable Perpetuating Factors: Head-forward posture with hunched shoulders. (Check spontaneously taken photos for a posture reality check.) The weight of a strap from a heavy bag, purse, or backpack carried on one shoulder can initiate and maintain these TrPs, as can repetitive or continuous overhead work. Chest surgery, especially mastectomy, can initiate these TrPs. Idiopathic scoliosis, asymmetrical or rotated pelvis, leg length inequality, and/or short upper arms can perpetuate them. For patients with heavy breasts that may contribute to symptoms, reduction mammoplasty can significantly reduce disability, muscle weakness, and pain in the middle and lower trapezius and the rhomboids (Chao et al. 2002).

Hints for Control (Patients): Ensure adequate lumbar support with some backward slope during any extended sitting. Avoid overstretching these muscles during therapy. Manage these TrPs with tennis-ball compression, learning how to keep the ball against the wall. Find a safe surface—even a soft tennis ball can damage drywall with repetitive use. These TrPs can also be worked when lying on your back on the floor, with a tennis ball between the rhomboids and the floor, but all the associated TrPs can't be reached as well from that position. Cane-type therapy aids can be very helpful for self-treatment. When driving long distance, change the position of the hands on the wheel, and use a ball between your back and the seat.

Hints for Control (Care Providers): Patients with these TrPs tend to restrict arm movement while walking. In severe cases they may hold their arms up and forward in a static position. Unless the patient is auditioning as a T. *rex*, check for the presence of rhomboid TrPs.

Stretch: Drape your body over a stability ball, and hug the ball with your arms and the front of your thighs. This stretch includes the entire back line from the base of your head to your tailbone. If you gently rotate the ball in several directions, you can bring more oblique fibers into play. Stability balls are great for all types of dynamic stretching, and the curve of the ball can be used to maximum effect. It's essential to seek expert advice and initial supervision to ensure correct technique. When you stretch, include the arms, back, and shoulders.

Pectoralis Minor
Latin *pectoralis* means "relating to the chest."

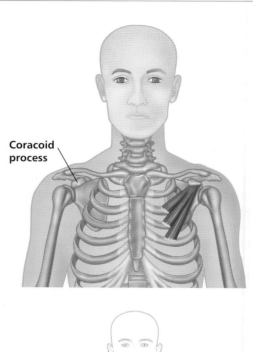

Coracoid process

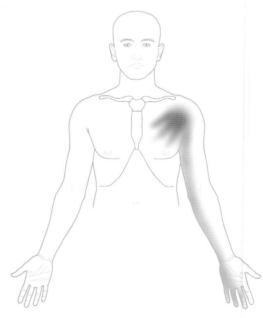

What It Does: Pulls down the coracoid process, which pulls the shoulder blade forward and down whenever you push, punch, or raise your arm out to the side (abduction) and return it to the starting position (adduction). The muscle helps produce shoulder blade rotation against resistance. When the shoulder blade is fixed, the pectoralis minor becomes an accessory muscle when inhaling during deep upper chest breathing, often during respiratory distress.

Kinetics Comments: This thin, flat muscle connects the ribs to the shoulder blade, and can be difficult to palpate, as it is under the pectoralis major. TrPs in the pectoralis minor have a distinct pattern. Tightness in this muscle causes problems when your arm is at shoulder level and you try to reach backward or forward, or forward and up.

Pain at the end of the ROM and restricted ROM are ways this muscle lets you know it's in trouble. Compensations in this muscle are common causes of thoracic tunnel syndrome, CTS, and frozen shoulder. When you hear these terms, think "probable TrPs," not "surgery." Blood vessel entrapment by TrPs in this muscle may contribute to some cases of Raynaud's phenomenon.

TrP Comments: Weakness of the lower trapezius may cause TrPs in the pectoralis minor; these TrPs can entrap nerves and blood vessels. TrPs in the scalene, pectoralis minor, and subclavius muscles can cause true TOS. Treat the TrPs and avoid unnecessary surgery. The last three fingers, or even the whole hand and arm, can become numb or tingly, especially if you are working hunched over, or lying on that side. Those areas may become cold and stiff after working on the computer for some time. The radial pulse can disappear because of arterial entrapment when the arm is raised into certain positions. TrPs in this muscle may cause cardiac arrhythmia, and the referral pattern may be mistaken for angina or heart attack. A well-aimed stretch and spray often eliminates symptoms immediately if they are TrP related. When in doubt, check it out. If hot, prickling jabs of pain are being referred to the pectoralis area, check for scar tissue TrPs in the coracoid attachment area. Failure to recognize TrPs in this area may needlessly have ended many an athlete's career, and caused disability in others.

Notable Perpetuating Factors: Paradoxical (shallow) breathing, head-forward posture, poorly fitted or overly heavy backpacks, heart conditions, using poles to pull yourself along when hiking or skiing, or prolonged use of crutches can perpetuate these TrPs, as can nursing an infant, prolonged cuddling of a child or pet in a hunched-over posture, carrying a heavy child, gardening, or sleeping curled up on the side with the lower shoulder forced forward. TrPs in this muscle may be initiated by malpositioning during surgery (Hsin et al. 2002).

Hints for Control: Check breathing and posture, and correct your workstation ergonomics. Check the pectoralis major, scalenes, SCM, and muscles in other areas for related TrPs. Even if "cardiac" symptoms provoked by these TrPs are temporarily eliminated by TrP therapy, if something is perpetuating them, an investigation of possible visceral initiators is warranted.

Stretch: Lie on your back on a stability ball, keeping your feet on the floor for stability. Hold a broomstick or similar stick in both hands. Starting from the belly button, lift and raise your arms over your head until you feel the point of bind; then return and repeat, each time trying to ease into a new ROM. Advancing in small steps is best—you can extend the ROM over time. Speed and repetitions are your enemies. For those people who would find the stability-ball stretch too difficult, try the stretch

lying on your bed with your head close to the edge, letting your arms and the stick fall back over your head: control "the fall." It is best to avoid trying these kinds of stretch when you are alone; if you have difficulty, you may need someone to come to your aid. Don't fall for the "if one is good for me then ten must be ten times better" error. Take your time, consider your limitations, and pace yourself. Listen to your body, and avoid pain, but expect a little discomfort as you encourage a new ROM. *Warning: Static stretching of this muscle may temporarily aggravate swelling, numbness, and tingling.*

Supraspinatus
Latin *supra* means "above"; *spina*, "spine."

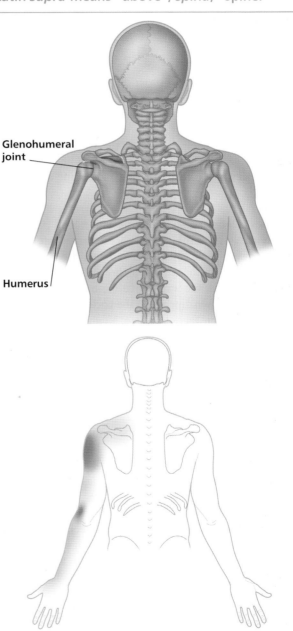

Glenohumeral joint

Humerus

Referral pattern from the upper supraspinatus and attachment areas.

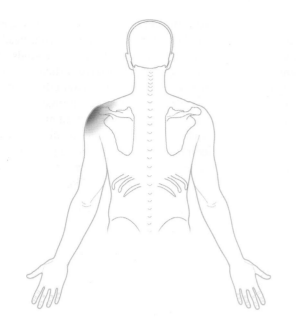

This referral pattern is from TrPs in the area of the supraspinatus tendon attachment to the glenohumeral joint.

What It Does: Helps stabilize the shoulder joint and rotates the arm to the outside. Works with the deltoid during sideways arm lifting, and rotates the arm to the side.

Kinetics Comments: This muscle, along with the infraspinatus, teres minor, and subscapularis, attaches to the upper arm bone (humerus) and is part of the rotator cuff. Tightness in the supraspinatus makes it difficult or impossible to lift the arm above the head. Women may not be able to reach zippers on the back; men may not be able to reach their faces to shave. Neither may be able to reach up and pull shirts over their heads. Even brushing teeth may initiate TrP pain. This muscle attaches high on the humerus, close to the joint. As the deltoid muscle contracts to lift the upper arm, the smaller supraspinatus pulls the head of the humerus into the shoulder joint so that the top of the humerus stays in the joint. A weak supraspinatus muscle places the entire shoulder joint complex at risk of soft tissue pain and injury.

TrP Comments: Lying on the outside of the shoulder blade, just above the teres major, the supraspinatus is easy to palpate. We suspect that TrPs in the periosteum may be the beginning of adhesive capsulitis, especially if motion is restricted due to pain. At rest, the pain of supraspinatus TrPs is usually a dull ache, which increases with movement. These TrPs can cause stiffness in the shoulder and a dull ache that disturbs sleep, and crunching and popping sounds when the shoulder is rotated. Calcified deposits can occur at the insertion of the tendon; TrPs here can be misdiagnosed as, or accompany, adhesive capsulitis or bursitis.

Notable Perpetuating Factors: Weak trapezius, sleeping with arms above the head, carrying heavy weights with the arms hanging at the sides (such as moving furniture or carrying heavy luggage), weightlifting, using rowing machines, sustained overhead work, being pulled along by a large, unruly dog, or repetitive sports such as golf and bowling.

Hints for Control (Patients): Warm showers and other sources of moist heat, followed by cooling, may be helpful, coupled with active dynamic stretching. Heat increases blood supply and flushes away noxious chemicals, which, in turn, can reduce irritation but may also increase the risk of inflammation. Finishing with cool or cold water reduces the risk of swelling and slows neural activity. Pressure tools such as cane-type knobbers carefully positioned on the top part of the shoulder blade can work these TrPs. Carefully warm up and dynamically stretch before any sports activities. Work on being able to perform a task or movement correctly, and subsequently on being able to repeat that task. Focus your exercise, not on the number of repetitions, but on the neuromuscular coordination of the movement. Give the supraspinatus a chance to replenish its blood supply between exercises.

Hints for Control (Care Providers): Assess other muscles in the area for TrPs, and check tendons as well. Calcification of the tendon responds to FSM; include the calcium oxalate crystal setting. Dry needling, ultrasound, and electrical stimulation can be useful.

Stretch: Hold a stick near one end with the right hand, and place it behind your back, pointing it up to the ceiling. Grasp the top of the stick with your left hand, and pull the stick upward as far as feels comfortable or until you feel a restriction—this stretches the supraspinatus fibers on the right side. At the same time, point the knuckles of the right hand towards the floor. Gently allow the arms to return to the starting position, and repeat the stretch on the left side, pointing the knuckles of the left hand towards the floor. The rhomboid stability-ball stretch is good for this muscle. Warning: *Don't stretch the supraspinatus if there is any suspicion of rotator cuff tears.*

Infraspinatus
Latin *infra* means "below"; *spina*, "spine."

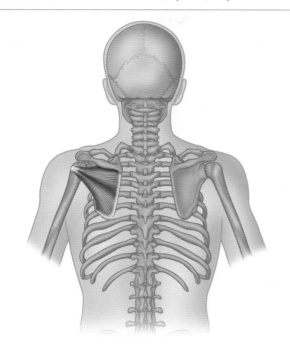

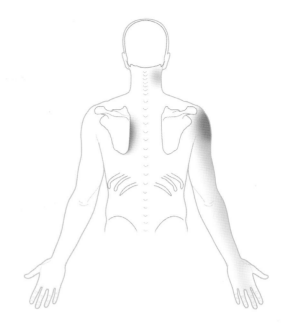

Common infraspinatus TrP referral patterns from the main portion of the muscle. TrPs in the attachment tendon of the infraspinatus cause a referral pattern along the interior shoulder blade edge, adjacent to and sometimes including the area of the TrP.

What It Does: Works with the teres minor to laterally rotate the upper arm and stabilize the shoulder joint.

Kinetics Comments: The infraspinatus is a component of the rotator cuff. It is important in shoulder blade positioning, and in decelerating internal rotation and shoulder flexion. If it hurts to reach into your back pocket, or to reach behind to hook up a bra or zip a back zipper, the infraspinatus and anterior deltoid are telling you they are restricted and tight.

TrP Comments: These common TrPs are often mistaken for adhesive capsulitis. They cause deep, throbbing pain in the shoulder joint and aching in the characteristic pattern. The shoulder may be noticeably weaker, with achy fatigue. There may be abnormal changes in skin temperature along the referral pattern. Grip strength may be reduced and objects may fall from the grasp. Even brushing the hair and teeth may hurt.

Notable Perpetuating Factors: Sudden extreme overhead reach, and any action that puts pressure on the infraspinatus. This muscle frequently pays for the "good-sport syndrome," when one ignores the body's signals to take it easy. Pain is a teacher to be ignored at your own risk. It will speak at an ever-increasing volume until you listen. These TrPs can be initiated when falling backward and using the outstretched hand to catch oneself. Some sources suggest sleeping on the uninvolved side with a pillow under the arm for support. However, there may be no "uninvolved side:" research indicates that patients with shoulder pain and infraspinatus TrPs on one side

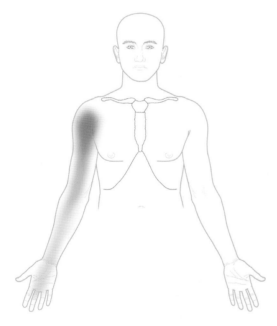

Common infraspinatus TrP referral patterns from the main portion of the muscle.

also have hypersensitivity on the other side as well (Ge et al. 2008a). Coexisting serratus anterior and related area TrPs may so sensitive that such use of a pillow is out of the question.

Hints for Control: Correct poor posture (including sleep posture), vary movements, and take frequent work breaks. Avoid pushing fatigued, chilled, or otherwise stressed muscles. Tennis-ball pressure or knobber devices can be useful. Try a hot, moist pack on the shoulder blade for 15 minutes before bed. Sleeping on the back with a properly fitted pillow providing neck support may allow better sleep. When checking for TrPs, don't neglect related tendons and ligaments. When dressing, put the most TrP-involved arm into the shirt first to minimize painful movement.

Stretch: Lie down on your back. Place your right hand, palm side down, under your bottom. Bend your knees at a 90-degree angle, and drop them to the right. Lean your body to the left until you feel a nice stretch. Then return to the start and repeat with the other side. Begin with the least involved side, and stretch both sides. This procedure stretches muscles associated with shoulder joint movement, as well as muscles and connective tissues that wrap around the upper body.

Teres Minor
Latin *teres* means "rounded" or "finely shaped"; *minor*, "smaller."

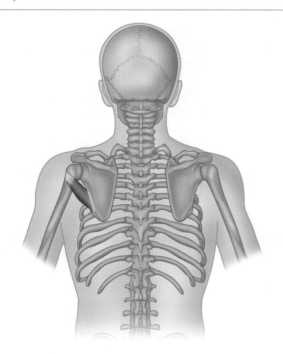

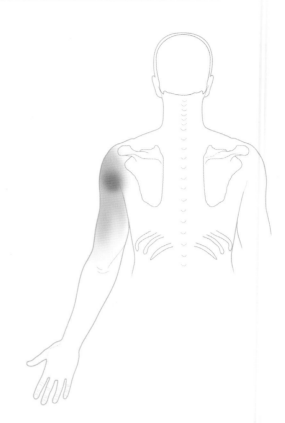

What It Does: Rotates the upper arm to the outside, away from the midline, and helps stabilize the shoulder joint.

Kinetics Comments: The teres minor is the smallest of the rotator cuff muscles, and symptomatic compensations in this muscle usually indicate that there are primary problems in other tissues. The shoulder is often left hanging out on its own, and that is not meant to be. The forces needed to support movement at the shoulder actually originate in the lower body—the *legs*. These forces must be translated through the low back-pelvic-hip area to the shoulder. When the core lacks neuromuscular integrity, it causes strain on muscles near the shoulder as they try to stabilize that joint. This leads to muscle overload, stiffness, fatigue, damage, and TrP formation. Improving core function and achieving a more stabilized sacroiliac joint will do wonders for restoring normal function to the shoulder muscles, and TrPs will melt away.

TrP Comments: These TrPs are often mistaken for bursitis or rotator cuff tendinitis. Numbness and tingling in the fourth and fifth fingers may accompany the characteristic sharply localized deep pain from teres minor TrPs. These TrPs may not be suspected until the infraspinatus is released, and they will then begin to scream. *Such a "new" pain doesn't mean the condition is worsening!* The muscle screaming the loudest has been soothed, and another one has taken up the call. Be patient—treatment is a process of unwinding that cannot be rushed.

Notable Perpetuating Factors: These TrPs are often secondary to or perpetuated by TrPs in the infraspinatus, subscapularis, latissimus dorsi, teres major, and pectoralis major muscles. Check ligaments and tendons around the shoulder girdle. (In anatomy, a "girdle" refers to any structure that acts like a belt. In this case, the shoulder girdle refers to the bony ring and surrounding connective tissues that attach and support the shoulder. It doesn't make the shoulder look thinner.) Other perpetuating factors include round-shouldered, head-forward posture; motor vehicle accidents (especially to the driver); compression of the arm while lying on the side; and repetitive overload from overhand sports such as swimming, rowing, tennis, or volleyball, or using exercise machines that require similar motions.

Hints for Control (Patients): Feel this muscle by reaching under your arm to the back portion of your armpit. If you rotate your arm to the outside on the side you are palpating, you can feel the muscle contract. As you return the arm to a relaxed position, the muscle will relax. Work on these TrPs with pincer palpation, pinching the TrPs and rubbing them gently between the thumb and fingers. These TrPs respond well to manual work, including stretch and spray, stretching while icing upward, and tennis-ball therapy. If sleep posture is a perpetuating factor, try hot, moist compresses before bed. If you sleep on your side, a flat pillow under your rib cage may take some pressure off the teres minor on the side closest to the bed. Another, fuller pillow in front of you may help prevent the upper arm from dropping down to the bed, and therefore avoid the muscle being held in an extended position.

Hints for Control (Care Providers): Teres minor TrPs can mimic ulnar neuropathy or C8 radiculopathy. These TrPs can be treated by local anesthetic injection, dry needling, and other therapies, but will not stay away until TrPs in other areas have been resolved and all perpetuating factors brought under control.

Stretch: Let the arm hang down by your side and bend it at the elbow to a right angle (halfway up for the geometrically impaired). Rotate the arm outward as far as feels comfortable, keeping your elbow close to your side. Go as far as you can, then rotate back inward until your hand touches your body. Repeat on the other side, and perform another set later in the day.

Subscapularis
Latin *sub* means "under"; *scapula*, "shoulder blade."

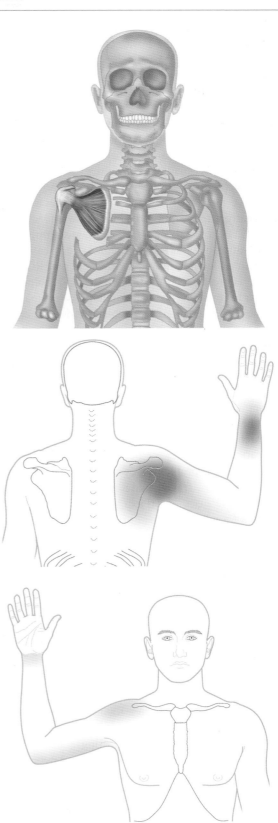

What It Does: Rotates the upper arm inward and stabilizes the shoulder joint, helping to keep the upper arm bone from being displaced upward during arm activity.

Kinetics Comments: A rotator cuff muscle, the subscapularis forms the posterior part of the underarm area. It takes up most of the space on the front of the shoulder blade, and is a prime suspect whenever "frozen shoulder" or "carpal tunnel syndrome" is mentioned.

TrP Comments: These TrPs can feel like a toothache in the shoulder, throbbing and aching relentlessly, both at rest and during motion. That pain, combined with wristband pain (usually worse on the back of the wrist), is the haunting cry of the wild subscapularis TrP, and may drive the owners of said subscapularis to despair. In the early stages, these TrPs may allow a reach up and forward, but not backward such as when starting to pitch a baseball or begin a serve in tennis. They can cause a maddening, bewildering underarm itch, and ROM may be severely restricted. It's difficult or impossible to raise the arm for brushing the hair; folding a sheet may leave you shaking with pain. If reaching across the chest to the opposite underarm is difficult or impossible, think of the subscapularis. TrPs in the subscapularis can join with TrPs in the pectoralis major, latissimus dorsi, and teres major to cause pseudo TOS.

Prompt attention to TrPs in the rotator cuff muscles might help prevent tears and subsequent surgery. If these TrPs aren't treated, there is a greater chance of upper arm dislocation. Once they've been active for a while, the microcirculation problems they cause can result in muscle atrophy (Simons, Travell, and Simons 1999, p. 602). Pain and stiffness caused by TrPs in the subscapularis may be mistaken for adhesive capsulitis, rotator cuff tears, CTS, bursitis, arthritis, or tendinitis. TrPs here can interact with cervical disc disease, or impair hand function due to inability to rotate the arm. When these TrPs yell, check for accompanying TrPs in ligaments and tendons in the area.

Notable Perpetuating Factors: Head-forward, slumped-shoulder posture; cervical disc disease; immobility such as prolonged use of an arm sling or driving long distances; and repetitive motions such as rowing, swimming the crawl stroke, or using exercise machines with similar motions. These TrPs are often found in golfers, patients with hemiplegia (due to overuse and awkward use of the arms), and volleyball players. Lifting a heavy weight out to the side may activate these TrPs. Any sustained shortening of the subscapularis can perpetuate TrPs.

Hints for Control: The subscapularis can be difficult to self-treat, as part of it lies under the shoulder blade. Tennis-ball pressure on the floor or against the wall may be helpful, as may knobber aids. Infraspinatus and teres minor TrPs may need treatment before the subscapularis TrPs resolve. Ice stroking during slow stretching may be helpful but requires help and education as to the proper method. Even after time, research indicates that less invasive techniques than surgery are indicated. Dry needling of subscapularis TrPs, combined with therapeutic stretching, resolved symptoms of shoulder impingement in athletes who'd been surgical candidates (Ingber 2000). Injection of a TrP in the medial scapular spine was extremely effective in restoring function to many patients with "scapulocostal syndrome" (Ormandy 1994).

Stretch: Hold a broom or yard stick in the palm of your right hand. Wrap your fingers and thumb around the top of the stick, and let it gently rest on your right forearm while placing it behind your back. Hold the other end of the stick with your left hand. Gently rotate your right arm outward, while your left hand pulls the stick forward to assist the motion. Slow down towards the end of the ROM or when you feel the point of "bind." Repeat on the other side. Avoid painful motion, although mild discomfort is acceptable.

Teres Major
Latin *teres* means "rounded" or "finely shaped"; *major*, "larger."

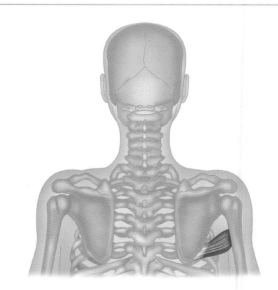

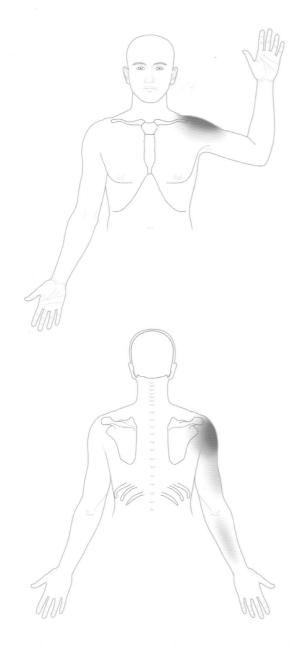

TrP Comments: When this muscle is tight, either the action of reaching straight up with the arm held close to the head causes pain, or that particular movement is restricted. Remember, TrPs are not always about pain, but also about changes in sensations. You're not being lazy avoiding jobs such as folding sheets and large towels—look for options, such as folding them across the bed. *Raising an arm in school or elsewhere may hurt too much.* Talk to the teacher, and find other options. Waving a backscratcher instead may not be the "in" thing yet; perhaps you can make it so. TrPs in the teres major may work with TrPs in the pectoralis major, latissimus dorsi, and subscapularis to cause pseudo TOS.

Notable Perpetuating Factors: Overuse with the arms upward and out; rowing, swimming crawl stroke, lifting weights overhead, or using exercise machines that repeat these movements; using a crutch; compensating with the arms for painful low back muscles; and driving a vehicle that requires heavy steering effort.

Hints for Control (Patients): Some of the most common teres major TrPs can be reached manually by pincer palpation or deep massage of the front surface of the back "wall" of the armpit. The muscle itself is located on the lower outside blade of the scapula, and rounds the upper rib cage as it heads towards the upper arm. Tennis-ball pressure on the floor can be a very helpful part of self-treatment, as can moist heat.

Hints for Control (Care Providers): FSM, injection, and/or dry needling may be especially useful. These TrPs may be activated during and after some breast surgery, and may be responsible for some treatable residual pain. Check for scar TrPs.

Stretch: Stand with the feet double hip-distance apart and slightly turned out, or lie on one side. The idea is to move the arm that you are stretching over your head so that your biceps makes contact with your head just behind your ear. Once you have reached as far as feels good, return the arm to your side. Then stretch the other side. Repeat, with a nice ebb and flow to the action, avoiding fast or jerky movements. If you have recently had a coronary episode or heart surgery, avoid raising both arms above your head at the same time. Try not to hyperextend your neck (i.e. avoid looking up at extremely high things). Stretching one arm at a time should be suitable, but check with your primary health care provider first.

What It Does: Along with all the other smaller muscles surrounding the shoulder joint, this muscle primarily rotates the arm inward, pulling it down and back.

Kinetics Comments: This muscle is attached to the outside of the shoulder blade and affects the positioning of that bone. A tight teres major pulls other muscles that attach to the shoulder blade out of position. This muscle attaches to the upper arm next to the latissimus dorsi and is therefore called the latissimus dorsi's "little helper." Comments regarding the interactive kinetic chain forces for the teres minor apply to the teres major as well.

Serratus Anterior
Latin *serratus* means "saw-shaped"; *anterior*, "before."

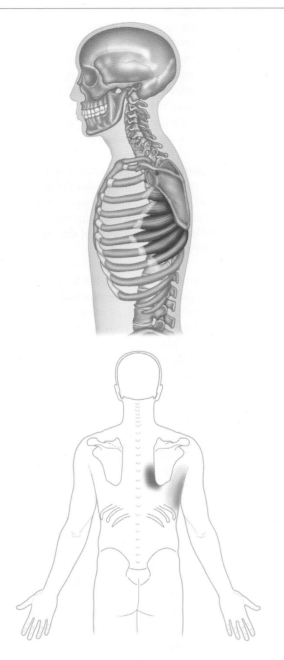

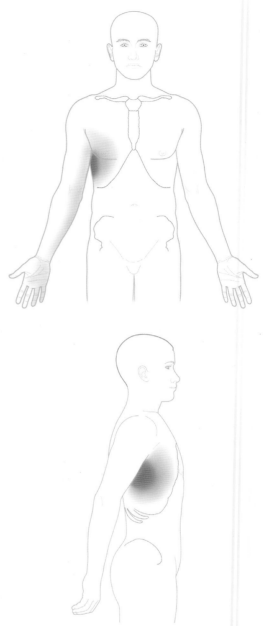

What It Does: Extends and rotates the shoulder blade to the side and helps stabilize it. This is the "boxing" muscle, used in pushing, punching, and thrusting. When it becomes weak, the shoulder blade "wings," standing away from the back like a wing. This large, flat muscle has finger-like projections; palpate them all carefully for TrPs.

Kinetics Comments: Tightness here can restrict breathing, as chest expansion and air volume can be radically restricted. This can be frightening, especially for people who already have respiratory or cardiac problems. The serratus anterior nerve supply may be entrapped by scalene TrPs.

TrP Comments: Shortness of breath may be the first sign that these TrPs are lurking, and a change of position usually doesn't ease symptoms. It hurts to breathe deeply when this muscle is being held tight by TrPs and is stretched beyond its restricted ROM. Attempts at running cause a "stitch in the side." With very active TrPs, there may be intense chest pain, even at rest. Singing, and even talking except in short gasps, may be impossible. These TrPs can cause air hunger, with mouth breathing or even panting in an attempt to get more oxygen into the body. This may be worse if coexisting FM or other oxygen-deprivation condition is part of the picture. If you get out of breath merely by talking, most of these TrPs had the last word. Look for the whole pattern, including breast pain and pain at the inner bottom edge of the shoulder blade. Check for these TrPs in developing COPD, emphysema, and other respiratory conditions. Keeping the respiratory muscles as flexible as possible may help minimize symptoms from coexisting conditions that affect breathing. Check the diaphragm and other respiratory muscles for TrPs.

Notable Perpetuating Factors: A chest cold, an allergy, or any condition causing repeated heavy coughing can activate these TrPs. Push-ups, chin-ups, overhead lifting, and machines that duplicate these motions will keep them aggravated. Sports activities such as swimming overhand stroke, playing tennis, and throwing a baseball can perpetuate these TrPs.

Hints for Control (Patients): Correct any paradoxical breathing. This muscle is thin and can be self-treated with sufficient experience in palpation skills and pressure release methods. Fingertip pressure works well on these TrPs. Lie on the less painful side with that arm above the head as you palpate and treat the muscle. Then switch to the other side and do the same. Standing treatment under a warm shower can be effective, but cool the area after treatment to reduce inflammation. Tennis-ball pressure against the wall is also useful.

Hints for Control (Care Providers): "Shoulder impingement syndrome" may be caused by nerve entrapment. If the shoulder blade is winging, check for serratus anterior or trapezius TrP entrapment of the long thoracic or accessory nerve. TrPs in these muscles must be assessed and treated, and all perpetuating factors brought under control before surgery is considered.

Stretch: Either standing or sitting up, place your hands behind your lower back. Hold the wrist of the right arm with the left hand. Pull the left arm gently towards the right until you feel the stretch on the left side. Depress your shoulders, while bending your right ear closer to your right shoulder. Return to the start. Rest a moment, and then switch sides. Breathe normally (assuming that you don't normally have paradoxical breathing!) You may find your ROM will improve rapidly, so do avoid getting over-zealous. See how you feel the next day before increasing the number of repetitions. Start with only a few repetitions, but if your body needs these stretches (and it will tell you if it does), do those few repetitions several times during the day.

Serratus Posterior Superior
Latin *serratus* means "saw-shaped"; *posterior*, "behind"; *superior*, "higher."

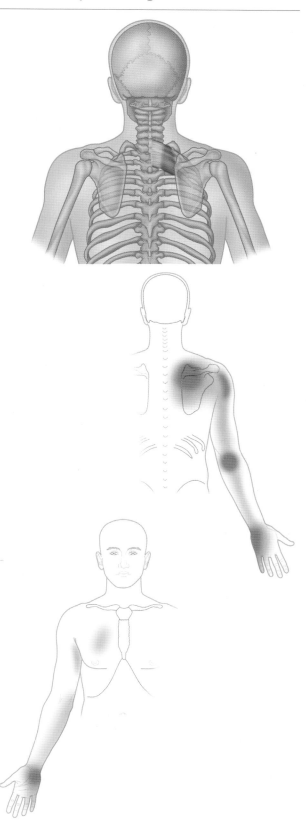

Right serratus posterior superior referral patterns.

What It Does: This muscle and its fascia are involved in proprioception (Vilensky et al. 2001). It may assist in shallow breathing by raising the attached upper ribs during inhalation, although this has been disputed in at least one study (Loukas et al. 2008).

Kinetics Comments: Healthy breathing is deep "belly" breathing. When someone continually breathes shallowly, such as in mouth breathing, these little muscles quickly become overwhelmed. The serratus posterior anterior is a thin flat muscle with "fingers" on one side that attach separately to individual ribs. When it's unhappy, it spreads its misery a long way. These TrPs most often live in the attachment area of the muscle, pinched between the shoulder blade and either rib bones or tight intercostal muscles. If referral pain gets worse when you lie on your side, when a shoulder strap or a heavy bag compresses this area, or when you reach forward with your arms, think about this muscle. These common TrPs are often overlooked.

TrP Comments: TrPs here cause a steady deep *ache*, even at rest, that may include tingling into the little finger. This may be mistaken for CTS. The complete complex pain pattern is important to help differentiate TrPs in this muscle from TrPs in others. This muscle is often combined with other muscles in CMP, and may be hidden until the others are treated. The TrPs are covered by the shoulder blade, and the related taut bands may be under several muscles as well.

Notable Perpetuating Factors: Paradoxical breathing; sustained head-forward posture, especially when using too high a surface such as a kitchen table for a desk; repetitive coughing from a lower respiratory infection, asthma or chronic lung conditions; and stress and related structural deformities such as scoliosis. There are often multiple perpetuating factors.

Hints for Control: Paradoxical breathing is the most common perpetuating factor for TrPs in this area, but it is correctable in motivated patients if deep breathing is possible. The first step is an assessment for TrPs in all respiratory muscles; those TrPs must be released for deep breathing to be fully possible. Paradoxical breathing may have perpetuating factors of its own, which must be brought under control. In patients with chronic lung disease, deep breathing may still be optimized but TrP assessment and treatment must be as chronic as the disease itself. FSM or stretch and spray is extremely helpful with these deep-seated TrPs.

Stretch: While hugging a stability ball, stand and keep your feet flat on the floor, double hip-distance apart; rotate your torso from side to side.

Serratus Posterior Inferior

Latin *serratus* means "saw-shaped"; *posterior*, "behind"; *inferior*, "lower."

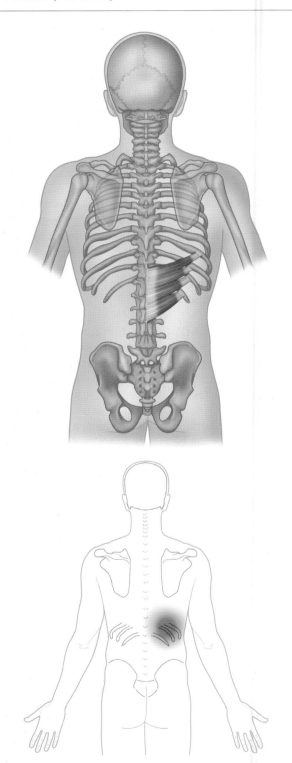

What It Does: It may be primarily a muscle of proprioception. It also acts as a supporting structure for the lower back, stabilizing the four lower ribs and assisting in pulling them down and back.

Kinetics Comments: This muscle works in conjunction with the ilicostalis, longissimus thoracis, and quadratus lumborum. It may also work with the serratus posterior superior as a spinal stretch receptor system or kinesiological monitor (Vilensky et al. 2001). Tightness in this muscle tends to be overlooked during an exam, which may give the muscle an inferior-ity complex.

TrP Comments: TrPs in this muscle may cause an uncommon local ache radiating over and around the muscle. This may extend across the back and over the lower ribs, even continuing through the chest to the front of the body. It's a nagging ache that remains after other TrPs have been inactivated; until that occurs, serratus posterior inferior TrPs may remain undiscovered.

Notable Perpetuating Factors: These TrPs are usually initiated by acute back strain in company with the strain of other muscles in the region. Perpetuating factors include paradoxical breathing, sagging and unsupportive mattresses (e.g. sleeping on a sofa or water bed), chairs with insufficient lumbar support, body asymmetry, and herpes zoster infections.

Hints for Control: Control perpetuating factors. Tennis-ball pressure, myofascial release, and other bodywork helps.

Stretch: Cross your forearms just above the wrist, at about chest height. Inhale deeply as you slowly raise them up until the area where the arms cross is level with your forehead. Now lower the arms as you exhale. Do this once or twice, allowing for a brief rest (a few breaths) before repeating. Do this exercise set several times a day.

Levator Scapulae
Latin *levare* means "to lift"; *scapulae*, "of the shoulder blade."

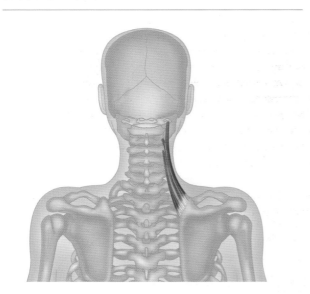

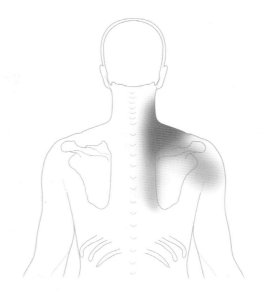

What It Does: Elevates the vertebral side of the shoulder blade.

Kinetics Comments: This muscle is involved when you shrug your shoulder; it is also affected if you feel as though you have the weight of the world on your shoulders. The levator scapulae lives under, and works with, the trapezius. Together they elevate and retract the pectoral girdle and keep it elevated against a downward push. Contraction of the levator scapulae on both sides causes the neck to extend; contraction on one side causes the other side of the neck to flex. These muscles help stabilize the shoulder blade. It's attached to the upper neck vertebrae, and TrPs here may be involved with vertebral misalignment and subsequent disc deformity.

TrP Comments: Although often caused by whiplash or static muscle overload, these TrPs have many possible initiating or perpetuating factors. TrPs in this muscle result in a stiff neck and reduced ROM, and may contribute to headache and/or shortness of breath. When severe, these TrPs can cause pain, even when the muscle is at rest. TrPs can tighten this muscle so much that a shoulder-bag strap slides right off. These TrPs can cause what is described as "wry neck," but if the head is tilted strongly to one side, the culprit is more likely to be SCM TrPs.

Notable Perpetuating Factors: Neck immobility; watching television or reading with the light displaced to one side; using a cane that is too high for the body; using the neck to hold a phone to your ear; postural stresses of computer work or other static jobs; emotional stress; head-forward position; hiked shoulders; inadequate vision correction; using too many pillows or a pillow that is too thick; drafts blowing on the neck; swimming overhand for too long, especially when the muscles are tired and the water is chilly; carrying a heavy shoulder purse or bag (letter carriers often develop these TrPs); short upper arms; watching a long tennis match; neck trauma; body asymmetry; and gait irregularity. In the early stages of a respiratory or other area infection (oral herpes, tonsillitis, tooth abscess, etc.), this muscle is much more vulnerable to TrP activation. The period of sensitivity may start several days before symptoms set in, and last for weeks.

Hints for Control (Patients): Avoid keeping the neck turned one way for any length of time. Pace your work, and stretch frequently. Correct posture defects, and avoid neck drafts. Ensure that your pillow and furniture fit and support. Any cane *must* be fitted to the user. As a general rule, turn the cane upside down and stand next to it: the cane tip should reach wrist level. If the cane promotes a hiked shoulder on that side, it doesn't fit. Levator scapulae TrPs are common and tend to recur. It's a wise patient who becomes adept at recognizing TrP activation and can self-treat them. The use of a cane knobber tool can be very effective, but be careful to treat both sides, even if only one hurts, to prevent reactive cramping. Start with the side that hurts the least or not at all. Be vigilant in controlling perpetuating factors. Moist heat may be relaxing to this muscle. Find a type of mind work—such as meditation, visualization, and/or prayer—that helps, and that you will continue to use. Look for ways to reduce stress. Combinations of mind and bodywork such as t'ai chi can be helpful.

Hints for Control (Care Providers): Tightness in the levator scapulae may cause or aggravate Chiari's syndrome, cervical radiculopathy, or narrowness in the dural tube, especially when the head is turned or the neck is flexed, thus increasing nerve compression effects. There is a significant association between the levator scapulae and disc irregularities at C3–C4, C4–C5, and C5–C6 (Hsueh et al. 1998). One study revealed that in over 50% of cadavers, a bursa existed between the shoulder blade, the serratus, and the levator scapulae (Menachem, Kaplan, and Dekel 1993). Check the omohyoid for TrPs, as their referral pattern may mimic levator scapulae.

Stretch: Start with your neck flexed and rotated laterally away from the side you wish to stretch. The collarbone must be stabilized. Keep the shoulder of the involved (or most involved) side stable and down by holding on to a chair with the hand of the (most) involved side. Bring your ear closer to your shoulder until you feel a mild stretch. Then return your head to a neutral (face forward) position, and stretch the other side. Repeat the stretch once or twice on both sides.

Pectoralis Major and Sternalis

Latin *pectoralis* means "relating to the chest"; major, "larger"; *sternalis*, "relating to the breastbone" (from Greek sternon, meaning "chest").

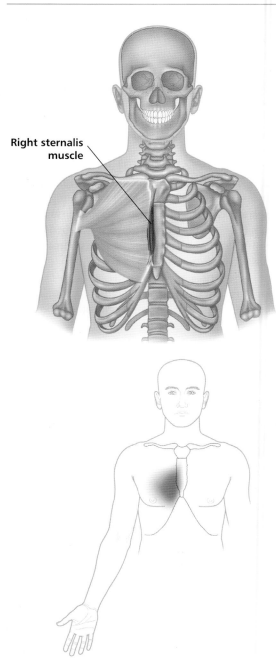

Right sternalis muscle

Pectoralis major.

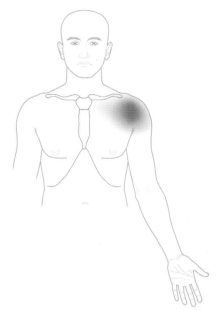

Sternalis.

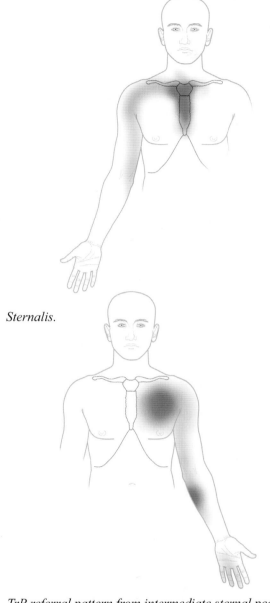

TrP referral pattern from intermediate sternal pectoralis major.

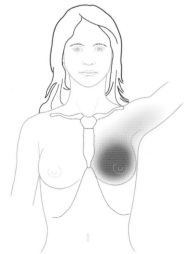

Lateral free margin.

TrP referral pattern from clavicular pectoralis major.

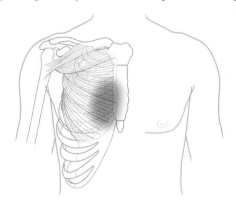

TrP area capable of causing cardiac arrhythmias.

What They Do: The pectoralis major elevates the chest in deep breathing, such as during respiratory distress. It helps stabilize the shoulder and rotate the upper arm medially (turning the palm facing inward), pulls objects down from above, and moves the arm forward and across the body (as when scratching the opposite elbow). The sternalis is a muscle remnant and continuation of the rectus abdominis.

Kinetics Comments: The pectoralis major is a climbing muscle, working with the latissimus dorsi to pull the body upward when the arms are overhead. It works hard during many martial arts, when pushing, punching, and throwing. Lymphatic drainage from the breast usually travels in front of, and around, the pectoralis major muscle to the axillary lymph nodes. Symptoms and signs of entrapped lymph vessels are often relieved by manual work on the pectoralis major. The sternalis isn't present in most of us, but occurs frequently enough to cause confusion in manual examinations and imaging, especially mammography. This muscle lies on top of the pectoralis minor, and, depending on its shape, can be mistaken for pathological masses in the chest. Its shape is exceedingly variable; it can occur on only one side of the breastbone, or on both, and may be of any length.

TrP Comments: TrPs in the sternalis cause symptoms that result in many unnecessary tests for breast, heart, and lung disease. These TrPs can cause soreness over the breastbone and also deep pain beneath it that is intense enough to disturb sleep. They may be activated by a heart attack, and cause lasting pain until they're treated. Their pain may be mistaken for a heart attack or angina. TrPs in both the pectoralis major and the sternalis can engage in a dangerous dance with cardiac disease, each worsening the other. TrPs on the right side of the pectoralis major, near the sternum, can be associated with cardiac arrhythmia, and successfully treating the TrPs may stop the arrhythmia. They usually cause pain as well as arrhythmias. TrP pain is usually more variable than angina in response to activity. TrPs do not exclude cardiac disease, and the reverse is also true. Tightness in the pectoralis major contributes to the round-shouldered, head-forward posture, and is often combined with weakness in the upper back muscles. TrP-shortened pectoralis major muscles can profoundly pull on the SCM. Release the pectoralis TrPs first, and the SCM may be easier to treat.

Any TrP that persists in spite of adequate treatment has a perpetuating factor, and some perpetuating factors are potentially deadly. When in doubt, check it out. Patients, take this book to the Emergency Department with you, as some care providers are still unaware that TrPs can mimic cardiac and other visceral problems. The issue may be in the tissue, not "all in your mind." Such an episode presents an opportunity for you to educate, and this book may ensure that you are taken seriously now and in the future. TrPs in the pectoralis major may work with TrPs in the subscapularis, latissimus dorsi, and teres major to cause pseudo TOS. The pectoralis muscle is made of many layers, each of which may hold multiple TrPs. Depending on where they are, these TrPs cause pain in the characteristic pattern, including severe breast pain and hypersensitivity, golfer's elbow, tennis elbow, and/or chest tightness. These TrPs must be handled carefully and, when active, treated thoroughly and as needed so that they don't aggravate other conditions. The presence of these TrPs and TrPs in other areas may become apparent when a patient is put on CPAP or other respiratory assistance. The sudden expansion of the chest cavity after prolonged restriction can cause frightening pain and muscle soreness unless the reason for it is understood and expected.

Notable Perpetuating Factors: These TrPs can be activated by chronic illness in the chest, seat-belt trauma from an automobile accident, paradoxical breathing (and any coexisting condition that encourages this), immobility of the arm or arms, prolonged sitting, hunched, head-forward posture (and workstations or prolonged emotional states that promote this posture), prolonged keyboarding, large breasts, wearing a tight or an underwire bra, and doing repetitive exercises such as the bench press (or using machines that duplicate this motion). Rowing, excessive poling in skiing or hiking, or using machines that reproduce these motions can initiate and maintain these TrPs, as can holding or supporting oneself with handrails while on a treadmill. The use of walkers can initiate and perpetuate these TrPs, initiating and maintaining a cycle of respiratory shallow breathing and worsening health.

Hints for Control (Patients): Control perpetuating factors. Avoid sleeping with the hands folded over the chest or over the head. Treat both sides of the sternalis with finger pressure and cold compresses. Breast and nipple hypersensitivity are often noticed through intolerance to clothing rubbing against these areas; treating TrPs in the side border of the pectoralis major may relieve the problem. We suggest that women avoid the use of underwire bras and try soft sports bras or undershirts. Creative clothing choices may be sufficient for some.

Hints for Control (Care Providers): Generally, TrPs that cause arrhythmia are found between the fifth and sixth ribs on the right side, midway between the breastbone and the nipple (Simons, Travell, and Simons 1999, p. 822). Careful spraying with vapocoolant, or ice stroking, may moderate pain and other symptoms enough to buy time and lower the anxiety level, but this is true even of pain of cardiac origin. The fact that pain can be relieved by nitrites does not indicate that it is cardiac pain and not TrP related (p. 832). Nitrites dilate the peripheral circulation, and may temporarily help TrPs and Raynaud's phenomenon as well. If cardiac pathology has been ruled out and these TrPs have been treated, continue to search for perpetuating factors and check for TrPs in the paraspinals on the same level as the pectoralis major, especially in the multifidi. If TrPs and cardiac disease coexist, treating the TrPs may minimize the symptoms. Pain control is of vital importance, as pain itself can be a potent vasoconstrictor. If coronary artery disease and TrP blood vessel entrapment are part of the picture, the complete treatment of all of them is critical to patient quality of life. Patients may be comforted to know that there is one more avenue available to treat their symptoms.

Stretch: To begin the in-doorway stretch, stand in a narrow doorway with your forearms and hands flat against the doorjambs. Don't grab and hang on—keep your arms and hands flat. Place one foot in front of the other, with the forward knee bent and your feet pointed straight ahead. Avoid the head-forward posture—keep the head lifted and suspended, as if it were hanging from a sky hook. Bend the front knee slowly and gently, until the knee is above, but not over, the tip of the toe. Move just enough to feel the tension in your chest and shoulders, breathing out as you stretch. Withdraw slowly to the starting position, breathing in as you do so; then stretch the other side. This dynamic stretch can be varied to work different areas of the muscles by moving the hand placement on the doorjambs up or down, targeting the entire muscle. Stretch each segment, not just the tightest areas.

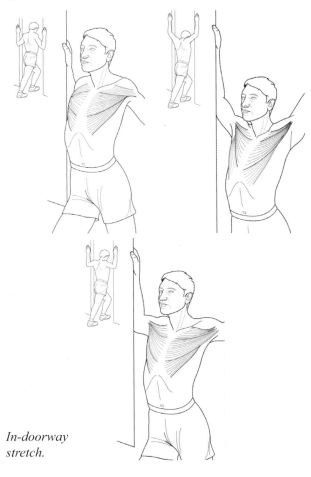

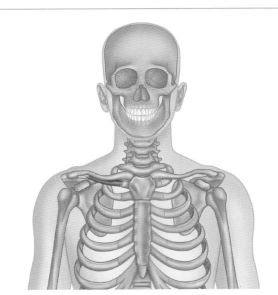

In-doorway stretch.

Subclavius
Latin *sub* means "under"; *clavis*, "key."

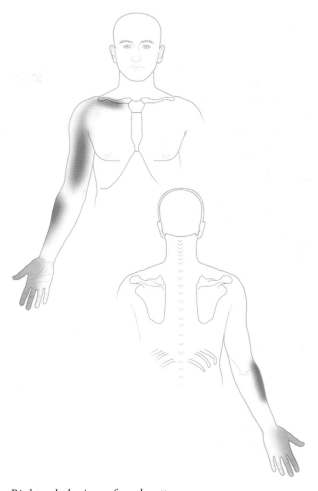

Right subclavius referral patterns.

What It Does: Stabilizes the clavicle (collar bone).

Kinetics Comments: If this muscle is tight, check the pelvic girdle for weakness, and ensure that the shoulder blade is properly positioned; either can lead to subclavius problems. A tight subclavius may pull back the collarbone, creating a more extreme angle than normal.

TrP Comments: These TrPs cause pins and needles in the shoulder, arm, and hand. The referral pattern may include the front and back of the thumb and next two fingers. The clues to the location of TrPs are not only where the pain is, but where it is *not*: this helps eliminate other TrPs. When this muscle is tight, avoid overuse, especially when it's fatigued or chilled. These TrPs can cause pain that may be mistaken for CTS. When TrPs and coronary artery disease coexist, TrP entrapment of blood vessels can interact with it. The coronary specialist needs to understand that this potential exists, as sudden activation of entrapping TrPs can cause immediate unexpected worsening of blood vessel occlusion that may be speedily (if temporarily) remedied by stretch and spray. This knowledge may save a life.

Notable Perpetuating Factors: These TrPs can be initiated by trauma, a heart attack or other visceral episode, arm immobilization such as a cast or sling, or overuse. This may come in the form of a new exercise regime, clearing snow from the sidewalk, or getting rid of junk from the attic. Stress is placed on the tissues by heavy lifting while reaching out in front, a slumping posture, and sustained lifting in a flexed posture such as when using a chain saw. Rather than trying to do big chores in one session, pace yourself.

Hints for Control (Patients): Control all possible perpetuating factors. Frequent use of the in-doorway dynamic stretch is recommended (see Pectoralis Major). Try a soothing, around-the-shoulder, moist heating pack.

Hints for Control (Care Providers): TrPs in the subclavius, pectoralis minor, and scalenes can produce true TOS. The shoulder blade is pulled down by the tight subclavius, impinging on the subclavian artery and vein as they pass over the first rib. Surgery should not be the first choice—not even the second or third. Assess for and treat TrPs and deal with perpetuating factors. Explain to the insurance company how much pain and misery and cost you are saving. Assess all tissues that attach to, or affect, the collarbone for possible TrPs and other pathology.

Stretch: Make a fist and bend your arm at the elbow to a right angle. Abduct your arm to shoulder level, until your fingernails face the floor. Take your elbow back as far as you comfortably can, and then reach the same arm out in front of you, punching the air. Return to neutral position, and stretch the other side. This stretch can be progressed to the in-doorway stretch, or used as an alternative; it can be fine-tuned with a subtle head rotation away from the side you are stretching, breathing in through the nose and out through the mouth as you stretch. Visualize breathing out the pain.

Latissimus Dorsi
Latin *latissimus* means "widest"; *dorsi*, "of the back."

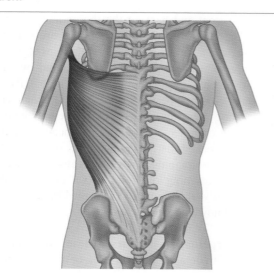

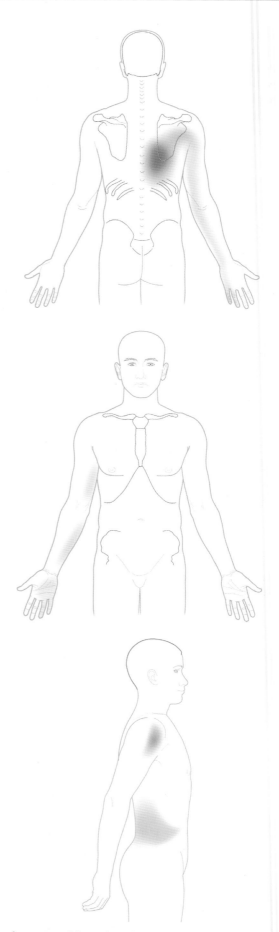

The location of the referral pattern often gives a clue to the location of the latissimus dorsi TrPs.

What It Does: Extends the flexed arm. When the upper arm is fixed in relation to the shoulder blade, it retracts the chest girdle. It rotates the upper arm medially at the shoulder joint. It's a climbing muscle and helps the pectoralis major pull the trunk upward. During deep breathing, it raises the lower ribs.

Kinetics Comments: This large, wide, flat **core muscle** covers much of the back. It twists around the teres major and meshes with it before attaching at the shoulder joint. It attaches to the hip, as well as to the vertebral column between the bottom level of the shoulder blade and the base of the spine. If the pelvis is tilted or rotated, this muscle adjusts, causing compensatory rotation above. It compresses the thorax and abdomen during a hard sneeze or cough. Parts of this muscle are (perhaps too) frequently removed and used as surgical replacement for other missing or damaged tissue, thus upsetting the kinetic chains. When this muscle is tight, stretching may offer little relief, and pain from pressure of the body on the muscle may interrupt sleep.

TrP Comments: Latissimus dorsi TrPs cause a constant ache that won't change much with position or activity. TrPs in this muscle are felt during sneezing and coughing. If it hurts to use your arms to get out of a chair, or pull something down from overhead, these TrPs may be calling for help. They may be misdiagnosed as chest disease, and can be associated with C3–C4, C5–C6, and/or C6–C7 disc problems. Check other muscles for the many satellite TrPs that these TrPs can launch. Lax and pendulous abdomen, shortness of breath, and stitch in the side can involve TrPs in the area between the top of the hip and the armpit on the side of the body. TrPs in the latissimus dorsi may work with TrPs in the pectoralis major, subscapularis, and teres major to cause pseudo TOS. Lower mid-level TrPs may refer pain down the arm.

Notable Perpetuating Factors: Latissimus dorsi TrPs can develop when the arms are overused to compensate for a painful low back. They may be initiated by lifting overhead weight, such as when using heavy tools at shoulder level. Downstroke motions may be perpetuators. Gymnastics, prolonged use of crutches, tennis, golf, or other repetitive motion sports can perpetuate these TrPs, as can any activity that requires repetitive extension, adduction, and internal rotation of the shoulder. The patient is often unaware of the activity that caused the TrPs. Even a tight bra may be a perpetuator, as it restricts circulation and oxygenation of the muscle. This can be compounded by episodic interstitial edema, such as may occur in metabolic syndrome or FM.

Hints for Control: Stretch and spray, tennis-ball pressure (include TrPs on the sides of the body), a cane knobber tool, moist heat, and stretching can be effective. Ensure full ROM.

Stretch: Standing with your feet together, raise both arms over your head in a neutral position. To stretch the left side, grasp the wrist of your left arm with your right hand. Breathe in comfortably as you bend to the right, going as far as feels comfortable. Exhale normally on the return to neutral. Switch the arm grasp and repeat this dynamic stretch on the other side. To add to the stretch, you can gently raise the arm upward using the hand that is grasping the wrist. Pay attention to unwanted movement such as the pelvis rising during the stretch. If you have a difficulty with balance, keep your feet wider apart. If you can't raise your arms over your head, try this exercise lying down, but tell your bodyworker.

Deltoid
Greek *deltoeides* means "shaped like the Greek letter delta."

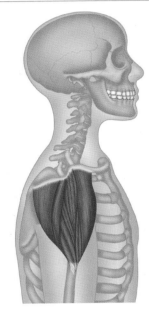

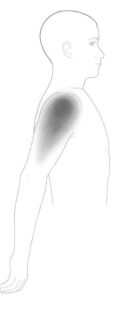

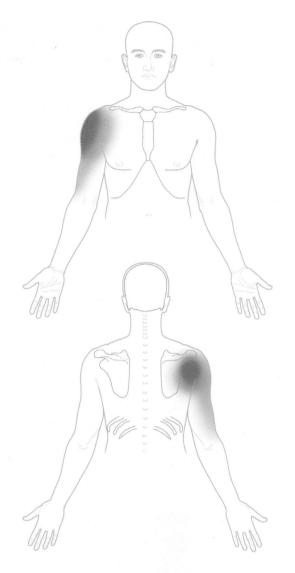

TrP Comments: There may be many TrPs in the layers and segments of this thick muscle. When this characteristic referral pattern pain occurs as the arm is raised to wave, it's probably the voice of the deltoid complaining. Shoulder pain in this pattern that occurs when the deltoid is at rest most likely originates in another muscle, although deltoid TrPs may exist as well and contribute to shoulder weakness. Many muscles refer to the deltoid area, so look at the whole pain pattern, with the understanding that there may be a composite pain pattern. Deltoid pain may radiate down as far as the elbow, but is generally local to the TrPs. The dull, deep ache of deltoid TrPs usually occurs when the arm is moved or contracted, and may be mistaken for rotator cuff injury. Deltoid TrPs are often satellite TrPs.

Notable Perpetuating Factors: Overuse in any task that requires repetitive overhand, underhand, or sideways arm movement; using a computer keyboard that is too high or too low; continued use of a tool at shoulder height; and repetitive lifting or prolonged carrying of a weight (e.g. child or heavy books) in one arm. These TrPs may be initiated by trauma from, for example, a high-velocity sports injury or motor vehicle accident. A TrP cascade can be initiated if a vaccine or other irritant is injected into a deltoid TrP. Static work positions, such as those of a surgeon or dental hygienist, perpetuate these TrPs.

Hints for Control: Tennis-ball or knobber-tool compression and manual therapy such as massage can be helpful. Ensure that the shoulder is warmed up before sports and work activities.

Stretch: From a neutral position, take the arm forward and backward until you reach a comfortable end range. Gently swinging the arm is acceptable, provided you slow down at the end of the range. The middle fibers of the deltoid are almost impossible to stretch without the help of a therapist.

What It Does: The deltoid is a triangular muscle forming the rounded shape of the shoulder. The anterior, posterior, and middle fibers of the muscle raise the arm and stabilize it in the shoulder joint. The anterior fibers, attaching to the collarbone, raise and internally rotate the arm. The middle portion assists the supraspinatus in raising the arm to the side. The posterior fibers are attached to the shoulder blade and work with the latissimus dorsi and teres major to raise and rotate the arm externally.

Kinetics Comments: When the **core muscles** are weak or otherwise deficient, many of the shoulder muscles compensate. **Core muscle** stability must be assessed and treated so that the deltoid area muscles can be successfully restored. The deltoid allows forces that are generated in your legs and torso to migrate into the upper limb, linking the shoulder blade and collarbone to the arm so that a specific movement or task can be accomplished. When the deltoid is tight, it hurts to reach into your back pocket. Keeping this muscle supple and free of tightness may help avoid chronic rotator cuff tears and/or OA of the shoulder (Berth et al. 2009).

Biceps Brachii

Latin: *biceps* means "two-headed"; *brachii*, "of the arm".

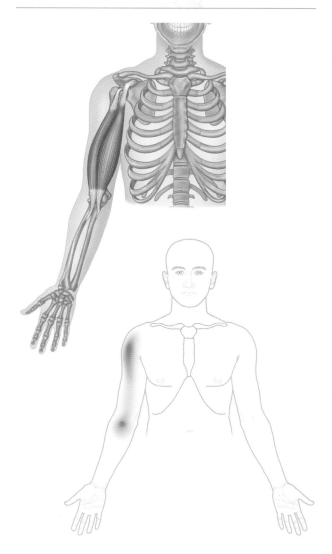

What It Does: Flexes the elbow and shoulder joints and assists in turning the forearm palm up (supination). It also assists in shoulder stabilization and, with the triceps brachii, promotes elbow stabilization.

Kinetics Comments: The two heads of the upper end of this muscle attach to the shoulder blade. The lower end attaches by a 90-degree twisting tendon to the back of the radial bone of the forearm. This muscle therefore affects both the shoulder and elbow joints. We use this muscle to pick up a cup, open a beverage bottle, or move food to our mouth.

TrP Comments: These TrPs are often mistaken for tendinitis or bursitis. They cause weakness, but seldom pain, when you raise your arm above your head. The ache from these TrPs feels superficial and is often accompanied by restriction of arm extension and by upper arm weakness. It may persist when the muscle is at rest and worsen when the arm is raised. Unlike infraspinatus TrPs, biceps TrPs seldom prevent lying on the affected side. The biceps brachii signature is notable by the pain in the inner area of the elbow (anticubital space). For as long as these TrPs refer pain to that area, it's best to avoid giving blood or having blood drawn in that region for testing. If this is unavoidable, tell the person drawing the blood about TrP referral pain and the possibility of a TrP cascade, and discuss options on pain control, including (but not limited to) the application of a cold compress afterward.

Notable Perpetuating Factors: These TrPs may be initiated by a sudden overstretch in a sports injury or other trauma, or lifting heavy objects with the arms outstretched, especially with the hands up. Immobilization during surgery or from wearing a cast can activate these TrPs, as can overusing or working muscles before they are warmed and pliable. Carrying heavy loads, such as multiple school books, with a bent arm can perpetuate these TrPs, as can any motion that requires bending the elbow the same way over and over, such as shoveling snow, operating factory machinery, playing some musical instruments, or carrying out repetitive work with the arms flexed, such as constant use of screwdrivers or computers. Even sleeping with the arm bent fully can maintain these TrPs, as can repetitive exercises such as chin-ups and weightlifting curls, or machines that imitate the same movements.

Hints for Control (Patients): When carrying objects, ensure that they are not too heavy and turn your palms down. Learn and use good body mechanics for lifting. Vary work and stretch the muscles frequently. Avoid perpetuating factors. Ensure that any keyboard or workstation that you use is ergonomically adjusted.

Hints for Control (Care Providers): The thickness of the fascia varies at different locations: for example, it is thin over the biceps brachii and thicker where it covers the triceps brachii and the epicondyles of the humerus. This is important knowledge for therapists, particularly those specializing in TrP dry needling. Immediately below the medial midpoint of the arm there is an opening in the deep fascia. This opening transmits the basilic vein and some lymphatic vessels and should always be avoided during dry needling.

Stretch: Stand with your back to a table that is no higher than the top of your pelvis. Place the palms of both hands on the table, keeping your back to it. Retaining contact with your hands flat on the table, step forward on one leg and gently lunge or squat so that you feel a stretch on both arms up through the biceps brachii. Then return to the start. Avoid letting your knee stick out over your toes, as this leads to ankle instability and increases the risk of injury. Keep your kneecap in line with the middle toe.

Coracobrachialis

Greek *korakoeides* means "raven-like" (here "shaped like a raven's beak").
Latin *brachialis* means "relating to the arm."

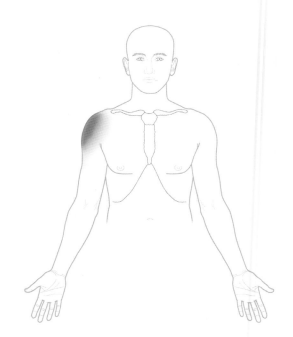

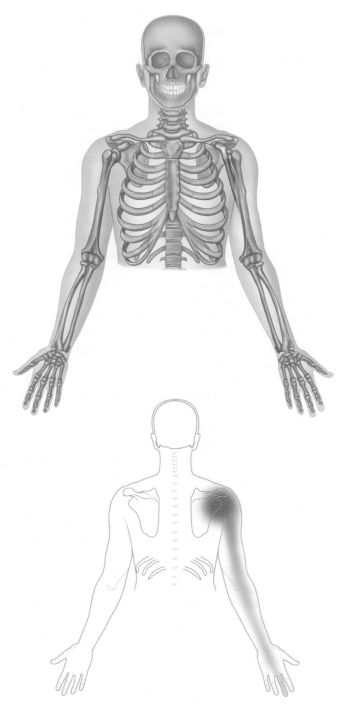

What It Does: Adducts and flexes the arm. It moves the humerus forward (shoulder flexion) and towards the body (shoulder adduction), but rarely gets attention. The pecs and biceps seem to get all the credit and blame.

Kinetics Comments: The coracobrachialis links the chest, shoulder blade, and arm through its tendinous attachments. An overexercised, hypertrophied coracobrachialis may compress the musculocutaneous nerve that passes through it; this has been noted in athletes (Colak et al. 2009). In some cases, due to anatomical variation, the median nerve may also be compressed by tightness in this muscle (Tatar et al. 2004).

TrP Comments: TrPs in this muscle have a big referral pattern. The pain worsens when reaching behind the body across the low back. These TrPs aren't obvious until you have released others that share parts of this referral pattern. They rarely occur alone, and can cause disabling pain but little restriction in ROM. The coracoid process should be checked for attachment TrPs (Karim et al. 2005).

Notable Perpetuating Factors: Lifting heavy objects with the arms outstretched in front. (Keep the elbows close to the body.) Overuse can come from a variety of sources, from keyboarding to heavy practice in shooting a hockey puck.

Hints for Control: Local moist heat before or after passive stretching will minimize post-exercise soreness.

Self-treatment: The idea that we can stretch all the muscles in the body using classical stretching is, in our opinion, erroneous. The best way to get length into the coracobrachialis (and many others that are almost impossible to stretch) is to have the care provider or the patient use their hands, fingers, and thumbs to glide along the muscle to release adhesions, reduce hypertonicity, and create free gliding of fascia and skin.

Brachialis
Latin *brachialis* means "relating to the arm."

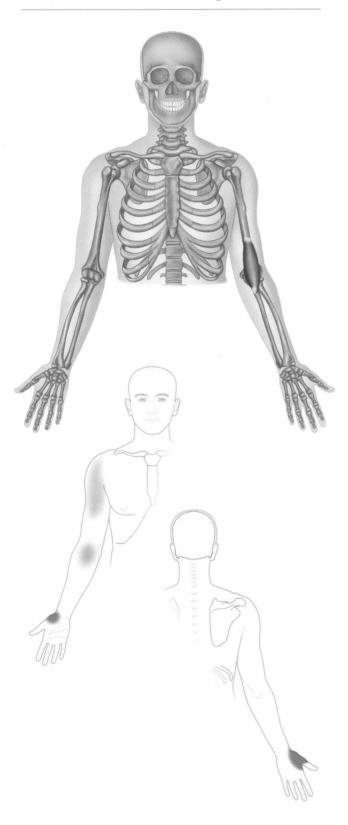

What It Does: Flexes the elbow, and helps control arm extension due to gravity.

Kinetics Comments: The brachialis links the upper arm with the lower arm. Tightness here can entrap the radial nerve, causing numbness or a variety of nerve pains and sensations that can be misdiagnosed as CTS; it can also cause entrapment of the median nerve (Bilecenoglu, Uz, and Karalezli 2005).

TrP Comments: These TrPs can cause pain, numbness, and tingling of the arm and thumb in the characteristic pattern, with secondary pain along the arm up to the shoulder area. They can cause or contribute to "tennis elbow." The area inside the elbow (a few inches above the antecubital or elbow fold area) may be painful. Referral areas may be hypersensitive to touch or other sensations. The pain may increase when the elbow is bent, but can also occur at rest. Odd sensations, called "dysthesias," including tingling, hypersensitivity, and numbness of the thumb, are common and due to nerve entrapment. Pain at the base of the thumb may also be caused by supinator, brachioradialis, or adductor pollicis TrPs.

Notable Perpetuating Factors: Overload of the forearm such as from repeated "chinning" movements, weightlifting, prolonged holding of the sharply flexed elbow (e.g. during a phone call or ironing), using crutches, carrying heavy loads or holding a heavy purse or bag over the forearm with the elbow bent, carrying groceries, or prolonged finger work on a violin or guitar.

Hints for Control: Small pressure tools are helpful for addressing these TrPs. When lifting, ensure the palm is turned up. During the night place a pillow in the angle of the elbow to prevent sleeping with the arm tightly folded. Avoid perpetuating factors.

Stretch: Start with the target arm bent at the elbow, with the palm facing away from you. As you extend your arm, begin to rotate your hand so that the palm faces forward. Allow the arm to extend at the shoulder to ensure full ROM. Return to the start, and repeat on the other side. As symptoms improve, this stretch can be intensified using your other hand to extend the fingers and wrist of the target arm, with the elbow extended. Keep it dynamic.

Triceps Brachii

Latin *triceps* means "three-headed"; *brachii*, "of the arm."

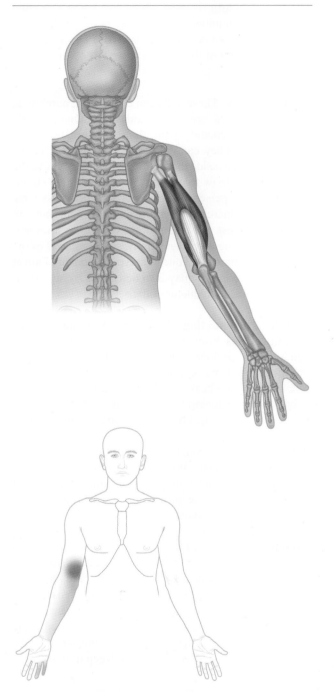

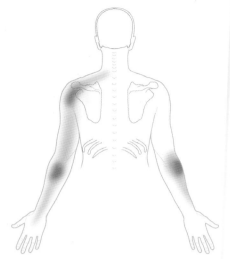

Referral patterns from TrPs in the central portion area of the left long head and from TrPs in the central portion of the right deep medial head.

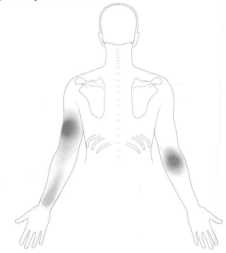

Referral pattern from TrPs in the area of the left lateral border of the left lateral head and from the right musculotendinous attachment area deep under the tendon.

What It Does: Extends the elbow, straightening the arm. It works with the latissimus dorsi to extend the shoulder joint. The three heads join at the elbow. The long head stabilizes the shoulder joint, adducts the arm, and extends it from the bent position; the medial head retracts the capsule of the elbow joint when the arm extends. The lateral head is commonly the area of this muscle where the radial nerve is entrapped, although entrapment can occur at any place along the nerve.

Kinetics Comments: This is the big muscle in the back of the upper arm. It works in opposition to the biceps: when one stretches, the other contracts. The three heads merge into a thick tendon, and, as with many muscles, multiple heads enable it to do different tasks, depending on where each one is attached. The triceps works hard for martial artists—in pushing, punching, and chopping moves. Cross-country skiers use it when poling, and

Referral pattern from TrPs in deep medial border of right deep medial head.

tennis players use it for backhand serves. Baseball pitchers depend on it, as do weightlifters, golfers, and American football quarterbacks. Gymnasts give it a workout on the parallel bars and the rings. It puts the "up" in "push-up." It helps us to lower and raise our bodies into and out of chairs, and use a cane or stick when walking. It allows those of us in wheelchairs to spin our wheels.

TrP Comments: TrPs in the region of each of the heads have their own referred pain pattern; all may be mistaken for arthritis. Some triceps TrPs are called tennis elbow or golfer's elbow, but the pain doesn't originate in the elbow and you needn't play these sports to have them. Hypersensitivity can be extreme with these TrPs: even touching the elbow to any surface may produce severe pain. Those TrPs that send pain to the back of the upper arm, and sometimes to the front of the forearm may have a referral pattern including the fourth and fifth fingers. These TrPs can also entrap the radial nerve, resulting in tingling and numbness over the top of the lower forearm, wrist, and middle finger. Triceps brachii TrPs may combine to produce a vague, hard-to-localize pain in the back of the shoulder and upper arm. They may also cause a distracting itch instead of pain, and this can be severe enough to disrupt sleep. Patients with these TrPs tend to keep the arm slightly flexed and away from the body to minimize pain.

Notable Perpetuating Factors: Use of crutches or a cane that is too long, short upper arms, and prolonged sitting with the elbow forward in front of the plane of the chest or abdomen, such as in an airplane or automobile. Triceps TrPs may also be perpetuated by doing needlepoint or other fine work, or writing without proper elbow support. These TrPs are usually due to overload stress of the muscle and repetitive activity (e.g. racket sports or weightlifting), poling such as in cross-country skiing, use of a walking stick, or machines that duplicate these motions.

Hints for Control: Deep massage and passive stretching, and ball, tool, or finger pressure may be helpful. Don't neglect the backs of the arms during stretching. When typing, writing, and reading, keep your upper arm vertical, and don't project your elbow forward. Modify activities and mechanical factors that stress the muscle. Avoid chairs with inadequate elbow support; keep the elbow behind the plane of the chest, and not projected upward. An armrest adjusted to the proper height should support your elbow whenever possible. Ice may sometimes relieve itching.

Stretch: Reach behind your back to the same-side shoulder blade, keeping the arm close to your head. Extend the stretch by pressing gently on the elbow with the other arm. Clenching the fist of the target arm will shorten the biceps brachii, allowing a full stretch of the triceps brachii without having to flex the elbow joint

further. A slight side-bend away from the side being stretched can make this stretch feel really good. Stretch each side.

Anconeus
Latin *anconeus* means "relating to the elbow."

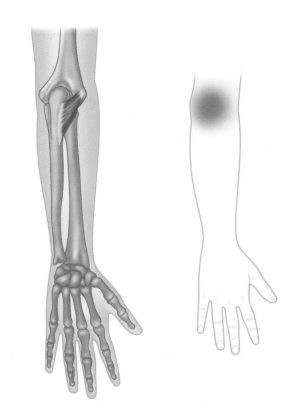

What It Does: Works with the triceps brachii to extend the elbow.

Kinetics Comments: This muscle is used when we push a door closed or reach out to touch someone.

TrP Comments: Active anconeus TrPs cause local pain, often called tennis elbow or epicondylitis. It hurts to bend the elbow or turn the forearm palm up. These TrPs can contribute to ulnar nerve compression; they are often satellite TrPs and may be mistaken for arthritis.

Notable Perpetuating Factors: Immobility, such as from a shoulder sling or bent arm cast, and repetition of movement. The anconeus can compensate for reduced core strength or for muscles in other areas weakened by TrPs. Use of crutches or overuse of this muscle in sports can perpetuate these TrPs.

Hints for Control (Patients): Loosen your grip on a tennis racket, golf club, or pen. Use soft felt-tipped pens or soft pencils (#2 or softer). Stretch frequently during repetitive tasks, especially writing or computer work.

Hints for Control (Care Providers): Treatment of ulnar nerve compression in cases of anconeus TrPs should be treatment of the TrPs, not surgical excision of the muscle; prevention is even better. Implementation with reimbursement requires education of insurance companies.

Stretch: This stretch targets the muscles and fascia associated with the back of the elbow. Sitting or standing with your back stretched out, point the fingers of your right arm up towards the ceiling. Keep your elbow straight and your right biceps close to your ear. Bend the right arm at the elbow so that your right palm touches your right shoulder blade (or as close to it as you can get). Keep the flat portion of your elbow facing forward. You can support this elbow with the left hand, gently pushing or directing the arm back to feel the stretch. Make a fist of your right hand and then release. Return to the start and repeat with the other side.

Forearm Flexors and the Wrist Retinaculum

(flexor digitorum superficialis and profundus, flexor pollicis longus, flexor carpi radialis and ulnaris)
Latin *flectere* means "to bend";
retinacula, "rope."

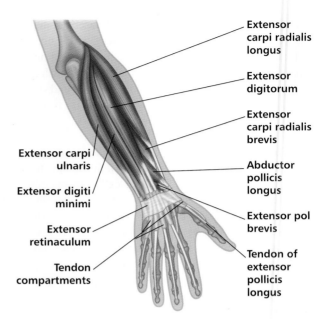

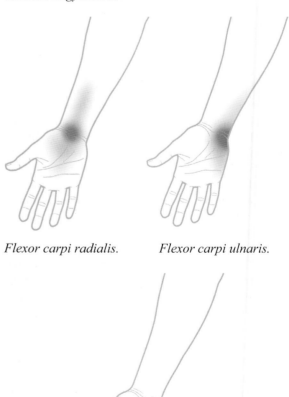

Although the extensor retinaculum is an extensor rather than a flexor, the retinacula are placed together here. TrPs in the extensor retinaculum seem to be more common in computer users. Those in the flexor retinaculum are more common in gymnasts.

Flexor carpi radialis.   *Flexor carpi ulnaris.*

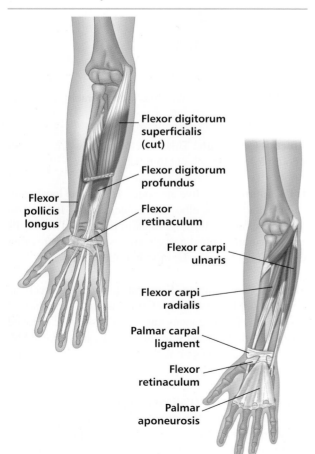

Flexor pollicis longus.

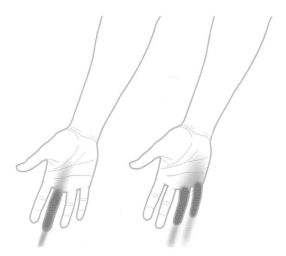

Flexor digitorum super-ficialis and profundus (radial head).

Flexor digitorum super-ficialis and profundus (humeral head).

What They Do: The forearm flexors primarily flex the wrist and fingers. The flexor carpi radialis, working with the flexor carpi ulnaris, turns the wrist away from the midline (abduction); the flexor carpi ulnaris, working with the flexor carpi radialis, turns the wrist towards the midline (adduction). The flexor carpi radialis and flexor carpi ulnaris are wrist (or hand) flexors and help stabilize the wrist joint. The other muscles in this group are the finger flexors. The retinacula secure the wrist tendons and supply proprioceptive functions.

Kinetics Comments: The forearm flexors are grouped together; they are treated the same way and have much in common. Their actions affect the wrist and fingers, but their referral patterns are different. When the core is weak, the forearm muscles in general become short and tight. The retinaculum is a strong fibrous net of thickened deep fascia that keeps the majority of the forearm tendons close to the wrist bones in spite of the variety and force of possible wrist movements. Tightness of the retinaculum due to TrPs causes loss of wrist flexibility, at which point the wrist cannot be moved smoothly in a circle. Circling movements are jerky and uneven, depending on how many TrPs are involved and where they are.

TrP Comments: TrPs in these flexors all create pain that centers on the underside of the wrist crease, but each reference zone is a bit different. The flexor digitorum superficialis and profundus refer pain to the fingers, and *beyond*. The pain seems to shoot out beyond the fingers! It's similar to the phantom pain of amputation, but without a missing digit. The superficialis muscle lies over the profundus; TrPs that occur in the area of these muscles upward of the little and ring fingers refer pain to the palm in a line to those fingers and beyond. The area of these muscles closer to the thumb side of the palm refers pain to the palm, the middle finger, and the area

beyond that finger. The flexor digitorum superficialis can entrap the median nerve (Bilecenoglu, Uz, and Karalezli 2005). Entrapment of the ulnar nerve can be caused (or aggravated) by TrPs in the flexor carpi ulnaris, digitorum superficialis, or digitorum profundus. Nerve entrapment associated with the cubital (elbow) tunnel is often called "tunnel syndrome." Treatment of the cause of the pain or altered sensation can often be accomplished with manual modalities if done promptly. Symptoms often begin with altered sensations, including burning pain or numbness of the fourth and fifth fingers.

Flexor pollicis longus TrPs send pain to the thumb, especially to the last joint and beyond. These TrPs may be first noticed as weakness when opening (or not being able to open) jars. If the TrPs worsen, they will scream as soon as you try. You may scream with them. Even wringing out a wash cloth may cause intense pain, and the cloth remains soggy because the muscles are weak. Finger flexor TrPs often affect fine motor control of the fingers, resulting in clumsiness and weakness of grip. They cause difficulty gardening, brushing hair, or using scissors to cut heavy cloth. They can also be associated with "trigger finger" and "trigger thumb." This is a painless locking of the finger or thumb, which is then stuck in a bent position until forcibly straightened.

As this is written, as far as we know, this is the first published work on retinaculum TrPs, although it's known that the extensor tendon may be impinged by the extensor retinaculum (Khazzam, Patillo, and Gainor 2008; VanHeest et al. 2007). I (Starlanyl) have seen over a dozen people with retinaculum TrPs. Extensor TrPs seem to be more common, but this may be due to the nature of the patients, most of whom had CMP with FM. Those who did not have FM were artisans or farmers, and had multiple TrPs in the arms. None of these patients required surgery, although in two cases there was palmar bowing of the flexor retinaculum before treatment. Several had been diagnosed with CTS and were considered surgical candidates.

TrPs in the retinaculum are palpable as discrete bead- or pearl-like nodules, referring pain across the retinaculum in a wristband or half-wristband distribution. Owing to the nature of the fibrous retinaculum, taut bands are often difficult to discern. The pain can be intense, and the pattern varies according to the placement of the nodule. Pressure on the TrPs can send a thin flash of pain down the hand. They can be mistaken for CTS or tenosynovitis. One study found hypoechoic (less reflective on ultrasonography) reticular areas that simulated tenosynovitis (Robertson, Jamadar, and Jacobson 2007); this finding may have been due to retinacular TrPs. Pressure from retinacular TrPs can restrict fluid flow and cause fascial inflammation that can be mistaken for arthritis of the wrist. More research is needed.

Notable Flexor Perpetuating Factors: Repetitive twisting or pulling actions, or any motions that require a prolonged tight handgrip, such as chronic scissors use, chopping wood, hammering nails, archery, motocross, prolonged motorcycling, lengthy keyboarding sessions, and driving for extended periods. Sudden strong flexion, such as a fall on an outstretched wrist, can initiate forearm flexor TrPs.

Notable Retinacular Perpetuating Factors: Chronic or acute overload of the wrist, especially if forearm TrPs are present. Prolonged repetitive work with the hands—such as manual therapy, writing, keyboarding, pottery, sculpting, fine carpentry, some farm work, and sustained use of vibrating tools—and prolonged equine dressage are perpetuating factors.

Hints for Control (Patients): Feel the forearm layers as you slowly extend the hand. Separate the muscles, and palpate (see Chapter 14) until you find a TrP. Use gentle finger pressure combined with stretching. It's important to treat all the TrPs. Electrical stimulation, stretch and spray, and other therapeutic modalities can be beneficial. Avoid using a clenched grip whenever possible, and try not to lean on a table or desk with a bent wrist to provide stability while working on the computer or doing other tasks.

Hints for Control (Care Providers): Neither trigger finger nor trigger thumb responds to exercises. They may respond well to injection into a spot deep in the tendon sheath, proximal to the metacarpal head. Using modalities such as electrical stimulation, ultrasound, or FSM (tendon) before manual therapy can help soften the tissue. Strengthening the flexors cannot proceed while TrPs are active in the **core muscles**.

Retinaculum TrPs are suspected to be satellite TrPs by one of the authors (Starlanyl), and the primary TrPs and perpetuating factors must be brought under control. These TrPs can be worked by gently separating the tissues and promoting fluid transport through the area, but they may require dry needling or TrP injection. Pacing and varying tasks are important. Similar retinacula occur in places such as the knee and the ankle area, and research concerning connective tissue TrPs is greatly needed. These are tissues that require the intervention of a qualified therapist with the skills to place their thumbs on the styloid process of each bone and gently separate them. This stretch is usually performed after the ulnar and radius bones are gently compressed, providing a slack to occur in the interosseous membrane.

Stretch: The forearm flexors are targeted best with the elbow extended. Take the fingers of the forearm to be stretched, palm facing forward, and cover them with the fingers of the opposite hand. Draw the fingers of the targeted hand into extension until a nice stretch is experienced. Return to the start position and repeat with the other arm. Stretching the hand both ways helps keep the forearm flexors and surrounding tissues supple. Keep the stretch dynamic. See Pronator Quadratus for illustration of stretch.

Abductor Pollicis Longus
Latin *abductor* means "a leader away from"; *pollicis*, "of the thumb"; *longus*, "long."

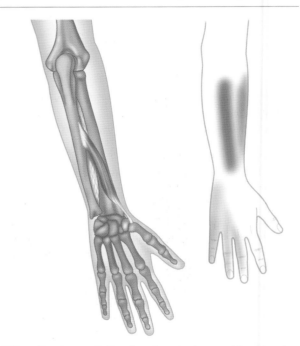

What It Does: Puts the thumb into mid extension away from the fingers, works with the extensors to help them extend the thumb at the wrist, and works with the abductor pollicis brevis to move the thumb away from the fingers.

Kinetics Comments: This muscle can reduce endurance in the finger and forearm and dysfunction here causes loss of thumb control.

TrP Comments: These TrPs can cause weakness, stiffness, and pain in the characteristic pattern, as well as cramps that can startle you out of sleep. They can cause fumbling and loss of coordination, and may be mistaken for arthritis or de Quervain's tenosynovitis.

Notable Perpetuating Factors: Any task that overuses this muscle and tendon, from constant microtrauma such as in volleyball to the relatively new perpetuating factor of texting, which also stresses the upper trapezius, abductor pollicis brevis, and opponens pollicis.

Hints for Control (Patients): Palpate this muscle while the thumb is extended. Finger or TrP tool pressure can be effective, as can a variety of manual methods. Soaking the arm in moderately hot water before stretching and manual therapy may ease the way.

Hints for Control (Care Providers): Even though the pain resembles arthritis and de Quervain's tenosynovitis, and follows C6, C7, and C8 dermatomes and superficial radial nerve distribution, assess for TrPs first. This may save a lot of pain, time, and resources.

Stretch: Move the thumb towards the second finger, and then away and a little backward. Moving the wrist into and out of flexion and extension while doing this extends the stretch.

Pronator Quadratus and Pronator Teres

Latin *pronare* means "to bend forward"; *quadratus*, "squared-off;" *teres*, "rounded" or "finely shaped."

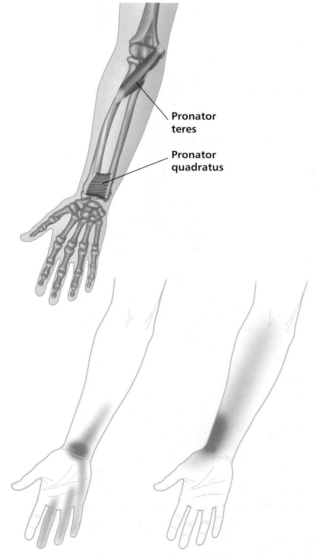

Pronator teres

Pronator quadratus

Pronator quadratus referral pain pattern.

Pronator teres referral pain pattern.

What It Does: The quadratus initiates pronation (rotation of the forearm so that the back of the hand faces forward). The teres pronates and flexes the arm at the elbow.

Kinetics Comments: The quadratus is deep. If you apply firm pressure between the long flexor tendons, you can feel it as it contracts against resistance. It's approximately rectangular in shape (and thus "squared-off"), and has a superficial and a deep head. The teres has two heads, with the median nerve passing between the heads. The nerve can become entrapped at that location—by musculotendinous tissue or by fascia, as the anatomy varies considerably.

TrP Comments: Pronator Quadratus: It's said that two heads are better than one. These two muscle heads may partially account for the two distinct TrP referral patterns. TrPs in parts of the muscle closer to the thumb side tend to refer to the middle and ring fingers. TrPs on the part of the muscle closest to the little-finger side tend to refer pain to the wrist and little fingers. TrPs cause more than pain—they cause dysfunction, which often manifests here as weakness. Attempts to strengthen this muscle before resolving the TrPs will worsen them and further weaken the muscle.

Pronator Teres: These TrPs cause characteristic pain and difficulty cupping the hand or supinating the palm while extending it.

Notable Perpetuating Factors: These TrPs may be initiated by acute overload, but are commonly due to repetitive use such as prolonged lifting of heavy bags, using a screwdriver, handcrafting, or assembly-line work. One of the most common and avoidable perpetuating factors is inappropriate exercise. Any TrP means contracture, even if it is too small or too deep to see. Repetitive strengthening exercise such as with weights, bands, or machines is counterproductive.

Hints for Control (Patients): Finger pressure may be helpful (Annis 2003). A compression bandage may relieve some pain temporarily, but that is a trade-off as it impairs circulation to some extent and shouldn't be used continually. Moist heat followed by manual work on muscles in the area may help the pronator quadratus release.

Hints for Control (Care Providers): Stretch and spray, neuromuscular therapy, and other forms of manual TrP treatment may be effective, but perpetuating factors must be brought under control. You can't strengthen a muscle that has TrPs. When muscles are weak, find out why. Nerve entrapments from the pronator teres and subscapularis muscles are often treated surgically, although research indicates that much of this surgery could be successfully replaced by myofascial neuromuscular therapy. (Hains et al 2010)

Stretch: The finger-extension stretch (see Forearm Flexors and the Wrist Retinaculum) is helpful for all the hand and finger muscles. Ensure that the arm being stretched is supported.

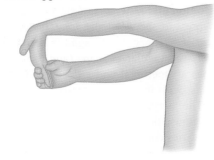

Abductor Pollicis Brevis

Latin *abductor* means "a leader away from"; *pollicis*, "of the thumb"; *brevis*, "short."

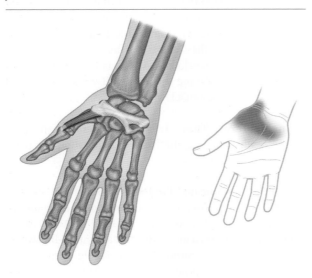

What It Does: Moves the thumb away from the fingers (abduction).

Kinetics Comments: The abductor pollicis brevis is the hitchhiking muscle: we don't advocate hitchhiking, but the term is descriptive. It's the largest muscle forming the mass of tissue at the base of the thumb—the thenar eminence. It functions with the rotation of the wrist, and helps give us the advantage of an opposable thumb.

TrP Comments: TrPs in the abductor pollicis brevis cause pain in the characteristic pattern and weakness of the muscle, which poses a problem opening jars and performing other tasks that require grip strength. These TrPs cause stiffness that may be mistaken for arthritis, and loss of fine motor control and coordination in the thumb. The characteristic pain pattern may be described as the perpetuating factor, such as "weeder's thumb" and "texter's thumb." TrPs in this muscle may be mistaken for CTS. The muscle may atrophy (lose tissue mass) if TrPs persist.

Notable Perpetuating Factors: Repetitive motion, and impact to the thenar area from a fall. Common perpetuating factors include video games, texting, writing, sewing, and crafting.

Hints for Control: This depends on what is perpetuating the TrPs: for example, if writing contributes to the TrPs, use ergonomic pens or felt tips or a vocal computer interface (if throat TrPs allow). Soaking the hand in moderately hot water may help before stretching. Stretch and spray, ultrasound, finger pressure, and hand tools may help melt the TrPs. Massaging this meaty area of the hand works well.

Stretch: Take the thumb towards the second finger and then away and a little backward. The correct hand and finger placement is vital to ensure that the joint at the base of the thumb is not stressed, so do investigate various grips to find the one that works best for you.

Abductor Digiti Minimi

Latin *abductor* means "a leader away from"; digiti, "of the finger"; *minimi*, "smallest." (This term can also apply to the little toe.)

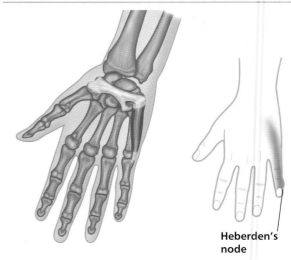

Heberden's node

What It Does: Moves the little finger out and away from the ring finger.

Kinetics Comments: This finger plays an important part in grasping large objects with the fingers outspread. When it becomes tight, the finger feels stiff and awkward.

TrP Comments: These TrPs cause referred pain on the outer edge of both sides of the little finger, accompanied by weakness and stiffness. TrPs in this muscle are often mistaken for arthritis, and Heberden's node may be associated with long-term TrPs. Buttoning clothes and grasping large objects may be difficult. Contracture of muscles due to TrPs may upset the alignment of bones, causing extra wear. Prompt attention to these TrPs may delay the onset or progression of OA.

Notable Perpetuating Factors: Chronic repetitive motion such as that of factory workers, mechanics, gardeners (weeding), bowlers, and golfers.

Hints for Control: Explore optional ways of doing tasks. Modify a pincer grip by relaxing the grip and shortening the duration of the muscle contraction. When using the hand, periodically rest it by allowing the arms to relax at your sides. Gently shake and flutter your fingers. After any work involving the fingers, soak the hand in moderately hot water and gently stretch it. When working one hand with the other, care must be taken to avoid overusing the massaging hand.

Stretch: This muscle usually requires little or no stretching due to its anatomy. When this muscle (and its associated fascia) becomes tight and stuck, it does so usually within its anatomical ROM. If you attempt a stretch, avoid straining or stressing the joint at the end of the little finger.

Brachioradialis
Latin *brachium* means "arm"; *radius*, "staff" or "wheel spoke."

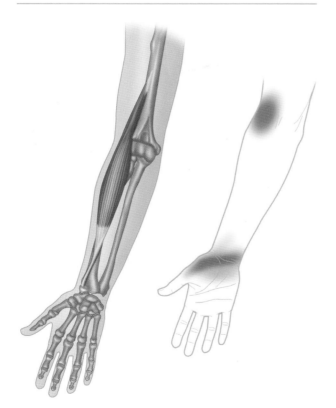

What It Does: Bends the arm at the elbow joint and helps return the forearm to the midline after twisting in supination or pronation (palm up or down). It does this by pulling the fascia above the elbow downward while pulling the fascia below the elbow upward.

Kinetics Comments: You can feel this superficial muscle pop up when you make a gentle fist. The brachioradialis bridges the upper and lower arm, and helps prevent upper limb bones from separating at the elbow during abrupt movements.

TrP Comments: These TrPs not only cause pain in their characteristic pattern, but also lead to grip failure. Spilling soup and dropping objects may be part of these TrPs' special effects. They are often associated with writer's cramp or tennis elbow, and may be mistaken for arthritis of the wrist. Many of these TrPs refer to the elbow and/or wrist areas; they are often satellite TrPs or exist in combination with other TrPs. Assess all muscles in the muscle's kinetic chain.

Notable Perpetuating Factors: Forceful or repetitive trauma such as from prolonged keyboarding, sports with wrist extension during pronation, writing, percussion (e.g. hammering), and twisting motions (e.g. prolonged use of a screwdriver).

Hints for Control: Depending on perpetuating factors, the use of an ergonomic wrist rest or elevated mouse pad, along with a careful pacing of work with frequent breaks, may help ease the TrPs. They are most easily palpated when making a gentle fist. Feel the upper third of the muscle for taut bands and TrPs. Press the TrPs, hold, and release. Try barrier release (see Chapter 14).

Stretch: Lie down on your back, with a pillow under your head and another across your chest. Place the arm that you're not stretching across the pillow, with the elbow bent to 90 degrees and the palm relaxed. Next, rest the elbow of the arm that you are stretching onto the curve made by the wrist and forearm of the other arm. Allow the elbow of the target arm to relax and straighten, with your thumb pointing up. Bend your wrist so that your thumb is pointing away from you. Point the thumb and bend the wrist as far as feels comfortable. Return to the beginning and repeat with the other arm.

Extensor Carpi Radialis Brevis

Latin *extendere* means "to extend"; *carpi*, "of the wrist"; *radius*, "staff" or "wheel spoke"; *brevis*, "short."

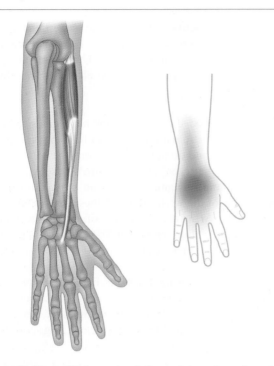

What It Does: Helps extend the wrist, and works with other muscles to move the wrist away from the midline.

Kinetics Comments: Wrist extensor muscles affect grip strength by helping control the flexor digitorum superficialis and profundus. This muscle is short, but its lower tendon is very long.

TrP Comments: TrPs in this muscle or tendon can cause a painful, weak grip that eventually fails; they may cause numbness or a "pins and needles" prickling sensation. They may also entrap parts of the radial nerve. Finger stiffness and/or loss of fine motor control may be part of these TrPs' symptoms. Pain from these TrPs may be called tennis elbow or tendinitis.

Notable Perpetuating Factors: Wrist curls and machines that duplicate them, and a prolonged tight, curled grip such as used in water skiing, writing, knitting, or crocheting. Some athletes, long-haul drivers, manual bodyworkers, and gardeners may develop these TrPs.

Hints for Control: Avoid repetitive use and vary tasks. Stretch and massage often between tasks. When applying finger pressure, barrier release, or other treatment, check the long lower attachment tendon for TrPs too. Tendon (attachment) TrPs often respond better to cold than to heat, while the muscle part may feel better with heat. If you suspect inflammation, end with cooling to avoid compounding the inflammation.

Stretch: Under normal circumstances, these muscles are virtually impossible to stretch, mostly because of the anatomy of the wrist. If these extensor muscles are short or tight we advise, as with all muscles, that you don't force the muscle to lengthen. This can cause harm. Overworked forearm extensors respond well to a gentle reintroduction to normal range movements—use your opposite hand to provide the movement of flexion at the wrist, with the elbow extended. Using the opposite hand, cover the back of the target hand at the base of its fingers and flex this wrist until a *mild* stretch is experienced. Release the stretch and repeat on the other side.

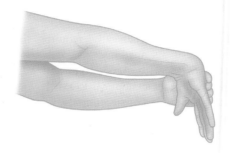

Extensor Carpi Radialis Longus

Latin *extendere* means "to extend"; *carpi*, "of the wrist"; *radius*, "staff" or "wheel spoke"; *longus*, "long."

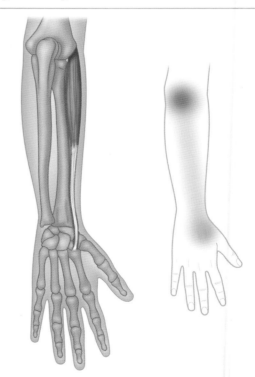

What It Does: Extends the wrist and tilts it away from the midline of the body (abduction).

Kinetics Comments: This muscle is called longus because it is longer than the extensor carpi radialis brevis. It has a long tendon, although the one on the brevis is longer.

TrP Comments: These TrPs cause a weak grip and loss of hand coordination. Food and drink may not reach their intended destination, becoming unexpected decorative effects instead—not a recommended way to lose weight. This TrP pain is often called tennis elbow or epicondylitis. There may be intense burning that doesn't stop even when the muscle is at rest.

Notable Perpetuating Factors: Weeding (especially with a trowel or deep weeder), ironing clothes, or using a resistance band strengthener.

Hints for Control: This pain is too often "treated" with rest and anti-inflammatory medication: the TrPs becomes latent and the pain goes, but muscle weakness remains, and when the resting is over, the TrPs activate once again. They require treatment. Moist heat can be effective for the muscle portion, and cold may ease the tendon attachment. Finger pressure on the TrPs may help: gently flex the hand (towards the palm) while pressing, and work slowly down the muscle and tendon, allowing each barrier to release before progressing to the next one. Check the tendon too.

Stretch: See Extensor Carpi Radialis Brevis.

Extensor Carpi Ulnaris
Latin, extensor means "to extend"; carpi, "of the wrist"; ulnaris, "of the elbow."

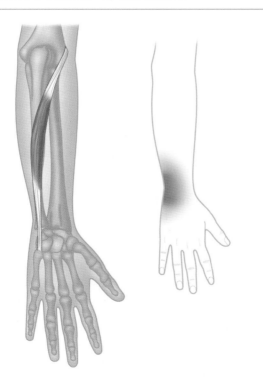

What it Does: Extends the wrist, working with the extensor carpi radialis muscles. It also works with the flexor carpi ulnaris to adduct the wrist and to pick things up, such as a coffee cup.

Kinetics Comments: This muscle is important to the dynamic stability of the wrist. The lower tendon attachment of this muscle passes beneath the wrist extensor retinaculum. It helps produce a powerful grip.

TrP Comments: TrPs here cause the characteristic referral pattern and add to a painful weak grip, and contribute to loss of fine motor control. Check for primary TrPs elsewhere.

Notable Perpetuating Factors: TrPs that develop in the ECU are usually secondary to trauma, "frozen shoulder", immobility of the arm, or satellite TrPs from other muscles. Check for static positions such as in long distance drivers or professional musicians. Dart-throwing and other repetitive actions can also perpetuate these TrPs. Use of repetitive exercises such as wrist roller or reverse wrist curls or machines that produce the same action should be avoided.

Hints for Control (Patients): Change position of arms frequently, and look for primary TrPs. Look to your history to see what is initiating and maintaining these TrPs. A hot pack on the wrist may ease the pain temporarily. If keyboarding is one of your perpetuating factors, find a lighter weight computer mouse or use an alternative.

Hints for Control (Care Providers): Cubital tunnel nerve compression is more likely to be part of TrPs at the head of the flexor carpi ulnaris. TrPs in this muscle may be misdiagnosed as de Quervain's, osteoarthritis, or tenosynovitis, although these conditions may coexist with the TrPs. Treat the TrPs and see what symptoms remain.

Stretch: These TrPs are often worse on the dominant hand. If you are right handed, with your hands in front of you, use your right hand to gently press your left hand slowly from a fingers-straight-out position to a position in which the hand and fingers point towards the floor. Then bring the hand back to a neutral position. Repeat with the other hand. If you are left handed, start by stretching the right hand. Do this several times during the day.

Finger Extensors
(extensor digitorum and extensor indicis)
Latin: *extensor*, to extend; *digitis*, finger; *indicis*, the forefinger.

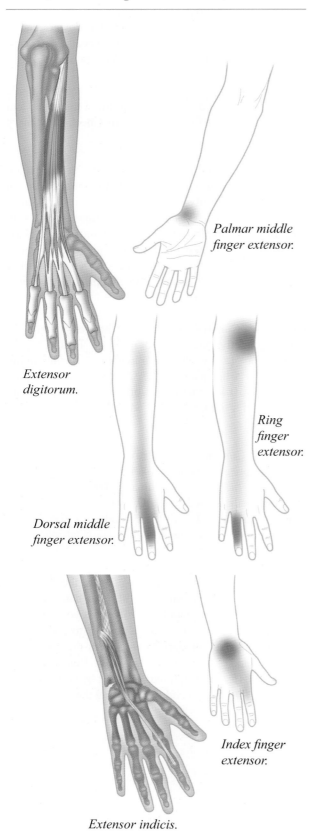

Palmar middle finger extensor.

Extensor digitorum.

Ring finger extensor.

Dorsal middle finger extensor.

Index finger extensor.

Extensor indicis.

What They Do: Extends the fingers primarily at the metacarpophalangeal joints. They also help to extend the entire fingers, and the hand at the wrist joint. They also contribute to forceful finger flexion. They are involved in grasping and gripping motions. When you lift your arm and pull your hand back and wave hello with your fingers, you are using these muscles.

Kinetics Comments: Notice how most of the finger extensor muscles are joined in one muscle, sometimes called the extensor digitorum communis. The tendon branches out to individual fingers. The index finger has its own muscle and tendon, and there are frequently anatomical variations in the tendons. Individual finger movements depend on the lumbrical, interosseous and individual finger flexor muscles. Impaired finger flexion may be due to TrPs in the finger extensors. Weak grip from TrPs in these muscles can be due to inhibition of muscular contraction by TrP contracture or through spastic activity of antagonistic muscles resulting in TrPs . These muscles work as a group. Unless they have TrPs.

TrP Comments: These TrPs are often mistaken for arthritis, because their pain patterns cover so many joints. They often occur in addition to arthritis. TrP location usually responds with the finger(s) or other areas experiencing symptoms. TrPs in the finger extensors can also cause tennis elbow. They cause pain in their characteristic pattern, along with tenderness, stiffness, soreness, cramping and weakness, in addition to loss or dysfunction of grip, grasp, and/or fine motor control. The pain usually stops before the ends of the fingers, with the nail bed and the ends of the fingers without pain (from these TrPs). TrPs are usually found in more than one of these muscles. Symptoms are worse when the muscle is in use, as during shaking hands, opening jars, of turning a doorknob. Dropping objects are part of life for those with these TrPs. Radial nerve entrapment may cause numbness and tingling over the back of the hand. TrPs in these muscles can be especially disabling for those who use them for work, such as writers, musicians, or for those who communicate by sign language.

Notable Perpetuating Factors: Repeated or forceful gripping any object such as during weeding, writing, massage, trigger point or other manual body work, carpentry, some sports such as tennis or darts or archery, frequent playing of some musical instruments such as piano or other stringed instrument, repetitive use of rubber band exercisers, extensive mobile phone use, frequent computer mouse use, or sleeping with the wrist and hand curled up under the chin or under a pillow.

Hints for Control (Patients): Avoid overloading these muscles. Learn to shake hands by offering your palm up with your hand slightly extended. When you open jar lids, use a jar opening device or ask someone else to do this if you have a choice. Control your perpetuating factors. For instance, if you play golf or tennis frequently, have your grip assessed and changed if required. Don't continually test painful muscles to see if they still hurt. If you have or think you have arthritis, check for TrPs. If you have TrPs and treat them, you may find that arthritis is not causing as much pain as you thought. If your arthritis has not been confirmed by radiological imaging or other testing, you may not have arthritis at all.

Hints for Control (Care Providers): When you suspect that your patient has arthritis, confirm it. They may have TrPs, and the TrPs require different treatment. TrPs often co-exist with arthritic conditions. The treatment for one condition may affect another, so proceed carefully. Keep an open dialogue with your patient. Check for TrPs in the supraspinatus, serratus posterior superior, supinator, extensor carpi radialis longus, extensor carpi ulnaris, supinator and brachioradialis if your patient has epicondylitis. The pain from these TrPs may be severe enough to disrupt your patient's sleep. Take them—both the TrPs and the patient—seriously. Stretch and spray from the tip of the fingers upwards can be helpful. The extensor tendons are heavily involved in rheumatoid arthritis, so checking these tendons for coexisting TrPs and treating those you find may reduce these patients' symptom burden.

Stretch: With your straight left palm side hand over the back of your straight right hand, let your left hand gently stretch your right hand into a more flexed position and curl your right hand into a light fist gently going through range of motion until you feel the "bind". Then use the left hand to gently straighten the right hand again. Change the hand positions and repeat.

Breathing gently will help you feel better. The secret to good breathing is to first breath out on a gentle exhale with pursed lips for as long as possible followed by holding your breath for as long as possible until you feel the need to inhale. This is a wonderful exercise to do in the morning and evening repeated several times, while increasing the time that you can hold your breath even if that is one additional second a week. Most adults should be able to hold their breath for twenty-five seconds following a complete non-forced exhale. Improved breathing will reduce pain states and pain sensitivity while increasing your energy levels and your sense well being.

Flexor Carpi Ulnaris
Latin *flectere* means "to bend"; *carpi*, "of the wrist"; *ulnaris*, "relating to the elbow or arm."

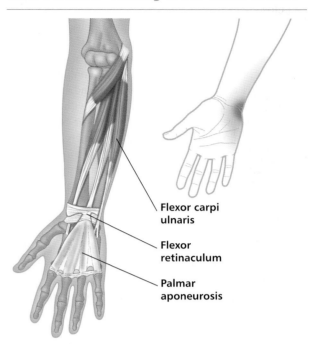

Flexor carpi ulnaris

Flexor retinaculum

Palmar aponeurosis

What It Does: Flexes the wrist, and works with other muscles to stabilize the area and move the wrist and hand away from the midline (abduction).

Kinetics Comments: Wrist extensor muscles affect grip strength by helping control the flexor digitorum superficialis and profundus.

TrP Comments: These TrPs cause finger soreness and decreased finger ROM. They can also cause numbness and burning in the third, fourth, and fifth fingers that may be mistaken for carpal or cubital tunnel syndromes, wrist sprain, neuropathy, arthritis, and other conditions, and may occur with these conditions. Weakness and tightness caused by these TrPs can lead to loss of fine motor control, causing disability; thus it is important to address these TrPs promptly.

Notable Perpetuating Factors: Repetitive motions such as performed by professional pianists, carpenters, skilled wood crafters, and computer users. Any prolonged gripping and hand twisting, such as in gardening and some handcrafting, can aggravate these TrPs.

Hints for Control: Learn to shake hands with the palm up, and be aware of how you use your arms and hands. Use the entire arm as a lever to protect finger and wrist muscles. Be attentive to sleep and resting positions. Avoid extreme curling of the hand and fingers, with the fingers resting on the chin or under the chin against the throat; this may occur during sleep, but can be changed. Awareness comes first, followed by intention to change, and then attention to change. Avoid gripping and hand-twisting motions, vary postures, and pace activities.

Self-treatment: A good dynamic exercise is to open and close your fingers, with full movement of the wrist included. Try using the thumb on your right hand to massage and compress this muscle on your left forearm. It makes no difference whether you move your thumb up or down: make the strokes long and continuous. Use a little water to grip the skin and fascia, and avoid going too deep. Eventually you can go deeper with the aid of a small amount of lubricant, such as a water-based oil or balm. If your fingers do not extend completely, straighten them out as far as you can. When you've reached the point where they won't go any further, hold that position and place the front of your finger pads against some immoveable object such as a tabletop. Then contract your finger muscles gently, trying to close or bend your fingers. After ten seconds, relax and take a deep breath, then close your fist completely. Immediately, but slowly, open the fingers to a new extended position. Repeat with the other hand. Keep the effort very light when contracting. If you use a more intense contraction, this technique will not work—less is more.

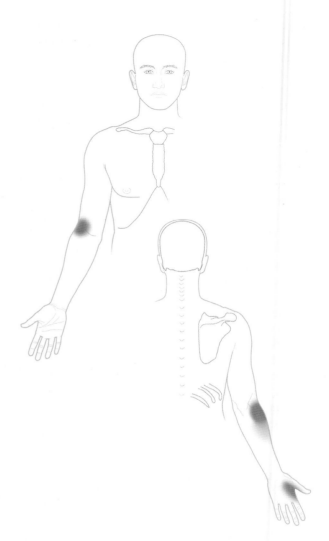

Supinator
Latin *supinus* means "lying on the back."

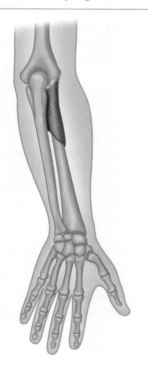

What It Does: Works with the biceps brachii to rotate the arm, primarily bringing the hand into a palm-up position when the arm is extended. It also assists in elbow flexion.

Kinetics Comments: This is a deep muscle almost totally covered by more superficial ones. If a powerful force is needed to supinate the arm and hand, the biceps brachii muscle is recruited to help when the arm flexes to about 120 degrees.

TrP Comments: These TrPs can cause the pain and weakness that may be called weeder's thumb, dog walker's elbow, or tennis elbow, depending on the examiner. There can be entrapment of the deep radial nerve at the elbow, as well as pain in the web of the thumb. When these TrPs are active, wringing out a washcloth or turning a doorknob can be incredibly painful, and the pain persists even when the muscle is at rest.

Notable Perpetuating Factors: Forceful or sustained supination (especially with the elbow straight), such as occurs with raking leaves, overturning a mattress, or walking unruly large dogs. Prolonged gripping motions, such as weeding, chronic use of a walking stick, or carrying heavy objects, may initiate or perpetuate these TrPs. If they are active, computer mousing can perpetuate them.

Hints for Control: Avoid overuse of this muscle, and find options for controlling the perpetuating factors, such as wearing a backpack or fanny pack (in Europe—a "bum bag") instead of carrying a heavy purse, or using mulch to cut down on the weeding.

Stretch: The effort to maintain ROM in the nearby joints should be the focus of attention, with the aim of restoring what has been lost. Place the back of your hands against your hips and move your elbows forward and backward gently. Gently compress the middle portion of this muscle: this will have a broadening effect on it and on associated fascia. This compression can be held for up to sixteen seconds, or you can compress for five to seven seconds, with a two-second break before another compression. This is a gentle compression with no pain and will increase the blood supply to the muscle. As long as there is no swelling in the area, this is a safe approach. If you are unsure about the possibility of inflammation being present, finish this stretch by cooling the tissue either under cold water or by applying a cold pack for three to six minutes. The ROM should be assessed both before you begin the compression and immediately after so that you can make a comparison—seeing an increase in ROM can be very motivational.

Adductor and Opponens Pollicis
Latin *adductor* means "toward", *opponens*, "opposing"; *pollicis*, "of the thumb."

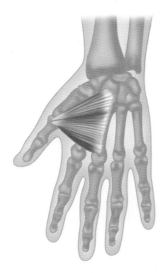

Adductor pollicis.

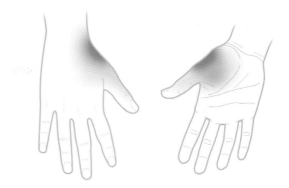

Adductor pollicis referral patterns.

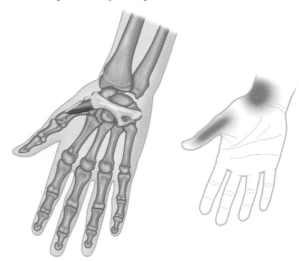

Opponens pollicis and referral pattern.

What It Does: Adductor: Brings thumb back to palm from abduction. **Opponens:** Draws the thumb towards the fingers so that the thumb tip can touch any fingertip.

Kinetics Comments: The three muscles that make up the thenar eminence are tightly bound together by fascia, and that fascia is tough. The opponens pollicis is covered by the abductor pollicis brevis and often partially fused with the flexor pollicis brevis. Palpation of the opponens pollicis is difficult, but don't be dismayed—you can treat them all at once! The adductor pollicis is a critical muscle used in gripping or pinching actions.

TrP Comments: These TrPs cause their characteristic pain patterns, along with clumsiness of the thumb, and a great deal of misunderstanding concerning the attention and care of the owner of that thumb. The ability to catch, grip and pinch may be compromised or lost. Handwriting becomes illegible without the need to attend medical school. Tasks requiring agility and control—such as buttoning, sewing, and painting—become difficult and frustrating because of muscle weakness and loss of fine motor control. Note that in the case of the opponens the muscle itself is in an area that is often free of pain, yet that area must be treated.

Notable Perpetuating Factors: Any pincer-type motion, such as weeding, sewing, opening jars, writing, texting, video gaming, computer keyboarding, or handcrafting, and any task involving excessive or repeated thumb pressure.

Hints for Control (Patients): Avoid rotational stress to the wrist such as that caused by repetitive use of a screwdriver. Pace tasks that use similar motions. Use the opposite hand when possible, and modify, delegate, or delete tasks when life allows. Avoid persistent grasping and pulling motions such as vigorous weeding. Use a soft felt-tipped pen for writing, and keep it to a minimum. These TrPs respond to stretch, manual finger therapy, and the use of small knobber tools. One of the authors (Starlanyl) uses a tool that is basically a marble-sized wooden ball with a small shaft on the end.

Hints for Control (Care Providers): Opponens TrPs may be mistaken for arthritis, carpal tunnel syndrome, C6 or C7 radiculopathy, de Quervain's stenosing tenosynovitis, or "unhealed" fracture. When pain remains after a fracture or the joint becomes "weak," check for these TrPs. Stretch and spray or light ultrasound can be extremely helpful. Avoid injecting hand TrPs, especially in patients with central sensitization (FM), as they can be extremely painful.

Stretch: A simple self-stretch for the opponens pollicis can be done using one hand to stretch the opposite thumb. Keep the fingers of the involved hand flat, and stretch the involved thumb gently through range of motion until you feel the first sense of bind then return to start and repeat. An easy self-stretch for the adductor pollicis involves filling a basin with moderately warm water and pressing the hand palm down with thumb and index finger widely spread on the bottom of the filled basin. As with all stretching the idea is to avoid unduly stressing the tissues while encouraging normal range of motion.

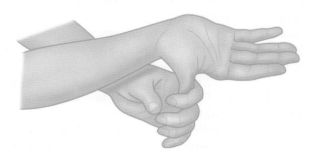

Palmaris Longus
Latin *palmaris* means "relating to the palm"; *longus*, "long."

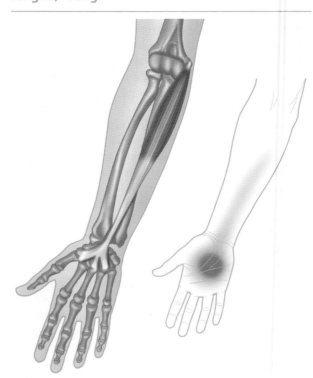

What It Does: This weak wrist flexor cups the palm and also contracts the palmar flexor.

Kinetics Comments: Due to its connection to the wide palmar tendon (aponeurosis), a progressive contracture may occur when this muscle tightens.

TrP Comments: These TrPs lie close to the skin. They cause a painful, superficial-prickling, needle-like sensation over the center of the palm and sometimes up the underside of the forearm, as well as palm tenderness. Pain can extend to the base of the thumb. In people who use strong repetitive movements with their hands, such as potters, the pain can cause a tightening of the muscles so extreme that the fingers are drawn up towards the palm. The palm feels tender, sore, and contracted, and there is loss of wrist power. This may worsen to the extent that the control of hand tools and even eating utensils is difficult. TrP contraction nodules may form in the palm. The TrPs must be treated as soon as possible to prevent contracture and fibrotic changes or even calcification. Some of these TrPs may be associated with trigger thumb, as the thumb locks in flexion lateral to the tendon of the pollicis longus.

Notable Perpetuating Factors: Trauma, such as a fall on an outstretched hand, and prolonged cupping of the hand or extensive grasping as with intense handwork such as pottery, sculpture, manual labor, power tool operation, use of a gardening trowel or deep weeder, and continually performing some manual bodywork.

Hints for Control (Patients): Perpetuating factors must be stringently controlled. After inactivation of the TrPs, stretch early mild-to-moderate contractures of the fascia under warm water, or after light ultrasound, and use tool therapy and frequent stretching. Check for TrPs in the triceps brachii.

Hints for Control (Care Providers): Ultrasound, stretch and spray, and barrier release are helpful. These TrPs may be mistaken for CTS or Dupuytren's contracture. There is presently no experimental data to tell how, or if, these conditions and TrPs are related, but we have seen repeated reversals of progression of mild-to-moderate contractures through treatment of TrPs in this muscle, the retinaculum (see Forearm Flexors and the Wrist Retinaculum), and the palmar aponeurosis. There is need for further research.

Stretch: Bend your right arm at the elbow and keep your palm facing forward, with the tips of your fingers facing towards the ceiling. With your left hand, take the fingers of your right hand and draw them backward, allowing your wrist to extend to facilitate the stretch. Always avoid pain and keep the stretch dynamic. This stretch will also target associated tissue and muscles, including the flexor carpi radialis, flexor carpi ulnaris, palmaris longus, flexor digiti minimi, and flexor digitorum muscles.

Lumbrical and Interosseous Muscles of the Hand

Latin *lumbricus* means "earthworm"; *inter*, "between" or "among"; *osseus*, "bony."

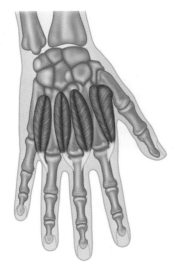

Interosseous muscles.

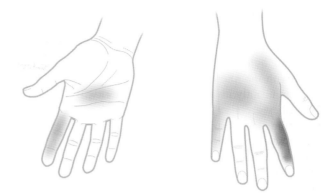

First dorsal interosseous TrP referral patterns.

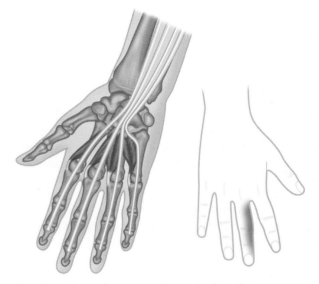

Lumbrical muscles.   *Second dorsal interosseous TrP referral pattern.*

What They Do: To readers who don't know medspeak—please be patient with the anatomical terms. You are learning about your own body. Your knowledge may prevent misery. The lumbrical muscles in both the hands and the feet pass between the flexor and extensor tendons and can be affected by them. The hand lumbricals work with the interosseous muscles (or interossei) to flex the metacarpophalangeal (MC) joints while they extend the interphalangeal (IP) joints on each respective finger. The interosseous muscles of the hand, like those in the foot, are separated into two divisions: the dorsal division is on the back of the hand, and the palmar is on the palm side. The palmar interossei move the thumb, index, ring, and little finger towards the middle finger. The first of the palmar interossei works with the flexor pollicis brevis to flex the thumb at the MC joint. The three other interossei work with the lumbricals to flex and expand the joints of the hand. The dorsal interossei abduct the index, middle, and ring fingers. The first of the dorsal interossei rotates the index finger at the MC joint, and may help the adductor pollicis in adduction of the thumb.

Kinetics Comments: As you can see from that simplified explanation, the hand is a very complex bit of engineering. The lumbricals are involved in coordinating movements involving both flexion and extension of the fingers. They work with the interosseous and thumb muscles, and all are significantly involved in hand dexterity. If they have TrPs, they are also significantly involved in all manner of spilling and dropping of different substances onto places where they don't belong, as well as in the creation of totally illegible writing. These muscles are richly innervated, which means that, if they have TrPs, they can cause an incredible amount of pain and other symptoms when you try to make them work.

TrP Comments: TrPs in the pointing finger (also known as the first dorsal interosseous) can send pain to the front and/or back of the hand, and even to the little finger. That's some coverage! The interosseous and lumbrical TrPs are similar in referral symptoms. The referral zone can include the back and palm of the hand, as well as either side of the fingers, depending on the location of the TrP. Finger stiffness is common, to the point of being unable to fully extend spread fingers. The most intense pain is usually felt in the last joint, where associated nodes may form. These nodes, or Heberden's nodes, are often considered part of arthritis, but are associated with interosseous TrPs. When the nodes first form they may feel very tender; this tenderness may be referred from TrPs. The nodes often harden with time and that pain can cease. Examination usually indicates no true joint-capsule or bony swelling. With these TrPs, you may have trouble buttoning buttons and grasping and holding objects. There may be active and latent TrPs in many of these muscles. They all need treatment as soon as possible, because even latent TrPs cause restricted movement, stiffness, and lack of finger coordination.

Interosseous TrPs may remain latent for years; when they activate, the pain may be blamed on arthritis or old age. Arthritic medications are not going to help these TrPs, and you may be needlessly damaging your internal organs by taking them. TrPs can be treated in a noninvasive manner, and the sooner they are treated the better. "Inactivating the related myofascial TrPs and the elimination of their perpetuating factors appear to be important parts of early therapy to delay or abort the progression of some kinds of osteoarthritis" (Simons, Travell, and Simons 1999, p. 792). Entrapment of the digital nerves by these TrPs is possible, causing numbness and/or parathesias such as tingling or burning sensations, but these effects disappear when the TrPs are properly treated. A condition of nerve entrapment called interosseous syndrome is often treated with surgery, but research has shown that it can be treated with conservative manipulation of the soft tissues (Saratsiotis and Myriokefalitakis 2010). Treat the cause: treat the TrPs.

Notable Perpetuating Factors: Any activity with prolonged or repetitive pincer grasps, such as weeding and other gardening work, computer and other electronic games, mechanical work, construction jobs, fine arts, and manual therapies, and prolonged playing of sports such as golf, lacrosse, or tennis. Trauma, or arthritis and other coexisting conditions in the area, can activate and perpetuate TrPs.

Hints for Control (Patients): Reduce the duration and force of the pincer grips controlled by the lumbricals and the interossei. Stretch these muscles frequently. Use pencils with soft graphite and other minimal-force writing implements. Some arthritis treatments, such as warm-wax therapies, may actually be working on TrPs, but other arthritis treatments, such as repetitious finger exercises, may worsen TrPs. Find out what you really have, and make sure your treatment is tailored to your condition(s).

Hints for Control (Care Providers): When there is pain in the palm, begin by checking the palmaris longus for TrPs, then check the first dorsal interosseous—they may both be involved. Mild ultrasound may be useful, but TrP injection of the hands may be extremely painful and should be avoided if possible. A flexion deformity of the fingers may occur with Heberden's nodes. Don't think arthritis unless definite inflammatory processes are evident: get confirmation. TrPs and arthritis may occur together. See what happens when you treat the TrPs. Catch them early enough, and, if there are no other perpetuating factors, your patients may be able to avoid the development or worsening of OA. We have no idea what kind of world it will be when all care providers can recognize and treat TrPs but they may prevent a world of pain.

Stretches: In a basin of warm water, press the palms of the hands down on the bottom of the basin, stretching the fingers and thumbs apart. For a different exercise, start with the palms and fingers pressed together in front of you. Then, while still pressing, move the fingers and thumbs out until only the tips are touching. Alternatively, treat yourself to a hand massage: it will stretch those muscles, and you will also find out where the "ouch" points are.

11 Muscles of the Hip and Thigh

Introduction

We use and abuse muscles without thought. We sit too long in awkward postures, using furniture that doesn't fit or support us. Many job stations are designed with the work rather than the worker in mind. The focus may be on doing as much as possible without moving, which may save time in the short term, but it doesn't save muscles. Muscles need movement, and a variety of movements at that. Then we may over-compensate on days off, failing to warm-up before and after unaccustomed activity. The muscles don't give up, but some may give out. The larger muscles that supply force for the kinetic chains are mostly found in this body region.

Regional Kinetics: Changes in one part of the body tend to start a cascade. Chronic low back pain creates changes in stride and in the recruitment patterns of the hip and thigh (Vogt, Pfeifer, and Banzer 2003). In addition, sacroiliac pain changes muscle recruitment patterns (Hungerford, Gilleard, and Hodges 2003). When we stand too long, the hip and back muscles form interactive stress associations as they try to support each other; these associations can cause low back pain (Nelson-Wong and Gallaghan 2010). Fatigue in the muscles of the thigh affects hip and knee mechanics, further impacting kinetics up and down the body (Thomas, McLean, and Palmieri-Smith 2010). Muscle imbalance at the hip may eventually cause or contribute to tears in the anterior cruciate ligament and other knee injuries. Correcting muscle imbalances may be the best way to prevent knee damage (Powers 2010).

Regional TrP Comments: When pain and dysfunction occur in the low back, hip, thigh, or knee, one should first check for tumors and other diseases that can cause the same symptoms as TrPs. That being said, it has been found that 96% of patients with low back pain have myofascial TrPs, and 48% of these have hip pain (Weiner et al. 2006). The most common cause of knee pain is TrPs in the muscles in the front of the thigh, and yet TrPs are rarely considered. Too often, knee pain eventually results in knee surgery; myofascial medicine is preventative medicine. Muscle imbalance may start at a very young age, yet infants and toddlers are not routinely screened for TrPs. For example, hip muscle contractures are often responsible for what is called "idiopathic scoliosis" in childhood (Karski 2002). If we identify and treat these contractures as early as possible, we can prevent further warping of the myofascial web, thus preventing many spine deformities, muscle compensations, and their subsequent imbalances.

This area contains many thick muscles, and deeper layers of TrPs are often difficult to access. If you have TrPs in the gluteus maximus and live in a cold climate or visit an ice rink, you—or your significant other—may have noticed that after prolonged exposure to low temperatures, your buttocks stay cold after the rest of the body warms. This slow rewarming may occur in any thick muscle and is a sign of impaired microcirculation often associated with TrPs and/or FM. Gluteus maximus TrPs can cause the muscle and the tissues above it, even the skin, to be extremely sensitive to microcirculation disruption. This region is also the site of many sports injuries. Kicking, jumping, running, walking, climbing stairs, and dancing use these muscles. They are our power muscles, and we use them to lift, support, and carry us on our way. They ask for our support in return.

Regional CMP Comments: When there are multiple TrPs in many of these muscles, as well as in the many layers of these muscles, it can be difficult to isolate the ones causing the worst pain. Pain can shift from one side of the body to the other with treatment: one TrP resolves only to have another activate. In CMP, TrPs are often part of an interactive cycle. Much of the research in regional pain is actually about TrPs, although the researchers are often unaware of this. For example, sciatic pain is associated with weakness of trunk and knee muscles, mostly on the sciatic side, as noted by Yahia et al. (2010). We don't know if patients in that study had TrPs before or after they developed sciatica, or even at all, but it is relatively safe to suspect they existed within that cycle. "Sciatica" describes any pain radiating from the buttock down the thigh. Sciatica and other leg pain can lead to gait changes which can initiate or perpetuate TrPs. TrPs can themselves cause sciatic pain and/or gait changes. Once established, the vicious circle has no discernable beginning or end. Although sciatica can be caused by pathology and that must always be ruled out, the most common cause is myofascial (Labat et al. 2009). In myofascial medicine, the origination of pain may not always be local. One of us (Sharkey 2008, p. 219) found that knee pain which was unresponsive to the usual therapy could be resolved by treating TrPs in the mouth.

All muscles are not made the same, and this is true from neurovascular and fascial viewpoints, among others. Therefore, muscles can be described independently by considering their circulatory supply networks, and the thickness of the associated fascia and its richness in proprioceptors. It's also important to distinguish the neural influences and neural physiology of the muscle fibers. For example, the gluteus maximus has significantly fewer proprioceptive units than even a small muscle in the base of the head, such as the rectus capitis posterior minor. If your gluteus maximus had the same number of proprioceptive units, you couldn't sit, as each attempt would cause a powerful gluteal contraction. This may also explain why certain muscles are prone to shortening, while others tend to become inhibited. "Inhibited," in this context, means the muscle response is slower. It is virtually impossible to find a patient with a short gluteus maximus that is caused by neural activity. If it is short and tight, it will probably be due to bone influences: the pelvis is tilting posteriorly, or the femur is sitting further back in the hip joint. The key is to find out what caused the pelvis to tilt—it could be a short psoas.

Example: A 46-year-old long-haul truck driver had suffered episodic low back pain for as long as he could remember. He saw a chiropractor regularly. He used a variety of OTC remedies for pain, and also took antacid tablets and consumed a lot of caffeine. When he was on the road, he often slept in his truck. He recently came home from a long trip and discovered his plowman had been unable to plow his driveway. He was already overtired and chilled, but shoveled over a foot of heavy, wet snow before he could park his pickup truck. After a sandwich and a few drinks, he fell asleep on the sofa. The next morning he had difficulty rising, with low back pain and stiffness in the hip and thigh. The right trochanter area was extremely sore, and he had sciatic distribution pain down the right leg. He'd been limping ever since, and could not sleep on his right side due to pain.

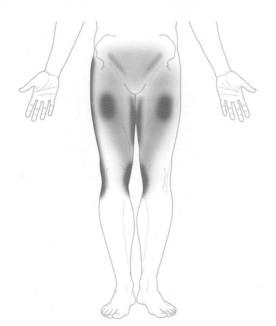

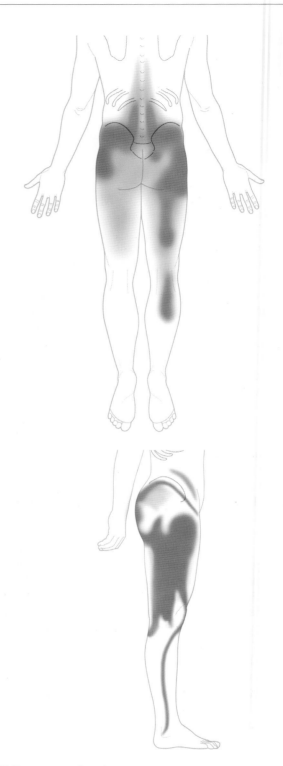

CMP patient referral patterns.

Examination revealed abdominal obesity with a lax, pendulous abdomen: he was 44 pounds overweight. TrPs were found bilaterally in the quadratus lumborum, low-level rectus abdominis, sartorius, gracilis, and piriformis; however, TrPs on the left side were mostly latent. TrPs on the right were found in the gluteus minimus, tensor fasciae latae, and the mid area of the vastus lateralis. When questioned, he admitted to occasionally having stinging pain inside his thigh, but he'd always been able to "walk it off."

The TrPs responded to procaine injection, non-manual thrust chiropractic therapy, cold and heat therapy, and stretch and spray. An MRI revealed some degeneration in the lumbar spine. He worked with his chiropractor to develop a stretch routine that he would follow; his chiropractor also provided instruction and handouts on body mechanics. He obtained an inflatable airbed mattress that would fit in his truck cab. He admitted he didn't eat balanced meals on the road, and questioning revealed that he didn't eat balanced meals at home either. He's working with his chiropractor to find nutritional supplements and healthy food options that work for him.

Regional Perpetuating Factors: Anything that impairs oxygenation of the muscle will be a perpetuating factor—muscles need to breathe. For example, COPD affects mitochondrial density in the thigh, decreasing oxidative capacity (Gosker et al. 2007). Those little energy factories—the mitochondria—don't work well in the absence of sufficient oxygen. This creates an energy crisis, setting the stage for TrP formation. Failure to stretch and warm muscles before strenuous use initiates and perpetuates TrPs. Big muscles, such as the gluteus maximus and hamstrings, are particularly susceptible. Postural overstretching of muscles, such as having one leg stretched over the other during sleep, can occur without thought. When muscles are overstretched, muscle fibers can tear. Snow shoveling and deep knee bends and squats are torture to these muscles. Exercise machines and most repetitive weight-training regimens can be perpetuating factors.

Immobility, including prolonged bed rest, can also cause microcirculation problems and damage the muscles. Bed rest can cause muscles to atrophy across the hip joint (Dilani Mendis et al. 2009). The phrase "move it or lose it" is a fact in myofascial medicine. Immobility includes restrictions such as casts: casted patients need to be checked for TrPs before casting, if possible, and certainly after the cast comes off. If a walking cast is placed on the foot, the other foot must have a shoe with an equally high heel or the stage will be set for TrP formation due to the resulting body asymmetry. High heels change the biomechanics of the knee joint muscles (Park et al. 2010), which then affects the hip and thigh. They compensate, twisting in attempt to balance shifting weight, which creates more havoc along the kinetic chain. Chairs are also major perpetuating factors in this region, because most were not designed for comfortable and healthy functional use, nor (with very few exceptions) were they made to fit the occupant. People come in all shapes and sizes. Look at an average classroom and the desks therein. This is a place where TrPs are made. One size does not fit all.

The unequal balance created by pregnancy puts a lot of strain on this region. During pregnancy, and immediately after, women have a greater chance of developing hip, knee, and foot pain, than at any other time, regardless of exercise (Vullo, Richardson, and Hurvitz 1996). Check men and women with abdominal obesity for insulin resistance, leaky gut, and the need for dietary changes. Abdominal obesity itself is unbalanced weight, which stresses muscles in that area, and often initiates and maintains TrPs in the abdomen, hips, and thighs.

Regional Hints for Control (Patients): If you have many hip and thigh TrPs, your care provider may decide to teach you basic stretch and spray techniques (see Chapter 14); ensure that you get a prescription for the spray and a detailed handout sheet for the muscles you need to treat. This may provide extra pain control to help you through the night and avoid an emergency visit. The direction and the order in which you spray the muscles are important, as is rewarming afterward. Ice massage of these muscles can provide temporary pain relief (Anaya-Terroba et al. 2010), but proper technique must be followed. Pregnant patients need to find a massage therapist who knows TrPs, and seek guidance on posture, exercise, and support. Lunge stretches, groin stretches, and muscle exercises are helpful, and tennis-ball and/or knobber-tool pressure can be useful. Once TrPs are under control, an exercise regime such as t'ai chi chuan may promote and improve stability, gait, balance, and coordination (Wu et al. 2004). Whatever the exercise, the teacher must be willing to learn basic TrP concepts and tailor any program to the needs of the specific student in order to avoid perpetuating factors. Needs may change as the patient improves or has setbacks. When physical flexibility is impaired, mental flexibility is required.

Regional Hints for Control (Care Providers): When there's pain in this region, check the sacroiliac, lower spine, and symphysis pubis. Upslip, or innominate shear dysfunction (upward displacement of an innominate bone in relation to the sacrum), is an important source of low back pain and groin pain (Travell and Simons 1992, p. 121). TrP development in the retinacular area of the patella is suspected, but has not been proved. Stretch and spray and other methods that can reach deep tissues are most helpful. Go cautiously. When tissue is stuck to the bone, as often occurs in this region, it's possible to free it, but this can be exceedingly painful. Injection therapy itself can cause explosions of pain. Be prepared for possible shock response by providing medical support, dimmed lightning, quiet, and warmth. This is more common if FM coexists, but it can happen to anyone, even with the most experienced care providers.

In releasing the adductors, release the hamstrings first. Then release the gluteus medius to minimize reactive cramping when the adductors are released later, but be prepared to treat the medius again during adductor release. Next, release the adductor magnus before the longus. After the longus, release the brevis, and then the gracilis and pectineus. *After treating each muscle, perform three passive full ROM stretches of the muscle.* Galvanic stimulation is ideal for deep muscles such as the adductor magnus. Avoid it on or near the gracilis or any muscle that is already causing burning and stinging pain. Empower your patients to do as much as they can with self-treatment. They spend more time with their own muscles than they spend with you.

Gluteus Maximus
Greek *gloutos* means "buttock."
Latin *maximus* means "biggest."

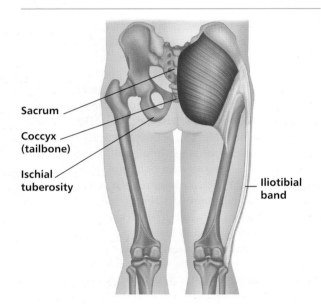

Sacrum
Coccyx (tailbone)
Ischial tuberosity
Iliotibial band

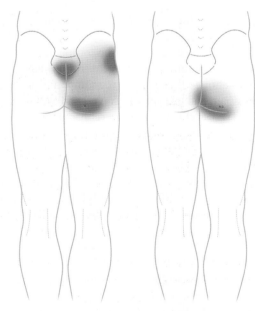

Referral pattern of TrPs in the lower midportion of the muscle, over the ischial tuberosity midpoint.

Referral pattern of TrPs in the lower area of the interior edge (medial inferior) of the muscle.

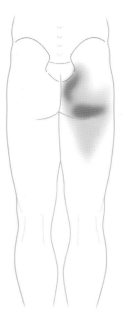

Referral pattern of TrPs along the sacrum area (superior medial) of the muscle.

What It Does: Rotates and extends the hip joint, extends the thigh (allowing us to walk up stairs and hills), and rotates the thighbone to turn the knee outward.

Kinetics Comments: The gluteus maximus is a **core muscle**, designed for maximum power and strength. It forms the thick outer layer of the buttocks and is the heaviest muscle in the body, as well as one of the strongest. It allows us to stand, run, and jump. Its attachments to the hipbone, sacrum, tendon attachment of the erector spinae, tailbone, thighbone, sacrotuberous ligament, and iliotibial band enable it to stabilize the sacroiliac and knee joints. Patients with low back pain recruit the gluteus maximus to help stabilize the pelvic spine during rotation (Pirouzi et al. 2006), but recruitment is delayed if there is sacroiliac pain (Hungerford, Gilleard, and Hodges 2003).

TrP Comments: These TrPs cause intense localized pain, with increased pain and restlessness after prolonged sitting, especially when there are TrPs just above the ischial tuberosity. Some gluteus maximus TrPs cause pain that feels as if a nail has been driven into the bone, making it difficult to sit. TrPs closer to the tailbone cause localized pain that increases when you sit, even without direct pressure on the TrPs. The TrPs in some areas can cause spillover pain on the back of the upper thigh, which perpetuate hamstring TrPs. There may be an increase in pain when walking uphill in a bent-forward position, and buttock pain on swimming the crawl or breaststroke. These TrPs may cause a staggering walk, mimic bursitis in the hip, or cause pain in the coccyx and gluteal crease. TrPs can cause this muscle and the tissues above it, even the skin, to be extremely sensitive to restrictions in microcirculation. If you are exposed to the cold and have

TrPs in the gluteus maximus, your buttocks may stay cold after the rest of the body has warmed. Immersion in cold water can cause cramp-like pain in these TrP-laden muscles, which can be life-threatening if it happens while swimming. This cramping has occurred in pools that were warm enough for arthritis therapy but not warm enough for TrPs. TrPs in this muscle may cause a limp or other gait irregularities that activate and perpetuate TrPs along the kinetic chain.

Notable Perpetuating Factors: Sports injuries, falls, failure to stretch and warm muscles adequately before strenuous use, low back or hip surgery, chronic low back pain, head-forward position, Morton's foot and other causes of hyper pronation, poor body mechanics especially while lifting, extended sitting, walking while leaning forward, walking uphill, sleeping on your side with the upper leg extended in front of the lower leg, and any inflammatory process such as arthritis of the hip, sacroiliac, pelvis, or knee. Gluteus maximus TrPs may be perpetuated by repetitive exercises, such as seated leg presses, stair stepping, and similar exercises using machines. These TrPs can be initiated by TrPs in the iliacus, psoas muscles, and gluteus medius and minimus. Good posture is important: a slumped posture causes weight to compress the gluteus maximus, while sitting up straight puts pressure on bones designed to support the weight.

Hints for Control: Check for any TrPs that refer pain to, or cause inhibition of, the gluteus maximus. Control perpetuating factors. For example, to avoid hyper extending the upper leg, place a pillow between the knees when sleeping on the side. Restrict uninterrupted sitting to 20 minutes. Stretch and spray helps these TrPs, but remember to rewarm the tissue promptly. Check for Morton's foot and other foot problems that may be perpetuating factors. Tennis-ball pressure release, manual TrP work, and the use of a knobber tool may help ease the TrPs. Sitting on "donut" rings will intensify the tailbone pain caused by these TrPs if the ring area is under the TrPs. The ring may help only if the TrPs are above the level of ring contact, or the ring can be situated so that the hole of the ring is under the TrPs. (A donut ring will not work if there are TrPs covering the entire gluteus maximus.) Although botulinum toxin injection has been suggested for relieving pain in the gluteus maximus after total hip replacement (Bertoni et al. 2008), we suggest that manual therapies and other alternatives be explored first. If these fail, TrP injection with lidocaine or procaine should be tried before more drastic methods are considered.

Self-treatment: From a neuromuscular viewpoint, it is virtually impossible for this muscle to become spastic and short. Because it rotates the femur, a short spastic quadratus femoris will give the gluteus maximus the appearance of being short. Not all muscles are designed the same. Patients commonly have a short psoas major, which, in turn, inhibits the gluteus maximus. In such cases, the last thing they should do is lengthen the gluteus maximus. It needs to be fired up! The best way to do that is to reduce spastic activity in the overpowering *psoas* muscle first and stretch it, and then ask the gluteus maximus to work.

Gluteus Medius
Greek *gloutos* means "buttock."
Latin *medius* means "middle."

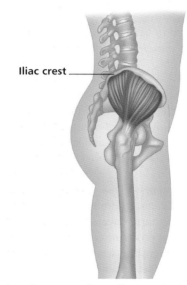

Iliac crest

TrPs in the gluteus medius often occur in a line along and below the iliac crest.

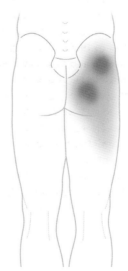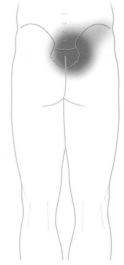

Referral pattern of TrPs usually found under the middle portion of the muscle along and under the iliac crest.

Referral pattern of TrPs usually found under the front portion of the muscle along and under the iliac crest.

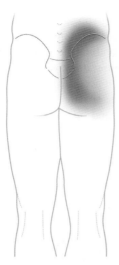

Referral pattern of TrPs usually found under the back portion of the muscle close to the sacrum, along and under the iliac crest."

What It Does: Moves the leg away from the midline of the body (abduction), rotates the hip mostly out (but can be involved with inward rotation), and stabilizes the pelvis. It also tilts the pelvis and keeps it balanced as we walk.

Kinetics Comments: This **core muscle** is mostly covered by the gluteus maximus. The lower portion of the gluteus medius, in turn, covers the gluteus minimus and shares some of its posterior fascia. The gluteal muscles have a close relationship: what affects one often affects the others. The gluteus medius may also interact with sacroiliac abnormalities. While the maximus provides running and jumping power, the medius propels us in walking and running, and also supports us during one-legged standing. It allows us to walk by keeping the pelvis even and balanced, supporting whichever leg is bearing all the weight during certain parts of the stride. Chronic low back pain may inhibit this muscle and can be a major perpetuating factor. When the muscle is inhibited, extra stress is placed on the knee.

TrP Comments: In general, these TrPs hurt most during walking, slouching in a chair, and lying on the back (compression of the maximus compresses the medius), or when the muscle is directly compressed. The pain can be intense enough to keep you awake, or wake you up if you roll over onto your side, compressing the TrPs. This can make sleep difficult if you have these TrPs on both sides, and you may yearn for zero-gravity. These TrPs could be mistaken for sacroiliac dysfunction, can be a reason for "failed surgical back," and may contribute to sciatica-like pain. Although TrPs in the gluteus medius tend to congregate near the tendon attachments, they can be found anywhere in the muscle. When the gluteus medius and minimus are weakened by TrPs, trochanter pain (in the area of the hip ball-and-socket joint),

sciatica-like pain and what some call "hip abductor pain syndrome" may result (Bewyer and Bewyer 2003). We believe that trochanteric bursitis may in some cases develop in response to uneven muscle contractures due to TrPs, and that TrPs may be a common contributor to the tendinopathy occurring in what some call "greater trochanteric pain syndrome" (Kong, Van der Vliet, and Zadow 2007).

Notable Perpetuating Factors: Poor posture, gait irregularity, Morton's foot, flat feet, repetitive sideways resistance exercises (including exercise machines or leg bands), body asymmetry, sudden falls, sports injuries, unequal weight distribution, hypermobile ligaments and tendons, bicycling in an upright position, injection of irritating substances into the muscle, running, playing long tennis matches, walking on soft sand, prolonged sitting with a wallet in your back pocket, or surgery in the area. These TrPs may act up if you stand on one foot for a long time or put more weight on one foot (such as when using a cast, cane, or crutches), carry a child on one hip for extended periods, or carry heavy school books on one side of the body. Gluteus medius muscles are so interactive with chronic low back pain that measurement of their activation patterns has been proposed as a test for predisposition to low back pain (Nelson-Wong et al. 2008). They are a common cause of low back pain in late pregnancy due to gait irregularity and uneven weight distribution, but may cause pain earlier if the patient is overweight or carrying twins, or has other perpetuating factors.

Hints for Control (Patients): It may be most comfortable to sleep propped by a pillow against your back. Avoid prolonged sitting in one position. Sit down to put on pants, socks, and shoes, to avoid falls and near-falls. Don't sit with your legs crossed (this is often a difficult habit to break). Using a rocking chair helps blood to circulate while sitting (it helped President John F. Kennedy treat his TrPs). These TrPs respond to tennis-ball work against a wall or on the floor, or use of a pressure tool, but beware: it hurts—a lot. At first, you may find it too painful. Remember, the pain created by the ball work is directly related to the amount of pressure you use, and will ease when you ease up on the pressure, although there may be residual pain if CMP and central sensitization (FM) are involved. It's more difficult to control the pressure on the floor, so start against a wall or press the ball against your hip with your hand. Go slowly and press briefly. See how you react to that session, and adjust the therapy the next day. Stretch before and after ball work—you may be able to stretch further afterward.

Hints for Control (Care Providers): Check for Morton's foot and other causes of hyper pronation. Teach your patients to avoid stretching through the joint if hypermobility is involved.

Stretch: Lie down with your hips on a padded surface such as an exercise mat or folded bath towel. Place a tennis ball under the gluteus medius. Stretch the muscle and identify TrPs by rolling the muscle and related areas over the ball. Perform tennis-ball pressure stretches too!

Gluteus Minimus
Greek *gloutos* means "buttock."
Latin *minimus* means "smallest."

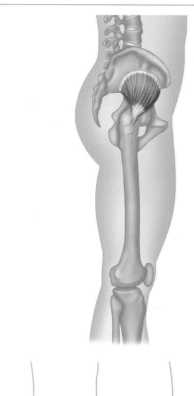

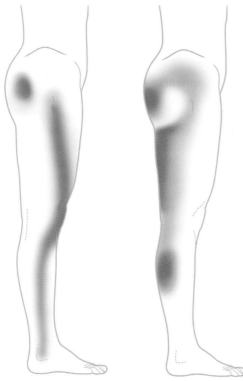

Anterior portion.   *Posterior portion.*

What It Does: Pulls the thigh laterally away from the body, and rotates the thigh medially (inward). This **core muscle** is a key link in pelvic stability. When you take one foot off the ground (as you do when walking), this muscle ensures that your pelvis on the standing leg side remains stable by reducing "sway."

Kinetics Comments: This deep muscle helps decelerate external rotation and adduction of the femur in the hip joint. It underlies the gluteus medius, supports the pelvis, and helps control pelvic motion. If you put a finger on the top area of the thighbone (greater trochanter), you can feel this muscle move as the leg is rotated inward. Anatomically, the term "leg" refers to only the knee and below; everything above the knee is the thigh.

TrP Comments: These TrPs may have a large referral zone, causing pain and/or numbness to the buttock, to the back and outside of the thigh, and even down to the top of the foot. TrPs in the posterior portion of the muscle cause pain further back that can extend down the calf to the ankle, and may be mistaken for sciatic pain or trochanteric bursitis. These TrPs can cause throbbing pain, as if the hip has a monstrous toothache. They can contribute to balance problems and be mistaken for clumsiness. Pain caused by these TrPs can be so severe that it interrupts sleep, especially if the patient rolls over onto the affected side. Travell and Simons (1992, p. 173) describe the pain as "excruciating." It may be mistaken for spinal nerve pain. If only one side is affected by TrPs, this can cause a limp or stagger during walking, and inability to cross the affected side over the other one while sitting. TrPs on both sides cause more than double the trouble. These TrPs may be accompanied by TrPs in the quadratus lumborum, iliopsoas, and other local muscles. The combination can be overwhelming, with no position bearable for long. Sleep can be difficult to gain and frequently interrupted. Unusual, altered sensations of pain or numbness may occur along the referral zone. TrPs here can be part of "failed surgical back."

Notable Perpetuating Factors: Overworking these muscles (including repeated exercise that keeps the weight on one leg for extended periods of time), crossing the legs and cutting off circulation, sleeping in the fetal position, injecting irritating substances into this muscle, sacroiliac dysfunction, obesity, quadratus lumborum TrPs, any gait disturbance (even that caused by a pebble in a shoe or a blister), and immobility. Avoiding immobility can be difficult, because with these TrPs you don't want to move—but you must.

Hints for Control: Frequent change of position helps. Wear flexible-soled shoes with good support. Check exercise routines carefully, and avoid repetition and overuse. Stand with the feet further apart to help stabilize stance. Stop frequently and stretch when driving or riding, or move about on a plane and do deliberate stretches.

Healthy sleep positions are crucial; a pillow between the knees and ankles can help sleeping if only one side is involved. Rolling over in bed or getting up after sitting may require assistance, and is a sign that aggressive (but not vigorous) intervention is required. Once the severe stage is over, take care to prevent activation by maintaining strict control over perpetuating factors. Treat these TrPs by tennis-ball pressure, but begin gently if pain is severe: you may have to start by rolling the ball against the side of the hip a few times. The use of moist heat before and after therapy may help reduce reactive soreness, but it's helpful to end the session with a cold compress for no longer than three to six minutes. Graduate to tennis-ball work against the wall, controlling the pressure. Don't overdo it—your body will guide you. Modify the ball pressure and duration accordingly.

Self-treatment: A short gluteus minimus muscle is short for a reason. This muscle is regularly inhibited and may not need stretching. We must first return normal neuromuscular efficiency, and improving core stabilization will aid in achieving this. Trying to "stretch it out" aggravates the muscle, compounding the issue in the tissue. Encourage dynamic ROM. Keep the core warm, especially the hip and low back. A gentle way to lengthen this kinetic chain is to stand with your feet hip-width apart and place your hands on the top line of your pelvis, with your thumb pads against your lower back. Gently arch your back until you feel the front of the hip stretching, and then return to the start position—repeat throughout the day. For those with coronary history, always avoid hyper extending your neck during this stretch. For people who would rather sit down, on the floor or a chair, a wonderful way to stretch this muscle is to bend both legs at the knee, keeping the soles of the feet on the floor. Gently allow the weight of each leg to fall "outward." When you reach the point of tension, bring the leg back to the starting position while squeezing your knees together; repeat the action as often as you like.

Tensor Fasciae Latae and Iliotibial Band

Latin *tensor* means "stretcher"; *fasciae*, "of the band"; *latae*, "broad."
Iliotibial means "connecting the *ilium* (flank) to the *tibia* (shinbone)."

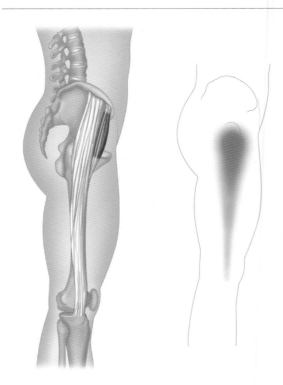

What It Does: This **core muscle** helps the hip to flex during the leg-swing stage of walking, and works with the gluteus maximus to create tension on the iliotibial band (ITB). This tension stabilizes and steadies both the hip and knee joints, especially during weight bearing.

Kinetics Comments: The tensor fasciae latae (TFL) controls force and motion rather than producing them. The ITB is a long, tapering band of fascia that emerges from the TFL and gluteus maximus fibers, forming a connection from the pelvis (the "ilio" part) to the knee (the "tibial" part). When the leg is bent and immobile for a prolonged period, the ITB shortens. When it becomes too short and tight, it may be difficult or impossible to straighten the leg. The TFL is a junction for many kinetic chains, so when its motion is restricted, multiple kinetic chains can be affected. It's often recruited to compensate for other weak hip flexors, and may be a key in same-side hip and knee pain. The ITB can develop considerable scar tissue that is painful to release.

TrP Comments: TrPs in this muscle and in the ITB cause hip joint pain that is often mistaken for trochanteric bursitis. It hurts to lie on the TrPs, flex the hip, or walk fast. It may be difficult to lie on the side without TrPs (if there is such a side) unless there's a pillow between the knees to help support the contractured muscle. These TrPs cause poor tolerance for sitting with the hip flexed. It's our opinion that persistent TrPs in the gluteus medius and TFL may in some cases lead to hip rotator-cuff tears.

Notable Perpetuating Factors: Poor posture, flat feet, Morton's foot, high arches, hyperpronation or hypopronation, compression of the area, sitting cross-legged (including yoga lotus position), asymmetry and balance compensation, sitting with knees higher than hips, sleeping in fetal position, repetitive motion with leg abductor exercise machines or resistance bands, some martial arts, walking or running uphill, and prolonged cycling, running, or walking on hard or crowned roads or other sloped areas. These TrPs can also be activated by sudden trauma such as landing after a jump from a height, or by hip replacement surgery.

Hints for Control (Patients): Chairs must be functional and comfortable and fit you, with an open angle at the hip. You may need a pad at the back of the buttocks to relieve pressure on this muscle, but this only works if you don't have TrPs in the back of the buttocks as well. Supportive shoes with flexible soles help avoid these TrPs, as does the use of a pillow between the knees during sleep if you sleep on your side. Warm up all muscles before exercising. A vibrating massager may help loosen a tight TFL and ITB before other self-treatment.

Hints for Control (Care Providers): Examine and treat the sides of the patient as well as the front and back, and use a patient symptom chart that includes side views. The Ober test will indicate contracture of the ITB. Iliotibial TrPs can affect contralateral sway due to defects in lateral knee stabilization. Keeping the TFL and ITB supple may help prevent lateral meniscus tears, anterior cruciate ligament damage, and/or hip rotator-cuff injury. When there is hyperpronation or hypopronation present, check for the *cause*. Multiple tissues may be contractured and in torsion because of these TrPs.

Stretch: Lying on the most involved side, extend and laterally rotate the uppermost hip. Breathe normally, allowing the hip and leg to relax with the exhalation. Then turn and stretch the most involved side. Advance this stretch by raising the upper arm and allowing it to gently fall above your head during the stretch.

Piriformis and Obturator Externus

Latin *pirum* means "pear"; *forma*, "shape"; *obturator*, "obstructor"; *externus*, "external."

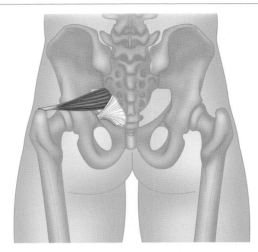

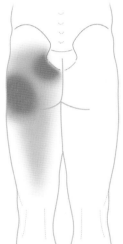

Piriformis anatomy figure (top) and pain referral pattern.

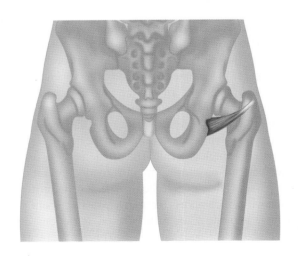

Obturator externus anatomy figure.

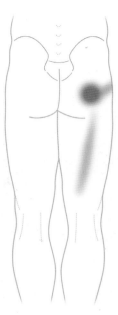

Obturator externus pain referral pattern.

What They Do: The piriformis rotates the thigh to the side and prevents it from over-rotating inward (medial rotation). As you sit, it moves the leg away from the midline. It also holds the head of the thighbone in its socket, and keeps us from falling when we shift weight from one foot to another. The obturator externus stabilizes the hip and rotates the thighbone to the side. During hip flexion, it pulls the top of the thighbone towards the midline.

Kinetics Comments: The five short lateral rotator **core muscles** are the piriformis, gemelli, quadratus femoris, and the obturators internus and externus. Piriformis weakness may become obvious when you attempt to get out of a car—you may need to use your arms and feet to help. This deep muscle also helps balance when you stand on a moving train or bus. A short, tight piriformis can rotate or tilt the sacrum, causing functional short leg. This is a perpetuating factor for dysfunction up and down the kinetic chains, including at the sacroiliac joint. The pudendal nerve leaves the pelvic cavity close to the lower border of the piriformis, and sticky piriformis fascia can trap the nerve there. Pudendal nerve entrapment is vicious; this nerve affects the genitalia, and sexual function may come to a screeching halt, or you may screech if it doesn't. Nerves that can be entrapped affect all sensations in the gluteals, much of the pelvic area, and the posterior thigh and calf. The sciatic nerve is usually underneath the piriformis, but in a goodly proportion of us it passes right through the muscle. As the piriformis tightens it can compress that nerve, causing sharp pain, tingling, numbness, or other altered sensations down the thigh, lower leg, and foot. This entrapment, or adherence entrapment as described above, is known as piriformis syndrome. Piriformis syndrome symptoms can be caused by other factors such as disc disease and tumors. The cause *must* be identified. The piriformis can

compress superior and inferior gluteal nerves and blood vessels, pudendal nerve and vessels, posterior femoral cutaneous nerve, and nerves supplying the other short lateral rotators except the obturator externus. When these nerves are entrapped, gluteal muscles and lateral rotators may atrophy.

TrP Comments: Hip pain, low back pain, groin pain, perineum pain, buttock pain, and pain radiating down the back of the leg, even to the soles of the feet, are all part of piriformis TrPs. The pain may be mistaken for OA. These TrPs can cause pain in women during sexual relations and impotency in men. Women may be unable to spread their thighs apart without severe pain. Piriformis TrPs can cause rectal pain, especially during defecation, and it's worse if constipation and straining are involved. These TrPs can cause or contribute to "failed surgical back." When you sit, these TrPs cause squirming and shifting of position. Chronic nerve compression from piriformis TrPs can give rise to intense pain and dysfunction (similar to that from a herniated disc) in many areas of the lower body. Besides causing piriformis syndrome, which should be enough for any TrP, they are often part of a matrix of TrPs in the hip and pelvis, and can entrap blood and vessels, causing swelling of the leg and foot. TrPs in this muscle can even lead to hyperpronation of the foot. The foot may feel numb, and proprioception may be affected, causing balance difficulties and a broad-based staggering gait. The obturator externus muscle is deep, and so is its TrP pain. Obturator externus TrPs can cause tenderness at the groin and/or sciatic nerve, but the pain may be so poorly localized that patients can't identify its origin. When the obturator externus has TrPs, the sacroiliac is often jammed.

Notable Perpetuating Factors: Prolonged flexing of the thighs with the knees spread (such as during medical procedures), sitting upright after a Cesarean delivery (Vallejo et al. 2004), chronic pelvic infections, arthritis of the hip, low back or hip surgery, sitting all day in one place with the hip flexed, prolonged seated positions in sports (such as rowing or cycling), quadratus lumborum TrPs, body asymmetry, Morton's foot, flat feet, sitting on one leg, sitting with legs crossed, gait irregularities, locked or otherwise dysfunctional sacroiliac joint, sexual activity, repetitive sports (such as running), squat lifts, twisting sideways while bending and lifting a heavy weight (such as stacking firewood or shoveling snow), and even sitting with a fat wallet in a back pocket.

Hints for Control (Patients): Control perpetuating and activating factors. Any work with massage tools, including tennis balls, must proceed carefully to avoid nerve compression. Keep these muscles in motion with the help of a rocking chair. Ice and heat can ease some of the pain. Ice often gives more relief than heat for nerve entrapment.

Hints for Control (Care Providers): Any of the short lateral rotators can interact with dysfunctions of L4 through S3 vertebrae. These TrPs generally mean a positive Pace Abduction Test. Proceed with care with any manual therapy and injection therapies to avoid nerve damage. Multiple nerves may be entrapped at multiple locations. Check for TrPs in the sacrotuberous and sacrospinous ligaments, the tendons, and other pelvic stabilizers. Obturator externus TrPs can be masked by coexisting pectineus and adductor brevis TrPs.

Stretch (Piriformis): Lie on a bed face down and bend both legs at the knees. Allow your feet to fall outward—this will rotate your thighbones and provide a safe dynamic stretch for all the short hip rotators. Return your feet to center and repeat a few times. Don't worry if you can't move your legs very far apart—those rotators can get tight! Once you can do this stretch comfortably, move your knees apart a little, increasing the stretch. Keep the stretch dynamic by keeping your legs moving slowly and not jerking the muscles. You can stretch all the internal rotator muscles with this simple stretch, but be sure to keep your hips down on the flat surface for the duration of the stretch. Loose, full rotation of hip muscles while standing (hula hoop optional) in a figure-eight conformation can help keep these muscles supple.

Stretch (Obturator Externus): Lie face down. Bend your knees and bring your heels close to your bottom. Allow your feet and thighs to rotate outward as far as feels comfortable. Keep the stretch dynamic and controlled. Return to the starting position. Repeat frequently during the day. You can also stretch this muscle sitting down on a chair. Cross one leg over the other and gently lean forward until you feel the stretch. Return to the starting position, and then stretch the other leg. Stretching the obturator externus will stretch associated fascia and short lateral rotator links.

Gemelli
Latin *gemellus* means "twin" or "double."

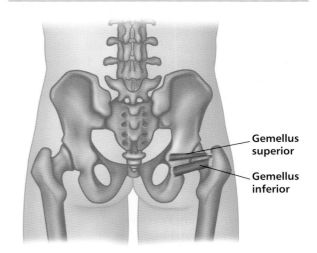

Gemellus superior
Gemellus inferior

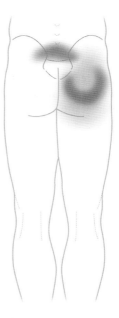

What They Do: Help the obturator internus stabilize and rotate the hip to the side.

Kinetics Comments: This pair of **core muscles** (superior and inferior gemellus) are short lateral rotators, which interact with dysfunctions of L4 through S3 vertebrae. The gemelli help to adjust for changes in the obturator internus as it turns. When they are tight and inflexible from TrPs, they lose the ability to compensate. Gemelli TrPs cause us to shift postures to *minimize pain*; these adjustments can cause distortions up and down the kinetic chains. Others may not understand why you need to move so often. Use this book to help explain that sitting on trigger pointed muscles can feel like sitting on broken glass or sharp gravel. How still would they be?

TrP Comments: TrPs in the gemelli cause *intense and relentless pain*. The muscles lie beneath the gluteus maximus, with nerves and blood vessels all around. We have no evidence in the medical literature, but we believe that the sciatic nerve can be compressed between the piriformis and the superior gemellus. These muscles have a high percentage of spindle cells, indicating a proprioception function. Do gemelli TrPs cause an inability to sense the true position of the hip joint? We don't know, but it's likely, and a good topic for research.

Notable Perpetuating Factors: See Piriformis.

Hints for Control (Patients): See Piriformis. Find a care provider who is superb in palpation skills and knows TrPs. That's what it takes.

Hints for Control (Care Providers): These short lateral rotators look so nice and neat, fanned out in anatomy illustrations, don't they? But anatomical variations are not uncommon among them, with split or double muscles, missing muscles, and, of course, myofascia sticking them together. The secret to separating them is palpation, palpation, palpation. Although these muscles can be palpated vaginally or rectally, they can also be palpated externally, and injected if the patient is in a hands-and-knees position, or knees-to-chest position lying on the side. Add some pelvic rotation. Dry needling helps, as does FSM, strain/counterstrain, electrical stimulation, and ultrasound. Check the pelvic floor, especially the levator ani and the coccygeus, for TrPs.

Stretch: See Piriformis.

Obturator Internus
Latin *obturator* means "obstructor"; *internus*, "internal."

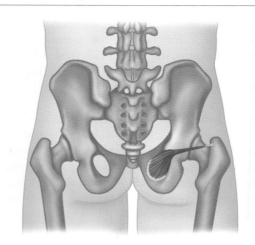

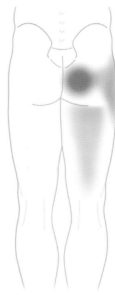

What It Does: The obturator internus helps rotate the extended thigh to the side, abduct the flexed thigh, and steady the head of the thighbone in the hip socket.

Kinetics Comments: This **core muscle** is one of the five short lateral rotator muscles, interacting with dysfunctions of L4 through S3 vertebrae.

TrP Comments: Obturator internus TrPs can cause the whole pelvic floor to ache outwardly to the hip. In addition to the deep characteristic pain pattern, TrPs in this muscle and adjoining tendons can cause sciatic pain (Murata et al. 2009; Meknas, Christensen, and Johansen 2003). These TrPs refer pain to the vaginal area and perineum, and around the anus and tailbone, with spillover pain to the posterior thigh. They can contribute significantly to vulvodynia. They may cause a full sensation in the rectum and limit sitting ability, and can cause backache in late pregnancy and early labor. They are associated with urinary hesitancy, frequency, burning, urgency, constipation, and/or painful bowel movements. Obturator internus TrPs may cause pudendal nerve entrapment, producing sharp pain, prickling, stabbing pain, burning, numbness, shivering sensations, or the sense of the presence of an internal pelvic foreign body. This nerve entrapment may cause male and female sexual dysfunction, anal and/or urinary incontinence.

Notable Perpetuating Factors: See Piriformis. Ligament prolotherapy can activate obturator internus TrPs (Jarrell 2003a).

Hints for Control (Patients): This is a deep muscle and hard to work. Sometimes you can catch it by sitting on a tennis ball, but be careful not to press on nerves and blood vessels. Be gentle and go slowly. Alternating cold and heat can help.

Hints for Control (Care Providers): These TrPs can be helped by FSM, stretch and spray, electrical stimulation, and ultrasound. The TrPs may be masked by piriformis TrPs (Dalmau-Carola 2005). When these TrPs exist, check for TrPs in the piriformis, iliacus, and psoas.

Stretch: See Piriformis.

Quadratus Femoris
Latin *quadratus* means "squared-off"; *femoris*, "of the thigh."

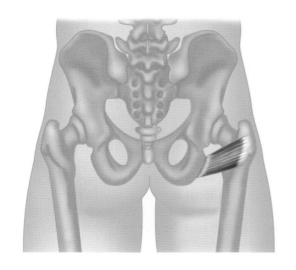

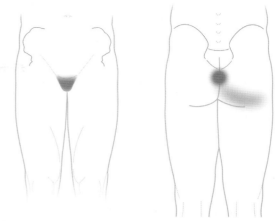

What It Does: Rotates the hip to the side. When the hip is flexed, it helps move the hip and thigh away from midline.

Kinetics Comments: The quadratus femoris is one of the short lateral rotator **core muscles**, which interact with dysfunctions of L4 through S3 vertebrae. Movement is the best indicator as to which lateral rotator is involved. This muscle may stick to the underlying obturator externus.

TrP Comments: These TrPs are often found in conjunction with other TrPs in the immediate vicinity, including the pelvic floor, hip, and thigh. Patients who have TrPs in this muscle have reported difficulty walking downstairs. These TrPs can cause pain that interrupts sleep.

Notable Perpetuating Factors: See Piriformis. Ballet dancers and gymnasts can activate these TrPs doing the splits. At least one member of an off-Broadway production of *Cats* extended a "hind leg" too far while "grooming." Cats we may portray, but cats we are not.

Hints for Control (Patients): See Piriformis. What helps one of these short lateral rotators helps them all.

Hints for Control (Care Providers): See Piriformis. When the quadratus femoris is tight with TrPs, there is a greater chance that tissue tears can develop and add to hip pain.

Stretch: See Piriformis.

Adductor Longus and Brevis

Latin *adductor* means "a bringer to"; *longus*, "long"; *brevis*, "short."

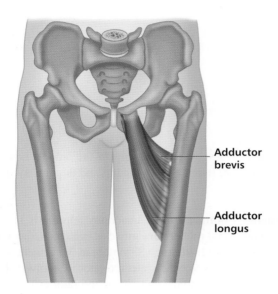

Adductor brevis

Adductor longus

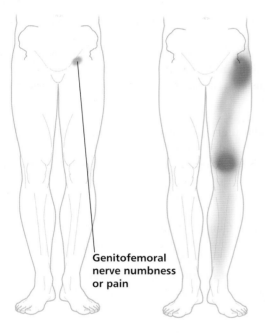

Genitofemoral nerve numbness or pain

What They Do: Both **core muscles** move the thigh towards the midline (adduction). The longus rotates the leg to the side, flexes the extended thigh, and extends the flexed thigh.

Kinetics Comments: The longus is connected to the back of the pubis and has a long attachment to the thighbone. Because of this attachment, there may be referral pain to the pelvic area, especially during intercourse. The location of the obturator nerve and adjacent blood supply indicates that nerve entrapment can occur (Harvey and Bell 1999). Tightness in the adductor longus interacts with traumas and diseases of the hip and pubic symphysis.

TrP Comments: Deep and often hard-to-localize pain and tenderness from TrPs in the longus can be mistaken for OA; these TrPs and OA may coexist. Deep groin and inner thigh pain may be most evident during vigorous effort, such as on twisting the hip while running up or down a hill. When the TrPs are very active, you aren't, as it hurts whenever you put weight on the muscle. Multidirectional restricted ROM from these TrPs may go unnoticed, even when extreme. This may be attributed to "old age," although it's reversible and can occur at any time of life due to TrPs. Although the pain referral pattern is the same as for the adductor brevis, adductor longus TrPs are less likely to refer pain below the knee. TrPs in the upper part of the longus can cause knee stiffness in addition to the characteristic pain. These TrPs are often the culprits in "growing pains" of the leg after growth spurts. We have seen leg swelling among athletes, especially cyclists, due to entrapment of the femoral blood vessels. This has been successfully resolved by TrP therapy on the adductor longus TrPs. Release of TrP-contractured adductor longus and magnus muscles may be accompanied by relief of unsuspected urine retention (Schnider et al. 1995). Brevis TrP pain is increased by sudden twists at the hip and by weight bearing.

Notable Perpetuating Factors: Overuse, especially in standing postures; trauma to the longus, pubis, hip, or thigh; coexisting diseases such as OA; vigorous twisting movements, especially if repetitive such as with exercise machines; prolonged immobility; slipping on icy surfaces; sideways stress such as with soccer kicks; crossing the legs while sitting (restricts circulation); and anything that changes the gait such as groin strain, hip replacement, or fracture. Leaning on the thighs while sitting, or resting a heavy weight (such as books or a computer) on the thighs, can also restrict circulation and contribute to TrPs.

Hints for Control (Patients): Any adductor stretching must begin with hamstrings stretching for complete release. To prevent reactive cramping, treat the gluteus medius muscles as well. Tennis-ball pressure, roller or knobber tools, and stretch and spray can be helpful, as can alternating hot and cold compresses. Use a tennis ball under the thigh to release the hamstrings during prolonged sitting. Change ball placement frequently. Pincer palpation (see Chapter 14) can work the TrPs in the lower attachment.

Hints for Control (Care Providers): Ensure that metabolic perpetuating factors controlled. For groin pain, check the inguinal ligament, adductor longus attachments, and muscles in other areas for TrPs, especially the pectineus. Successful release of the adductors can cause reactive cramping of the gluteus medius, so treat that first. Hamstring TrPs may inhibit adductor TrP release, so treat that before also. Ultrasound, FSM, and/or electrical stimulation can be effective.

Stretch: Standing, move your legs as wide apart as you comfortably can. Keep the leg to be stretched straight. As you slowly shift your weight to the other leg, gradually bend that knee, while allowing that foot to turn out slightly. Keep the kneecap in line with the middle toe of that foot, while keeping the knee over your heel bone. (Poking your knee out past the tip of your toes will cause instability to the ankle and possible injury.) Then return to the upright position, rest a moment, and stretch the other leg. At first you may need to hold onto a support. Lunge stretches, such as the t'ai chi chuan posture "Snake Creeps Down," are great for the adductors. The snake may not be able to creep down very far initially and may have trouble creeping back up—it may just want to curl up in a basket and sleep. Persevere.

Adductor Magnus
Latin *adductor* means "a bringer to"; *magnus,* "large."

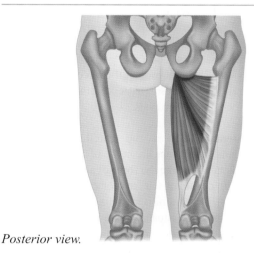

Posterior view.

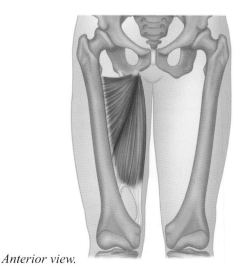

Anterior view.

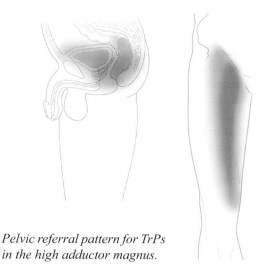

Pelvic referral pattern for TrPs in the high adductor magnus.

What It Does: Moves hip and leg towards the midline. The posterior portion helps extend the hip.

Kinetics Comments: This three-part **core muscle** is the largest and most posterior hip adductor. The upper fibers are sometimes fused with the quadratus femoris, and some of the lower fibers fuse with the medial collateral ligament. The femur attachment has multiple openings allowing passage of nerves and blood vessels—and creating possibility for entrapment. Tightness in this muscle and the lower tendon attachment can increase the likelihood of knee injury. These TrPs can interact with a tight TFL to cause gait instability. Healthy, supple muscles and attachments act as shock absorbers; tight ones can't.

TrP Comments: Adductor magnus TrPs can cause inner thigh pain that may extend to the knee, as well as symptoms that can be a diagnostic nightmare. That may be the closest that patients can get to a dream, because these TrPs may make it impossible to find a comfortable position in which to sleep or sit. TrPs in the middle region of the muscle and higher up can refer severe pain deep within the pelvis. This pain can vary, with a referral pattern that can include the pubic bone, vagina, rectum, and/or bladder. In some patients, the pain only occurs during sexual intercourse, which may lead to avoidance of sexual activity. TrPs high in the muscle can cause a diffuse, raw pain throughout the pelvis that mimics pelvic inflammatory disease or prostatitis. These high magnus TrPs can send a shooting pain into the pelvis that either explodes inside or drills up through the pelvis like a spear; they can also cause diffuse itch or other sensations in the pelvis. Adductor magnus TrPs can compress femoral blood vessels and/or entrap the popliteal artery and vein (Aktan Ikiz, Ucerler, and Ozgur 2009). Cold feet may be the least of your problems: adductor magnus TrPs can, in essence, block circulation to the lower leg, to the point where the pulse is absent at the foot and ankle. Active magnus TrPs can contribute to an unstable gait.

Notable Perpetuating Factors: Unaccustomed overuse; prolonged immobility; slipping on icy surfaces; sideways stressors such as soccer kicks; running, skiing, or hiking up or down hills (or stairs); use of adductor-strengthening machines; repetitious martial arts side kicks; trauma to the area; and anything that changes the gait.

Hints for Control (Patients): Any adductor stretching must begin with hamstrings stretching for complete release. Work on the gluteus medius muscle before adductors to minimize the chance of reactive cramp occurring in the medius. The adductor magnus is very deep and not easily accessible. Use a tennis ball under the thigh to release the hamstrings during long trips or meetings—or whenever you sit relatively immobile; this helps prevent stress to the thigh. Move the ball often, and treat each leg. Lie face down on the floor and roll a tennis ball between your thigh and the floor, from one side of the thigh to the other. Massage can be a great help.

Hints for Control (Care Providers): Check the pulse at the foot and ankle to make sure that blood is flowing properly. Control metabolic perpetuating factors. These TrPs may be secondary to psoas TrPs, so successful treatment of the psoas may allow the adductor TrPs to become latent. They aren't gone—so treat them. Ultrasound, FSM, and/or electrical stimulation or massage (and other forms of bodywork) can help to loosen these tight muscles. TrPs in this muscle can cause contracture after hip surgery. Adductor magnus and pectineus TrPs can interact with pubic stress symphysitis, as muscle contracture contributes to symphysis shearing.

Stretch: See Adductor Longus and Brevis.

Gracilis
Latin *gracilis* means "slender."

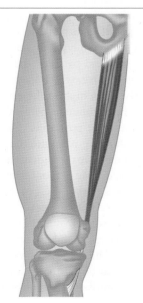

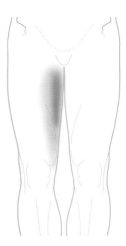

What It Does: Moves the leg towards midline, flexes the knee, and helps to rotate the leg at the hip so that the knee faces towards the midline (medial rotation).

Kinetics Comments: This long, thin **core muscle** attaches to the front of the pubis at its upper end and to the tibia at its lower end, crossing both the hip and knee joints. The lower tendons of the gracilis, sartorius, and semitendinosus muscles form a conjoined tendon called the pes anserinus (Latin for "goose foot") that may significantly stabilize and protect the knee in the upright posture. Gracilis tightness may contribute to fatigue fracture of the pubic symphysis.

TrP Comments: TrPs in the gracilis cause more superficial pain than those in most of the other thigh muscles. The pain can take the form of a diffuse achiness along the length of the muscle, and/or can have a hot and stinging quality like a burn. It's confined to the length of the muscle, and may be constant even when the muscle is at rest. Change of position, or stretching, usually doesn't affect the pain, but walking can relieve it. Check the muscles on both sides for TrPs.

Notable Perpetuating Factors: Prolonged immobility (such as when sitting in a wheelchair), acute or chronic overuse, trauma, restriction of circulation to the muscle (such as during horseback or motorcycle riding), slipping on icy surfaces, sideways stressors (such as soccer kicks), crossing legs while sitting, or anything that changes the gait.

Hints for Control (Patients): Walking can provide temporary relief of stinging pain, as can deep-water walking in a warm pool. The water may need to be warmer than that for arthritis patients (see Indirect Therapy in Chapter 14). Adductor stretches will work on the gracilis if the knee can be kept straight. If you are thin enough, you may be able to work on this muscle with pincer-like motions, pressing the muscle between the thumb and fingers and working from one end of the muscle to the other (see pincer palpation in Chapter 14).

Hints for Control (Care Providers): Gracilis TrPs may contribute to valgus deformities. Pincer palpation may be adequate for thin patients. Flat palpation and the barrier release method can be useful unless the patient is obese or the thigh is swollen or otherwise under extreme tension. Release hamstrings and other adductors first. Electrical stimulation may be problematic, as it can amplify burning- and stinging-type pain. Strain-counterstrain and other release techniques, stretch and spray, FSM, or TrP injections may be effective. Check the pectineus and the lower sartorius for TrPs. Tight clothing over the inguinal ligament can compress the genitofemoral nerve, causing pain or numbness in an elliptical area below the middle of the ligament.

Stretch: Stand with your feet double shoulder-width apart and your toes pointed slightly outward at a 45-degree angle. Keep your torso upright. Lunge towards one side, ensuring that your kneecap is in line with your middle toe and that your knee doesn't extend beyond your ankle. You will feel the stretch in your other leg, which remains straight. Return to the start and repeat with the opposite side. If you are not relaxed, or you find you are holding your breath, the intensity may be too great. Remember—sometimes, less is more.

Pectineus
Latin *pectinatus* means "comb-shaped."

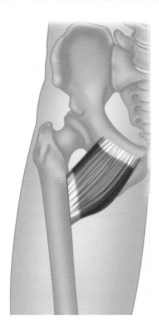

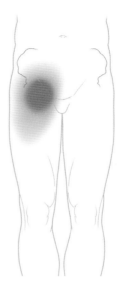

What It Does: Draws the thigh inward and forward and thus works as a deep hip flexor. The more the thigh is flexed, the more this muscle acts as an adductor.

Kinetics Comments: This **core muscle** helps us to walk in a straight line. It attaches to the lesser trochanter of the femur, so has a close fascial relationship with the psoas major and works with the iliopsoas to cross one leg over the other. When the adductor magnus and pectineus are rigid and shortened by TrPs, those TrPs can interact with pubic stress symphysitis, with the TrP contracture contributing to symphysis shearing.

TrP Comments: Pectineus TrPs cause deep, persistent, internal local pain in the groin area and hip, and slightly down the front thigh. The pain can feel as if it is coming from the joint. These TrPs are usually not alone, and may not become evident until after adductor, gracilis, and iliopsoas TrPs have been successfully treated. When those muscles are released—*Wham!* The pectineus TrPs say "Hel-lo": you may instinctively reply with just the first syllable.

Notable Perpetuating Factors: Groin strain, pregnancy, fracture of the femoral neck, gait irregularity, body asymmetry, total hip replacement, sexual activity, gymnastic exercises, sitting with legs crossed, and horseback or motorcycle riding. These TrPs can be activated or perpetuated by a fall, trauma from contact sports, prolonged sitting cross-legged, sitting with the knees higher than the hips, prolonged standing in a martial-arts horse stance, or doing repetitive side kicks. These TrPs can also be activated by stretching the muscle too far, such as by stepping into a shallow hole or onto a fallen tree branch or unstable stone.

Hints for Control (Patients): You can learn to palpate this muscle as you sit with your thigh rotated outward and your knee bent, such as described in the stretch

189

below. For palpation purposes, lean against a support (e.g. the front of a sofa), and keep the other leg relatively straight. Find the taut band and the tender lump(s) of TrP contraction nodule(s), starting close to the join of the leg to the trunk, then use the barrier release method (see Chapter 14). Equestrians should use Sally Swift's Centered Riding Technique, using legs and feet rather than thighs.

Hints for Control (Care Providers): Check for apparent asymmetry caused by ilial rotation, and correct it by mobilization and restoration of pelvic symmetry. Release the hamstrings, adductors, and gracilis first, and be alert for possible gluteus medius reflex cramping. Check the inguinal ligament for TrPs as well. Stretch and spray can be very useful for releasing these TrPs.

Stretch: Sitting up, gently bend your legs and rotate your thighs until the soles of your feet are together. Lean slightly forward until you feel the stretch—you don't have to go far. Then return to the start and repeat, making sure that you keep your back elongated. Pelvic tilts are good too. For those who prefer to stand, take your feet double hip-distance apart, with your feet facing straight out. Lean your body weight to one side while you bend the leg on that side at the knee. Turn the foot of the bent knee outward, and make sure your knee stays in line with your middle toe. Don't let your knee extend past your toes. The opposite leg will feel the stretch in the groin, including the pectineus. You can create a nice motion by rocking from one side to the other, providing a functional dynamic stretch, but avoid bouncing.

Hamstrings
(semitendinosus, semimembranosus, biceps femoris)
German *hamme* means "back of the leg." "Strings" refers to the string-like tendons that attach to the knee.

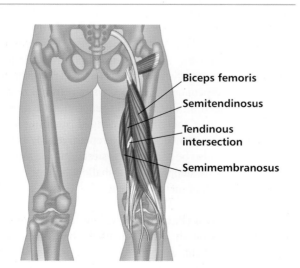

Biceps femoris
Semitendinosus
Tendinous intersection
Semimembranosus

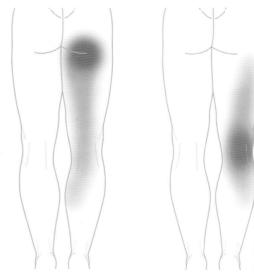

Semitendinosus and semimembranosus.   *Biceps femoris.*

What They Do: The semitendinosus (ST), semi-membranosus (SM), and biceps femoris (BF), together with their tendons, are called the hamstrings. These powerful **core muscles** work together to flex and stabilize the knee, and work individually to rotate the flexed knee. The SM and ST rotate the knee joint inward, and help rotate the hip joint inward when the knee is flexed. The BF rotates the knee joint outward, and helps rotate the hip outward when the knee is flexed. When the lower tendons are fixed, the hamstrings extend the hip joint. These muscles also help fine-tune pelvic balance. They may provide anterior and rotational stabilization of the tibia, supporting the work of the anterior cruciate ligament (Kwak et al. 2000). Hamstring tightness causes the rest of the body to accommodate up and down the kinetic lines, affecting the curves of the spine, the gait, and everything we do.

Kinetics Comments: These muscles cross the back of both the hip and knee joints. Hamstring anatomy can vary. Part of the SM may be fused with the ST or the adductor magnus, or may not be present at all. The long head of the BF may be attached to the sacrum, the tailbone, or the sacrotuberal ligament. These variations affect tissue interactions and potentially the muscles' resilience to stressors. The upper hamstring muscles attach to the pelvis. The BF attaches to the head of the fibula on its lower end, and the ST and SM attach to the back of the tibia. The pes anserinus, where the lower tendons of the gracilis, sartorius, and semitendinosus muscles conjoin, may be a significant stabilizer of the knee in the upright posture. If you can't touch your toes when bending forward, your hamstrings are probably part of the problem, although short and tight muscles in the foot, calf, or back can cause tight hamstrings. Tight hamstrings can contribute to posterior pelvic tilt, hip instability, and head-forward posture. Overtraining the quadriceps muscles leads to hamstring imbalance, and what author Carol Shifflett calls "bubble butt," often seen in young gymnasts. Hamstrings can tighten in response to weak gluteal muscles. When the hamstrings are tight, attachments and associated tissues, including the anterior cruciate ligament, are more susceptible to injury. Part or all of the pain that seems to come from the hamstring may be caused by TrPs elsewhere, including the obturator internus, piriformis, gluteus medius and minimus, vastus lateralis, popliteus, plantaris, and/or gastrocnemius. There are other causes of hamstring pain, but TrPs are often co-contributors. The ability to fully open the mouth is affected by tightness in the back of the leg, down to the sole of the foot! Amazing—isn't it?

TrP Comments: Hamstring TrPs are a cause of posterior pelvic tilt, and a key factor in many complaints of low back pain. Pain increases with marked knee bending, as when walking downstairs or performing similar exercises. SM and ST TrP pain tends to be sharper than the deep ache of biceps femoris TrPs, which is felt more on the side of the knee. These pains may be worse at night, and can often disturb sleep, especially BF TrPs. Hamstring TrPs cause pain during walking, and may contribute to a limp. These TrPs can be mistaken for sciatica—TrP pain must be distinguished from sciatic pain. It is not uncommon for the hamstring tendons to entrap the sciatic nerve, especially in athletes (Saikku, Vasenius, and Saar 2010). Hamstring TrPs put stress on the quadriceps and promote TrPs there. BF TrPs can cause muscle tightness so severe that it feels as if there's a bowling ball in the back of the thigh. Pain or discomfort when sitting is most commonly due to TrPs in the upper medial hamstring, above the tendinous inscription in the SM (Gerwin 2001), though they may also be found in nearby adductor magnus areas.

Hamstring TrPs are common in children, and frequently dismissed as "growing pains" (Travell and Simons 1992, p. 316). Children don't know what they should be feeling, and may suffer in silence; these TrPs should be treated promptly and perpetuating factors brought under control to avoid unnecessary suffering and central sensitization. Highchairs need footrests, since dangling feet may lead to TrPs. Support your children by supporting their feet, and check to see that your child's desk fits your child.

Hamstring TrPs may contribute to "failed surgical back." This may occur from hamstring overload as hamstrings attempt to compensate for weak QL and/or other weak muscles. When the hamstrings are riddled with TrPs, other muscles, including arm muscles, may be recruited to help get up from a chair or out of a car. This stress can initiate TrPs in compensating muscles. Hamstrings TrPs are common with low back pain, but do not necessarily cause it. Hamstring pain may result from TrPs in the obturator internus, piriformis, gluteus medius, vastus lateralis, popliteus, plantaris, and gastrocnemius. Hamstring TrPs in the part of the muscles used to cover

the end of an above-the-knee amputation stump can cause phantom limb pain.

Notable Perpetuating Factors: During prolonged sitting, feet should reach the floor or be placed on a support to prevent under-thigh compression. Fingers must be able to slide easily between chair and thigh. These deep muscles depend on good circulation. Short lower legs, short stature, and long torso compound this problem; in these cases footstools are a must. One of the most easily avoided perpetuating factors is inappropriate exercise. You can't strengthen a TrP-laden muscle. Avoid repetitious prolonged exercise such as leg curls, deep knee bends, complete squats, or repetitive stretches (including exercises using elastic bands, weights, or machines). Other perpetuating factors include body asymmetry, immobility, head-forward posture, soccer-style kicking, sprinting, gymnastics, and running up and down hills. Getting up from a chair after sitting with one leg crossed over the other, overtraining the quadriceps muscles, and bicycling with the seat too low (legs must be able to extend fully) are perpetuating factors. Postural problems may be revealed in photos of the body position during work, driving, and sports activities. Many TrP books suggest using a pillow under the knees to ease back muscles when lying down on the back. If there are hamstring TrPs, especially in the biceps femoris, such use of a pillow can cause painful compression. What helps one TrP may worsen another. Patients with low back pain may recruit the erector spinae, gluteus maximus, and hamstrings to help stabilize the pelvic spine during rotation exercises (Pirouzi et al. 2006). When the hamstrings are tight, check the gluteus maximus: if it isn't laden with its own TrPs, it may be lax and inhibited.

Hints for Control (Patients): During prolonged immobility, take frequent stretch breaks. Change position often. Use a tennis ball to stretch under the thigh, changing ball position often. Keep a pad under the back of your butt to elevate it, especially if you have bucket seats. Prevent under-thigh compression elsewhere with a foot rest, preferably one that angles up from the heel to prevent shortening of the calf muscles. Alternating heat and cold may help, and vibration therapy may subsequently allow deeper tennis-ball pressure. Dysfunction in other muscles, even distant ones, can affect hamstring tightness. For example, work done on the suboccipitals can ease tightness in the SM but not in the ST or BF (Aparicio et al. 2009). Stretching the hamstrings and associated muscles can help release the masseter and upper trapezius (Bretischwerdt et al. 2010).

Hints for Control (Care Providers): Remember, you cannot strengthen a muscle that has TrPs! Treatment must first focus on restoring neuromuscular efficiency and flexibility, and that can't be rushed. Hamstring TrPs may be hard to access through manual work when the muscles are very taut. Galvanic stimulation, ultrasound, microstimulation, FSM, stretch and spray, and/or moist heat and vibrational therapies may release the muscles enough to enable easier access for treatments such as barrier release. Hamstring TrP injection may cause an explosion of pain that can shock the CNS. Patients may require extra medication before and after injection, and care providers must be prepared to provide medical support if needed.

Begin treatment of low back pain with hamstring release, even if other muscles seem to be more involved. However, releasing tight adductors first helps release tight hamstrings (but if the focus is the adductors, release the hamstrings first). If they are all involved, go slowly, and release both thighs. Release of one thigh often results in at least partial release of the other. Symptoms from quadriceps TrPs can mask hamstrings symptoms, so the pain may seem to originate in the front of the thigh; nevertheless, you must release the hamstrings before the quadriceps can be released.

The term "growing pains" is a description, not a diagnosis. Find the source of the pain (often TrPs), and treat that. Children often respond well to stretch and spray, although this is not advised for all children, as cold spray can feel like needles and may add to the child's stress. Explain what you're going to do first, and be sensitive and ask for feedback. Manual work may be very helpful. Children may need pain control too, and often enjoy dynamic stretching. Teach them the correct way to stretch, and don't stretch hypermobile joints to their full ROM.

Stretch: The ball is your friend. Start with a softer ball or roller tool, and work up to a harder ball or knobber tool. Sit on the floor and roll the ball between the floor and the back of your thigh. You can also do this while sitting on a chair. Let gravity help release the muscles. Lengthening hamstrings takes time—they are bulky. Place one leg on a step or chair, with the extended leg lined up with your nose and navel, and your toes pointing straight up. If this feels too intense at the back of your knee, point your toes instead. Your hips should be squared and straight. Turn your upper body to one side and raise your arms, palms together, elongating your body. Then turn your body back to face your outstretched leg. Lean over slowly, bending from the hip, as you count (slowly) to five. Come back up just as slowly, and stretch the other leg. Then stretch the adductors. Repeat several times a day.

Sartorius
Latin *sartor* means "a tailor" (here it refers to sitting tailor-fashion).

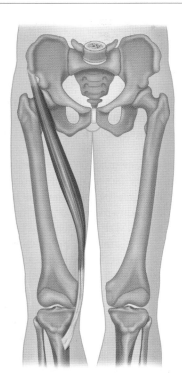

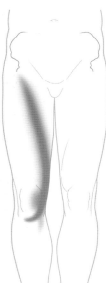

What It Does: Mainly flexes the knee, but also rotates the hip joint to the side. You use this muscle when you jump, or any other time you combine flexion of both the knee and the hip.

Kinetics Comments: This is the longest muscle in the body. Its tendon attachments may vary, and an attachment to the inguinal ligament or pubis can be reflected in the referral pattern. Some of its lower tendon fibers extend to the medial collateral ligament. A tight sartorius stresses the TFL and abdominal muscles. The lower tendons of the gracilis, sartorius, and semitendinosus muscles form a conjoined tendon—the pes anserinus.

TrP Comments: TrPs can occur anywhere in this muscle, and pain location varies accordingly although the whole muscle may be involved. Sartorius TrP pain can strike in heavy, superficial streaks or jolts, or may come as a severe burst of burning "electrical" pain on the side of (but not deep in) the knee, sometimes curling around the bottom of the kneecap with a fiery pain whenever one tries to kneel on the involved knee. Sartorius TrPs can contribute to pain and tightness in the ITB (as well as the TFL), with pain usually increasing when standing or walking. These TrPs are associated with a pendulous, flabby abdomen. Upper sartorius TrPs may entrap the shallow femoral cutaneous nerve, producing a condition called meralgia paresthetica. This can occur suddenly after repetitive motion (Otoshi et al. 2008), may become noticeable after a slowly worsening entrapment, or could be secondary to total hip replacement or other trauma. The nerve location may vary considerably (Ropars et al. 2009). The term "meralgia paresthetica" isn't a diagnosis: it merely describes either entrapment or crushing of the nerve leading to altered sensations on the side of the thigh. That area feels either hypersensitive to touch (even to clothes or a breeze) or numb, or may exhibit altered sensations, including that of water trickling down the leg or insects crawling under the skin. Symptoms tend to worsen when the thigh is extended, and ease when the patient is sitting down. The patient may be hesitant to describe these bizarre symptoms, but they're neurogenic, not psychological.

Notable Perpetuating Factors: Sports or dance injury, use of leg-band exercisers or adductor exercise machines, immobility, constricting garments, running on sloping surfaces, Morton's foot, sleeping in a jackknife position with the knees flexed, obesity, and any gait irregularity. Meralgia paresthetica is especially associated with the lax, pendulous abdominal wall often found in cases of insulin resistance, even if there isn't excess fat elsewhere. Meralgia paresthetica can occur during pregnancy or secondary to a lipoma. Sartorius TrPs can interact with other diseases of the knee or hip.

Hints for Control (Patients): Mobilize the tissue by moving it in as many directions as possible, using flat palpation techniques (see Chapter 14), massage, a broad vibrator appliance, or TrP tennis-ball compression. Start gently if meralgia paresthetica is present, working around the sensitive areas, while focusing on control of perpetuating factors. Use a pillow between the knees when sleeping on the side, with the upper knee slightly behind the lower one (the compression of one knee on the other may be too much to endure). If the nerves on both legs are entrapped, sleeping on the side may not be an option. Get that tissue mobile and blood and lymph circulating. Avoid prolonged hip flexion, such as walking or running uphill, sitting with the knees crossed, or using shoes that are excessively worn. Avoid the lotus position in yoga. If you have meralgia paresthetica, aim for healthy weight loss with adequate nutrition. Minimize excess carbohydrate intake, and ensure there is sufficient protein with every meal and snack. Protein shakes and food bars can help, but they must be healthy ones with adequate fiber and nutrition. Read the labels carefully.

Hints for Control (Care Providers): Check for hip, spine, and knee pathology. Mobilize tissue with gentle techniques. Teach your patients a daily home exercise regimen. Flat palpation and barrier release may help you creep up on the TrPs. You can't rush this process. Teach your patient ways to relax the taut bands; this often requires daily work and may need to be coupled with weight loss. Sartorius TrPs can entrap the lateral femoral cutaneous nerve, most likely in the vicinity of the nerve exiting the pelvis. Also check nerve sites along the spine, in the psoas, and in the abdominal cavity, remembering that anatomy varies from individual to individual and that the nerve may be entrapped in more than one area. Treat all TrPs and release the surrounding tissue. A lidocaine block of the lateral femoral cutaneous nerve may offer temporary symptom relief, allowing manual TrP release that otherwise might be too painful. Avoid friction massage or stripping techniques, especially if FM coexists. Surgery is only a last resort.

Stretch: We have seen patients who have come to harm through the best of intentions through inappropriate static stretching. Stretching must be prescribed with as much care as any other prescription. Not all muscles need to be "stretched" in the way most people think, and the sartorius is a classic example. Placing yourself in a position that will "stretch" this muscle will more than likely place you at a greater risk of injury. Stepping up and down using a secure platform is a good way to keep this muscle supple, but there are many components to this seemingly simple stretch. Step up by placing the entire foot onto the platform. As you step onto the platform, extend your body at the hip and open up the hip joint to the front as much as possible. Alternate each leg when stepping—just a few repetitions will suffice.

Vastus Medialis
Latin *vastus* means "vast"; *medialis*, "middle."

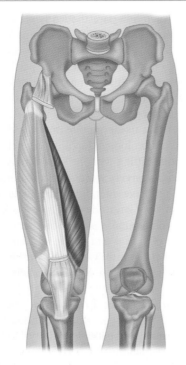

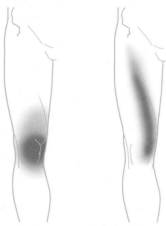

Referral pattern of TrPs in the lower muscle.   *Referral pattern of TrPs in the upper muscle.*

What It Does: Extends the knee joint.

Kinetics Comments: The vastus medialis is part of the quadriceps femoris (Latin for "four-headed" and "of the thigh") muscle group. All the muscles of this group, referred to simply as the "quadriceps," must work together for a smooth stride; they must be supple and coordinated for controlled knee action. Like the other quadriceps muscles, the medialis (including the vastus medialis oblique) is a shock absorber, and shock absorbers don't function when they are rigid and inflexible. The lower tendons of the quadriceps muscles join to form a single tendon in the knee area, supporting the kneecap. The quadriceps muscles tend to weaken considerably as we age.

TrP Comments: Vastus medialis TrPs cause pain in the knee, especially towards the inside, and in the inner thigh above the knee. It's a toothache-type pain, and can feel as if it's coming from deep within the knee joint; it can disturb or prevent sleep. These TrPs cause your knee to give out, or feel like it is going to, which is a particular threat to the elderly. Of course, if your knee gives out while you're on top of a ladder or in other perilous location, it's a threat to anybody. This dysfunction seems to occur more often when one is traversing uneven ground. Many of us don't use the interior of the thigh very much and it resents neglect. We tend to pay attention to muscles that cry out in pain, and this one cries very well. Buckling knee can originate from either the vastus medialis or the vastus lateralis (although the medialis seems more common) and most often occurs after the TrPs become latent. Vastus medialis TrPs occur frequent in children, and cause or contribute to accidents that may be blamed on a child being clumsy. "Clumsy" is easier to say than "vastus medialis TrPs," "vision impairment," or "proprioceptor dysfunction," but it may not be true and can be harmful. This applies to adults as well. Vastus medialis TrPs may restrict motion of the kneecap. A locked kneecap is usually the call of wild vastus lateralis TrPs.

Notable Perpetuating Factors: Body asymmetry, immobility, flat feet, Morton's foot, prolonged kneeling on a hard floor, sports and other activities that stress the knee and inner thigh, anything that places extra stress on the interior knee or causes gait irregularities, and trauma or disease to the lumbar spine, hip, or knee.

Hints for Control (Patients): Work on these muscles while seated. It's a good way to practice palpation skills, but be careful not to overwork the hands and fingers—stretch often, and use knobber tools and rollers to help. Tennis-ball pressure may be effective on the lower part of the muscle. Rocking chairs provide good exercise by keeping some muscles in motion. Avoid sitting with one foot curled up under the hip, sitting with the legs straight out in front, or sleeping with the legs strongly flexed. Ensure that shoes have low heels and flexible soles.

Hints for Control (Care Providers): Check for hypermobile joints and avoid stretching them to their full ROM. Hypermobile joints may not become evident until tight muscles have been treated. Check for lumbar spine, sacroiliac, or hip dysfunction. Stretch and spray, manual therapy (including massage), and electrical stimulation work well on these deep muscles. Start with the hamstrings and treat them simultaneously when you work the quadriceps, stretching them throughout the treatment, or the patient may experience reactive kickback. Check the other quadriceps muscles and the iliopsoas for TrPs. Check for weakness in the plantar flexors, as this may place undue stress on the quadriceps and help create TrPs. Treat pronation by treating the *cause*: a shoe insert may not be the answer, and one remedy won't help all causes.

Stretch: Stretching this muscle requires care and attention. Many people don't have the ROM in their back or hip to stretch this muscle using the traditional single-leg standing stretch. One problem associated with that stretch is that people use momentum to swing their foot into the hand of their extended arm. This can cause structural damage, including muscle tears. Stretch by lying on one side and flexing the hip of the targeted muscle. Once the hip is flexed, you're in a safe position to reach the hand of the same side around the front of the ankle. Now you can extend the hip until you feel the stretch. Squeezing the cheeks of your bottom can increase the effect without having to bring the limb through additional ROM. Use a towel or stretch rope if necessary. An alternative is to squat down while standing on both feet *just* until you feel a stretch, then return to standing. If you need to hold onto a wall or other support, do so. *Seek professional advice if attempting to complete this stretch (or any other) hurts your knees or back.*

Vastus Lateralis
Latin *vastus* means "vast"; *lateralis*, "side."

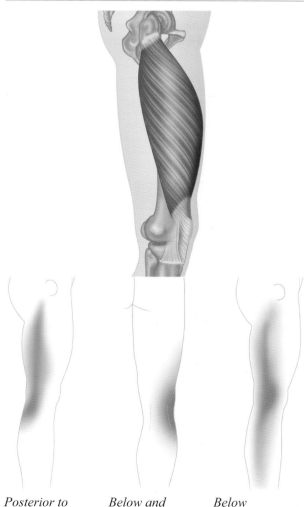

Posterior to Hornets' nest. *Below and posterior to Hornets' nest.* *Below Hornets' nest.*

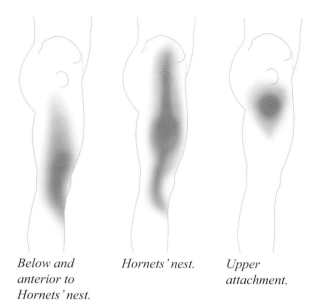

Below and anterior to Hornets' nest. *Hornets' nest.* *Upper attachment.*

What It Does: Extends the knee joint, and works with the medialis to stabilize the kneecap. If both muscles don't work in a coordinated fashion, more than the kneecap is in trouble.

Kinetics Comments: The vastus lateralis is part of the quadriceps muscle group—the part that forms much of the outside of the thigh. It has a broad tendon attachment on the upper side, with fibers that interact with the fascia lata. The lower tendon interacts with the ITB and the kneecap. Each quadriceps muscle is more active in a different stage of extension. See Vastus Medialis.

TrP Comments: This muscle harbors common TrP sites along the outside of the thigh, from the pelvis to the knee, and referral patterns may extend into and through the back of the knee. Symptoms are chiefly pain and muscle weakness. There may be multiple interacting TrP patterns from TrPs in layers throughout the muscle. The pain may disturb your sleep, and it can be impossibly painful to lie on your side. In some cases, a lightning-like jolt of pain may strike if you roll over onto the TrP or if something or someone presses it. If you experience this, alert your medical team to avoid pressure therapies in that area. This jolt of pain may strike when kneeling, and is responsible for this Episcopalian (Starlanyl) standing for prayer instead. For me, the culprit was most often a cluster of TrPs outside and slightly above the kneecap.

These TrPs usually hurt more during walking than sitting. TrP pain referral in the upper area is often mistaken for trochanteric bursitis. TrPs, most often those in the lower part of the muscle, can restrict motion of the kneecap and even cause the knee to lock when the leg is straight. With a locked kneecap, you may be unable to walk, or even sit comfortably unless the leg is extended. That, of course, will perpetuate TrPs in other quadriceps muscles. A locked knee can be frightening unless you know why it locked and what to do about it. Lateralis TrPs tend to become fibrotic. The whole muscle may feel tight and swollen. This often starts near the attachments, and complicates treatment.

Lateralis TrPs can cause deep knee pain that may wrap around the outside edge of the knee and under the outer half of the kneecap, or may spread around to the back of the knee. They often occur in clusters, and breaking them up can be difficult and painful. There's an area near mid thigh that Travell and Simons call the "hornets' nest." This cluster of TrPs can cause pain along the thigh and hip that may travel down to and curve around the bottom of the knee. Another cluster may form further towards the back to the thigh, on the same level as the hornets' nest. That group sends vertical pain down the thigh a bit further back. Unexplained thigh and knee pain in children, even in infants, is often caused by quadriceps TrPs.

Notable Perpetuating Factors: Body asymmetry, gait irregularities, poor posture, shoes or boots with high heels, instability of the pelvis or low back, immobility, trauma, use of knee-extension exercise machines, TrPs in the hamstrings and TFL, and tightness in the ITB. When you kneel or squat for a long time, you invite these TrPs. Avoid prolonged sitting with the legs out straight in front of you. Latent vastus lateralis TrPs may activate from insulin or other injections. Buckling knee can occur from medialis or lateralis TrPs.

Hints for Control (Patients): If you've experienced a lightning-like or nerve-type pain in this referral area, use care with any pressure therapy on this muscle. Use a *light* touch to palpate. See if you can feel the difference between the ITB (with the TFL) and the vastus lateralis. Stretch them both often, but not repetitiously. Try the gentlest therapy first, and control perpetuating factors. Do what you can to improve microcirculation in the area. Moist heat and cold, barrier release, and gentle manual work *around* the TrP areas may help loosen the tissues and get fluid flowing. You can work this muscle with your fingers while seated, but it can be difficult. The entire muscle may be riddled with TrPs—some may be extremely sore, and some may be in the tendon attachments and ITB. You may only be able to work TrPs in the top layers at first. Be patient and don't overwork your fingers. Try gentle vibration or a roller tool. If you can do so without undue pain, use knobber tools or tennis-ball therapy to help. If the TrPs are too tender, try a softer surface at first.

Hints for Control (Care Providers): Check for hypermobile joints and avoid stretching them to their full ROM. Hypermobile joints may not become evident until TrPs have been treated. Check for lumbar spine, sacroiliac, or hip dysfunction, and for ITB TrPs. This muscle tends to become fibrotic. This can be reversed, but proceed slowly and gently to avoid worsening central sensitization. If FM is already present, avoid more painful therapies. *Don't attempt to force the tissues apart!* Barrier release is still possible, but you may need moist heat, vibration, electrical stimulation (if meralgia paresthetica is not present), or stretch and spray to help break up fibrotic tissue, thus allowing further work to be done on these deep muscles. Injection of deep lateralis TrPs may cause an explosion of pain. Take precautions. The presence of coexisting conditions, other TrPs, geloid masses, calcifications, and scars complicates treatment. Be innovative, keep a dialogue open with your patient, and use a soft touch. Provide handouts for situations that would otherwise be considered emergencies, such as a locked kneecap. See Vastus Medialis.

Stretch: *The single-leg standing stretch often used for this muscle is ineffective and can even be dangerous.* The vastus lateralis, lying as it does on the most lateral aspect of the biggest bone in your body, is best stretched by means of massage and hands-on mobilization.

Vastus Intermedius
Latin *vastus* means "vast"; *intermedius*, "intermediate."

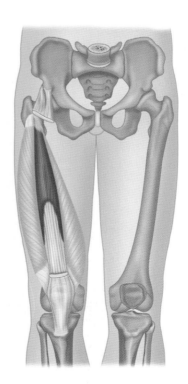
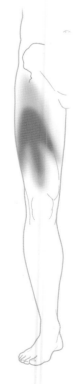

What It Does: Extends the knee joint, and thus extends the leg.

Kinetics Comments: See Vastus Medialis.

TrP Comments: These TrPs aren't as common as other quadriceps TrPs, and they often can't be felt because this muscle lies beneath the rectus femoris. Patients can feel the referral pain, especially when the muscle is in motion. The referral pattern is shaped like a dinosaur's claw, and you don't want it stomping on your leg. With these TrPs, after climbing one step, the leg may not want to straighten; after prolonged sitting or lying with that knee flexed and the muscle short, you may limp for a while. If TrPs are present both in the rectus femoris and high in the vastus intermedius, the hip can give out ("buckling hip syndrome"). You may fall, causing even more TrPs and more pain. Travell and Simons (1992, pp. 280–281) mention the possibility of severe "autonomic disruption" caused by the "explosive impact of injecting these TrPs." Those authors mostly wrote of minimal TrP situations in individual muscle chapters, and without the impact of interactive conditions such as FM. We now know that central sensitization can occur with chronic myofascial pain. We suspect that the "apprehensive patients" to whom Travell and Simons referred were patients with FM. TrP injections can be done on deep TrPs, but it may require intensive pain control—before, during, and after—to avoid further damage to the CNS. Pain management techniques include medication, craniosacral and other CNS-soothing work, adequate medications, prayer, meditation, and positive visualization.

Notable Perpetuating Factors: These TrPs are often secondary to other quadriceps and area TrPs. Good body mechanics aren't always enough to prevent them: for example, when the soleus is weak due to TrPs, the quadriceps muscles try to compensate for them during heavy lifting. It isn't just time that differentiates acute trauma from chronic trauma. The latter is often self-inflicted, and may occur through work-related repetitive motions, overdoing sports activities, poor posture, exercise machines, or doing excessive knee bends.

Hints for Control (Patients): Care options depend on what you are able to do, on what coexisting conditions you have, and on coexisting TrPs. You must go through the rectus femoris to reach the intermedius, and TrPs in the intermedius are often secondary to TrPs in the rectus femoris. If you have multiple TrPs in the thigh area, stretch and spray can be a blessing. Try to find a care provider who can teach you the basic safe technique for this region. You can then start to release one hamstring, move on to an adductor, progress to the quadriceps, and so forth. You can't do it all yourself, but you can do a lot. If the overlying tissues and the pain level allow, try a smaller, harder ball than a tennis ball to get to this muscle. Moist heat, a roller tool, and/or a wide vibration tool may help loosen the overlying tissue, and that may help loosen the intermedius as well. With time and attention, you can learn to differentiate the layers of tissue with palpation. This is your body—be patient. Anything that releases any of the thigh muscles can help.

Hints for Control (Care Providers): It's important to be aware of the effects of TrP injections (see TrP comments above). Vastus intermedius TrPs significantly impair knee flexion, and that may offer a clue to their presence. Seek the primary TrPs, including those in the iliopsoas, TFL, gluteal muscles, hamstrings, and other quadriceps: treat them and it will be easier to clear the intermedius. Check the intermedius for latent TrPs if muscles in other areas have been treated for TrPs and symptoms persist. Don't feel overwhelmed. Your patient is part of the treatment team, and there is more to self-treatment than stretching. Empower them. To those suitable, provide written handouts for techniques within their capabilities. These may include basic, safe stretch and spray for some patients (see Chapter 14). The education/handout approach may work with contract-relax methods, muscle energy techniques, and other procedures that you find useful as well. Investigate and treat the cause(s) of any hyperpronation. Even if care has been taken to exercise all the muscles, there may be hidden factors that lead to muscle imbalance: for example, the vastus intermedius fatigues at a significantly higher rate than the vastus lateralis (Watanabe and Akima 2010). Check for perpetuating factors that may be depleting the muscles of oxygen.

Stretch: Self-massage over this muscle is recommended for enhancing pliability and length.

Rectus Femoris
Latin *rectus* means "straight"; *femoris,* "of the thigh."

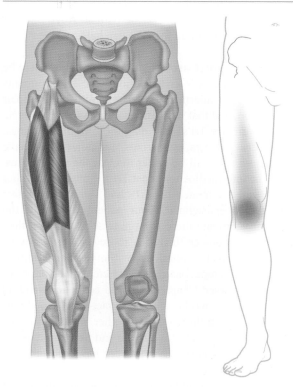

What It Does: This **core muscle** is part of the quadriceps muscle group, and the only one of these muscles that crosses both the hip and knee joints. In addition to the quadriceps action of extending the knee, this muscle also flexes the thigh, working particularly hard during straight-leg raises and any movement that combines hip flexion with knee extension.

Kinetics Comments: Everything this muscle does involves two joints, adding to the complexity of its interactions with other tissues and the kinetic chains. Any shortening or lengthening of the muscle affects many other muscles, tendons, and ligaments. The rectus femoris is activated during walking as the leg comes forward and the knee extends—the "swing phase" of the stride. Tightness due to TrPs in this muscle places additional stress on the cruciate ligaments of the knee, making them susceptible to injury. See Vastus Medialis.

TrP Comments: Rectus femoris TrPs can cause a sense of thigh and leg weakness, especially when going downstairs. The combination of TrPs in this muscle and in the vastus intermedius can cause the hip to buckle when both the hip and knee are extended. If the knee itself buckles, check for TrPs in the vastus medialis as well as in the tendon insertion area. Rec fem TrPs cause pain in the front of the leg and deep into the knee, especially noticeable at night. There's often a sense of knee weakness. The most common rectus femoris TrPs

occur at the upper end, although they send pain to the lower front thigh and knee, and especially to the kneecap. This pain can feel like joint pain; it's very deep, and intense enough to disturb sleep. Rectus femoris TrPs also tend to form just above the knee near the kneecap, and they refer pain deep into the knee. As with all muscles, TrPs can occur in any area. These TrPs are frequently associated with growing pains. Moreover, they can mask hamstrings symptoms. Though it may seem as if all the pain is coming from the front of the thigh, surprise!—it's not always the case.

Notable Perpetuating Factors: Prolonged immobility (a cast), flat feet, Morton's foot and other causes of hyperpronation, gait irregularities, misalignments of tissues in the leg, body asymmetry or torsion, tight hamstrings, falls, sleeping in fetal or other knee-flexed positions, or any activity that includes landing with the weight heavily on the feet (from parachuting and hang gliding to jumping over an obstacle). Activities that require frequent or repetitive knee stress (such as skiing, hockey, soccer, and gardening), repetitive knee exercises (including squats, kicks, jumps, leg presses, and knee extensions), prolonged sitting with a heavy weight on the lap (a child or computer), deep knee bends, or running hurdle races can activate or worsen these TrPs. So can disease, surgery or other trauma, or lumbar spine, hip, or thigh fracture.

Sitting with one foot tucked under the buttock is a common, yet avoidable, initiating or perpetuating factor of quadriceps TrPs; sitting with both feet under the buttocks isn't good either. High heels add stress to the whole body. Rectus femoris TrPs can be secondary to iliopsoas TrPs, and hamstring TrPs can initiate and perpetuate TrPs in any of the quadriceps. Latent rectus femoris or vastus lateralis TrPs may be activated by insulin or other injections. TrPs in one quadriceps muscle encourage the formation of TrPs in the rest of them. Growth spurts may initiate "growing pains" that are really treatable TrPs.

Hints for Control (Patients): Massage the TrPs, not the referred pain. Try a roller tool—it can work wonders. You can also treat this muscle sitting, using a bent elbow on the muscle, although you may need a knobber tool to get the high TrPs. If you can lie on the floor on your belly, you can work these TrPs with a tennis ball between the front of your thigh and the floor. If you sleep on your side, put a pillow between your legs to prevent the upper knee from overextending. When these TrPs are active, use your arms to assist you in getting out of chairs. Switch your usual reading or other entertainment furniture to a rocking chair that fits you.

Hints for Control (Care Providers): See Vastus Medialis.

Stretch: See Vastus Medialis

12 Muscles of the Lower Leg and Foot

Introduction

The legs and feet are the foundations upon which we stand. How small the feet are in comparison to the rest of us, and yet they hold us up! They also have the greatest density of proprioceptors, sensory receptors, and pain receptors (Lewit 2010, p. 21). They affect the entire locomotor system, and form a functional unit with the deep stabilizers in the pelvis (p. 294). Where this region of the body is concerned, we tend to prop it with stretch bandages and shoe inserts, and generally disregard warning signs that something is going wrong. It's time to change that attitude.

Regional Kinetics: Symptoms here may require treatment of structural problems elsewhere. For example, TrPs in the trunk and hip areas can cause mid-body stiffness that dramatically affects the ability of the legs and feet to keep the body upright and steady. They increase the compensation and energy expenditure needed by the legs and feet to maintain body balance (Gruneberg et al. 2004). Rotating the thighs inward can cause pain inside and below the knee, with compensatory outward leg rotation and hyperpronation. A zigzag pattern of muscles rotating inward and compensatory muscles rotating outward can trace the history of dysfunction in the kinetic chain, and often the TrPs that initiated it. Muscle dysfunction from TrPs in this part of the body set you up for problems elsewhere. Gastrocnemius tightness, for example, causes the gait to be unstable, and affects joint angles at the hip, knee, and ankle (You, Lee, and Luo 2009). This, in turn, upsets the rest of the kinetic chain, and can create TrP cascades affecting the whole body. The ankle retinaculum is similar to the one in the wrist—it's been relatively ignored in the medical world, often being regarded as an anatomical napkin ring for tendons. However, it may play a significant role in maintaining the stability of the ankle joint (Hatch et al. 2007). Changes in the retinaculum correspond to proprioceptive dysfunction, and therapy that focuses on this tissue can improve recovery (Stecco et al. 2011).

Regional CMP Comments: Plantar fasciitis is a common and often misunderstood problem. Plantar fasciitis is—of course—a description, and descriptions are "whys" that the wise must explore. Underneath layers of foot muscles lies the plantar aponeurosis—a long, flat tendon.

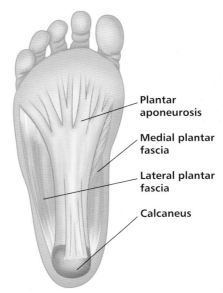

Plantar aponeurosis

Medial plantar fascia

Lateral plantar fascia

Calcaneus

There is also a *lot* of fascia. Plantar fasciitis is a description meaning inflammation in the plantar aponeurosis and surrounding tissues. When muscles anchored to the plantar aponeurosis are under increased tension, the aponeurosis tightens and thickens to protect the tender tissues. This process continues until it produces crowding and constricted circulation. The feet hurt, sometimes to the extent that you can no longer walk on them.

One of the most common causes of increased tension in this area is—you guessed it—TrPs in the surrounding muscles. The most common TrPs associated with plantar fasciitis are found in the intrinsic toe flexors, gastrocnemius, and soleus (Travell and Simons 1992, p. 510). One factor involved in the development of this condition is a tight Achilles tendon, often caused by TrPs. Plantar fasciitis itself activates TrPs and causes ripples of compensation up the kinetic chain. Massage of deep calf muscles can ease the pain of plantar fasciitis as they are all part of the same kinetic chain. Plantar fasciitis can be even more serious if it coexists with a metabolic condition such as diabetes (Giacomozzi et al. 2005); diabetics must also be extremely vigilant about TrPs due to the penchant of some TrPs for restricting circulatory flow.

Tarsal tunnel syndrome is similar to CTS, only it occurs in the ankle. When the foot bends upward, compressing the area in front of the ankle, serious pain results. The entrapped peroneal nerve (due to extensor hallucis brevis TrPs) may be treated surgically, rather than manually, if

TrP training is lacking. Bunions can also be TrP related, and may often be prevented if TrPs are caught early so that contracture in the adductor hallucis tendon and related muscles can be relieved and the toes (and bones) brought back into alignment. Bones follow muscles.

Example: A 48-year-old surgical nurse was on her feet constantly at work. She worked part-time because of FM, and spent time off at the cinema, or watching videos with her feet up. She enjoyed "movie snacks"—caramel popcorn, cheese puffs, and candy bars kept her energy level up. At work she drank coffee or cola, and kept candy bars at the nurses' station. Her pain level was under control, but her weight wasn't. She came back from a trip with "new" pain in her feet and legs, and fallen arches. The podiatrist whom she consulted was familiar with TrPs, and he knew she shouldn't have such deep indentations from stretch socks.

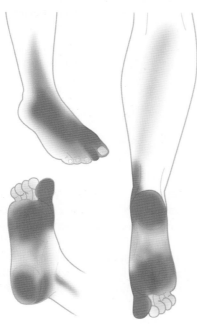

CMP patient referral patterns.

The podiatrist found bilateral TrPs in the toe extenders and flexors, and in the deep and superficial intrinsic foot muscles. TrPs in the retinaculum were the source of the new pain in the front of the ankle. Suspecting that there was more to the story, he referred the patient to a rheumatologist who specialized in myofascial pain. The rheumatologist discovered TrPs in every quadrant of the patient's body, with coexisting insulin resistance. After questioning the patient and uncovering many hypothyroid symptoms, he tested her: the result was low normal. He prescribed topical T3 cream and adjusted the dosage until symptoms were gone. He also prescribed major lifestyle changes, and got her involved with a local FM and CMP support group. She began working with a bodyworker who knew TrPs. In time, she got her arches and much of her life back.

Regional Perpetuating Factors: The presence of leg and foot TrPs signals the need for an assessment of foot structure and gait. A tight Achilles tendon can impair the energy efficiency of surrounding muscles, causing early fatigue (Lichtwark and Wilson 2007), which can contribute to energy crisis and more TrPs. Anything that restricts circulation in the leg or foot is a potential TrP perpetuating factor. Tight socks identify themselves by the indentation they leave on the leg after they are taken off. In cases of central sensitization states such as FM, and/or metabolic conditions such as insulin resistance or diabetes, interstitial swelling is common. Research now indicates that much of the interstitial swelling may be due to absorption of fluid and other materials by excess hyaluronic acid in the fascia. (Stecco et al. 2011). Swelling enhances circulation constriction and can add to a host of foot and leg problems.

Tightness in the fibular head is a frequent cause of pain and dysfunction in the lower leg and foot, and the release of this area is often overlooked. Another perpetuating factor is poor foot posture. Pointing the toes under the weight of bed covers or angling the foot down from a rung while seated causes the tissues in the bottom of the foot to contract. Keep feet in a neutral position.

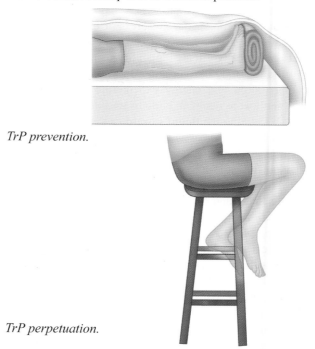

TrP prevention.

TrP perpetuation.

One of the most common TrP perpetuating factors in this region of the body is the use of poorly fitting or poorly designed shoes. High-heeled footwear causes increased work for the muscles and attachments at the hip and knee, as well as restricting the ankle flexors, which requires other muscles to compensate. In general, high heels can cause a tendency for musculoskeletal pain to develop (Esenyel et al. 2003). You may need to look for boots and shoes with heels of a maximum height of ¾" (about 1.9 cm). If you can only endure wearing shoes while you are sitting down, you're in denial, as well as in unsuitable shoes.

There's a type of Morton's foot that's a TrP perpetuating factor and is an anatomical variation occurring in about 40% of people—a structural configuration with a relatively short first metatarsal and a relatively long second one.

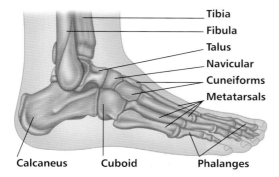

- Tibia
- Fibula
- Talus
- Navicular
- Cuneiforms
- Metatarsals

Calcaneus   Cuboid   Phalanges

The key isn't a relatively short first toe, but is instead a relatively short first metatarsal.

Morton's foot creates a mediolateral rocking motion from the heel to the head of that long metatarsal, causing foot instability. This can activate and maintain TrPs up the kinetic chain; it can also cause a typical callus development.

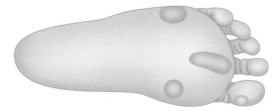

Some or all of these calluses maybe associated with the Morton's foot structure.

It can be difficult to find appropriate shoes that fit, especially if there is another foot variation. For example, when feet are wide in front and narrow in the heel, excessive heel movement inside the shoe leads to more calluses and more functional problems.

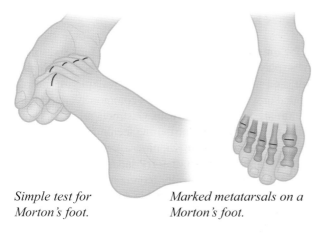

Simple test for Morton's foot.   *Marked metatarsals on a Morton's foot.*

Regional Hints for Control (Patients): Take inventory of your shoes and boots. Check for wear, support, flexibility, and heel height. If you possess shoes that are ill-fitting or worn, or have high heels, you're in a toxic relationship. Better to have one pair of shoes that won't contribute to the ruin of your body than to have a dozen that do. People who are uncomfortable in anything but high-heeled shoes or boots may have severely contractured calves that could require professional help to restore them to normal length. You may need boots and shoes with heels no higher than ¾" (about 1.9 cm)—see what works for you. If you have Morton's foot, purchase shoes with a removable insert so that you can replace it with your own. One of the authors (Starlanyl) uses a modified Travell insert made from a three-quarter length, flexible, arch cushion insert similar to that mentioned in Travell and Simons (1992, p. 390).

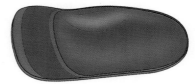

Sample shoe insert before modification.

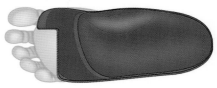

Sample shoe insert after modification. The area beneath the big (great) toe and the area immediately behind that toe must be very firm material, or reinforced.

Some people require additional support or height under the first metatarsal. Your shoe or insert needs to have good arch support and *must* be flexible. Your feet were designed to move, and move they must. Stretch the Achilles tendon and surrounding tissues using a stair step, with the toes and metatarsals of both feet on the step. Stretch the heel and middle of the foot below the step, holding the wall or handrail for support.

Regional Hints for Control (Care Providers): When prescribing a walking cast, ensure the patient has shoes with heels that are the same height as the cast. Otherwise the cast (and you) will become a major perpetuating factor for TrPs. In cases of adult-acquired flat foot, you can often feel taut bands stretching across the area where the arch should be. If they are more easily felt when the toes are extended or flexed, TrPs are advertising their presence. Work on toe extenders or flexors as well as the extrinsic foot muscles. This is often a reversible condition, but it takes time and commitment on the parts of the patients and care providers alike.

Note: TrP injections in the hands and feet may be especially painful, and should be avoided whenever possible.

Gastrocnemius

Greek *gaster* means "stomach"; *kneme*, "leg."
(A working gastrocnemius bulges out like the
stomach does on far too many of us.)

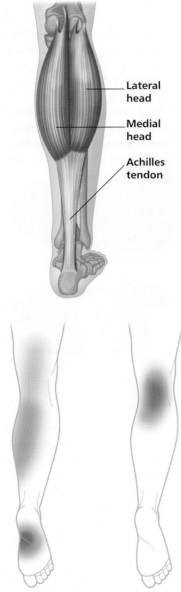

Lateral head

Medial head

Achilles tendon

*This referral pattern is
from TrPs in the area of the
upper medial head.*

*This referral pattern is
from TrPs in the extreme
upper medial head and its
tendon attachment.*

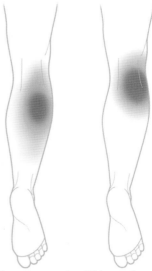

*This referral pattern is
from TrPs in the area of the
middle lateral head.*

*This referral pattern is
from TrPs in the area of the
upper medial head and its
tendon attachment.*

What It Does: The gastrocnemius and soleus muscles
are the primary plantar flexors of the ankle. They work
hard when you point your toes or stand on the ball of your
foot. The gastrocnemius also helps flex the knee during
the swing phase of the gait cycle, while one leg supports
body weight. The muscle supports a considerable amount
of our body weight when we stand, and adds stability to
the knee and ankle joints, as well as helping to maintain
postural balance.

Kinetics Comments: The gastrocnemius muscle bellies
create the shape of the calf. Because of its attachments,
the gastrocnemius spans two joints. The upper fibers of
the two muscle bellies cross the knee joint to attach to
the femur. At the other end, the gastrocnemius fibers join
with the soleus fibers to form the Achilles tendon, thus
connecting to the plantar fascia of the foot. Anatomical
variations of this muscle are not uncommon—for
example, some have three heads, and one anatomical
variation can cause popliteal artery entrapment at the
medial or lateral head (Rochier and Sumpio 2009). When
the gastrocnemius is tight, look for compensation along
the entire kinetic chain.

TrP Comments: Patients with gastrocnemius and soleus
TrPs may have a flat-footed, stiff-legged, clumping
gait, and may experience difficulty walking on uneven
ground or walking fast. The most common symptoms are
nocturnal calf cramps and pain. Gastrocnemius TrPs are a
common cause of, or contributing factor to, nocturnal leg
cramps (Prateepavanich, Kupniratsaikul, and Charoensak
1999). While you sleep, the TrP-laden muscles are still
awake and physiologically contractured—they don't
relax at night, so they get irritable. Nocturnal leg cramps
are called systremma, and can be caused by even latent

TrPs. Patients may be unable to straighten the involved leg while the foot is flexed with the toes pulled back (dorsiflexed). These TrPs can cause severe pain behind the knee when the muscle is active, but minimal or absent pain when the muscle is at rest. They can cause or contribute to post-laminectomy syndrome. They're often part of "growing pains" in children and adolescents (Leung et al. 1999). Nocturnal leg cramps are different than intermittent claudication, which is a type of peripheral artery disease. Leg cramps from claudication occur after walking a certain distance, and may interact with TrPs in the gastrocnemius and soleus.

Cramps can significantly affect both the quality and the quantity of the patient's sleep, and that of any bed partner. They are due to sustained immobility with the toes plantar flexed, which can occur while lying down or when seated with the foot hooked over the rung of a chair, or if the foot is hanging unsupported with the toes pointing downward. Cramp aftereffects, such as muscle soreness, can last for days. The most effective way to get rid of these cramps is to stretch the muscle. Be careful: walking stretches and contracts the muscle, and contraction can activate the TrP and the cramp again. Prevention of the TrPs is important. Other muscles may join with the gastrocnemius to add to the cramp.

Notable Perpetuating Factors: Short lower legs, short stature, ill-fitting furniture, hooking feet on the rung of a stool or chair, sitting in reclining chairs with leg rests, and anything that impairs calf circulation. Wearing high heels shorten gastrocnemius fibers, bringing the two sets of muscle attachments closer together. This shortens the muscle and reduces available muscle force. Prolonged or hard pointing of the foot is common in ballet and other dancers, swimmers, competition divers, and people who sleep on their backs. Growth spurts in children, even those under five years of age, can activate gastrocnemius TrPs. Viral infections often increase irritability of muscles (Travell and Simons 1992, p. 411), so be especially careful when you have a cold or flu. Cold environments and drafts significantly affect the stiffness of the gastrocnemius and Achilles tendon (Muraoka et al. 2008). Immobility (especially that caused by a cast), walking on uneven surfaces, walking or jogging uphill, overdoing calf raising or using a calf-raise machine, wearing smooth leather shoes on slippery floors, cycling with a seat set too low, typing for too long at a computer station, and using a stick shift are all perpetuating factors for these TrPs. Standing in one position while leaning forward for a sustained period, such as at a kitchen counter designed for looks, not function, and with no toe room, invites these TrPs. TrPs anywhere can be contributing factors for the formation of TrPs in other areas. For example, TrPs in the trapezius can affect biochemical components of the gastrocnemius muscle, predisposing it to the formation of TrPs (Shah et al. 2008). This characteristic is probably true of all TrPs and all muscles, although we simply don't have studies to show that every TrP can change the amounts of some of the inflammatory mediators, neuropeptides, cytokines, and catecholamines present in other muscles. Gastrocnemius TrPs are often interactive with sacroiliac dysfunction, Achilles tendinitis, and TrPs in the soleus, hamstrings, tibialis posterior, and long toe-flexor muscles.

Perpetuating factors for nocturnal leg cramps include TrPs, dehydration, lumbar spinal stenosis, electrolytic imbalance, some medications, metabolic acidosis (from vomiting), low serum magnesium or calcium, low potassium (from diarrhea), low parathyroid, heat stress, Parkinson's disease, and metabolic conditions such as diabetes or insulin resistance. There may be a CNS component to nocturnal leg cramps, which may make individuals with FM, IBS or migraines predisposed to these cramps. These coexisting conditions are also TrP perpetuating factors.

Hints for Control (Patients): If you have nocturnal cramps, check with your care provider. Ensure that you're getting adequate lower-leg circulation and that there are no other reasons for the cramps. Visualize a ballerina dancing en Pointe. Don't put your feet in that position for a sustained time. Place a pillow or rolled-up blanket under the bed covers beneath your feet to keep them in a neutral position while sleeping. Rocking chairs help keep these muscles active if you actually rock in them. Use a footrest if your feet, including the heels, don't reach the floor. Find out what height of heel is too high for you. Avoid immobility. If you are on a slippery surface, make sure your shoes have adequate traction. If you've been having nocturnal cramps, try moist heat on your calves before bed, followed by self-massage and gentle stretching of the gastrocnemius muscles. Remember, prevention is your best medicine. Check both bellies of the muscle for TrPs. You can use one bent knee to press on the gastrocnemius of the other leg, or work these muscles with tennis balls on the floor. Vitamin E 400 IU for two weeks may help the cramps (Travell and Simons 1992, p. 422).

Hints for Control (Care Providers): Be attentive to the possibility of other conditions, including posterior compartment syndrome, popliteal synovial cyst, or phlebitis. These TrPs may be mistaken for S1 nerve compression, but that may coexist. Look at the dermatome, and look for TrPs that coexist with arachnoradiculitis too. When these TrPs exist, check for TrPs in the soleus, hamstrings, gluteus minimus, and long flexors of the toes. Some medications, such as lithium or cimetidine, can cause or contribute to leg cramps. In many cases of intermittent claudication, the restricted blood flow itself is not painful: the pain is caused by coexisting TrPs, partly produced by the poor circulation (Travell and Simons 1992, p. 410).

Stretch: Use a tennis ball. When doing standing stretches for this muscle, keep your heels down and ensure that the foot is at the proper angle—straight or slightly turned in. If you wear orthotics, stretch with the orthotics in your shoes. Stretching or lightly massaging the symptoms is not the solution here and at best gives only temporary relief. The deeper muscles in the back of the calf are the ones that are often spastic and house TrPs requiring specific bodywork.

Tibialis Anterior
Latin *tibialis* means "relating to the shin"; *anterior*, "before."

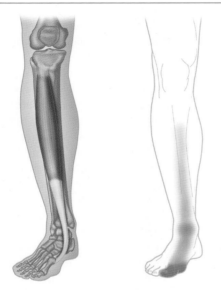

What It Does: Dorsiflexes the ankle joint; moving the front of the foot upward and towards the shin. It also inverts the foot; lifting arch and big toe off the floor while the small toe and outer blade of the foot remain flat. The tibialis anterior enables the ankle to have some horizontal movement, and helps the foot clear the ground during the swing phase of the gait cycle.

Kinetics Comments: The function of this muscle depends on what the leg is doing. After the heel first makes ground contact, the tibialis anterior controls foot placement and ankle stabilization during the contact phase of walking; during the swing phase, this muscle ensures that the foot clears the ground. When the foot is flat, it helps keep the leg vertical over the ankle, even when on rough ground, although that puts stress on the muscle. It maintains the body's balance on the foot, even as upper-body weight distribution realigns. Like all anterior calf muscles, the tibialis is covered by dense, tough fascia, which means that its tissues can't expand as easily as many other muscles can. Note how the muscle crosses the bony leg, and the length of the lower tendon.

TrP Comments: Tibialis anterior TrPs are responsible for many unexpected trips and frequent-flyer opportunities we could do without. They cause the pace that launched a thousand slips. Having read kinetics comments, think what happens when this muscle is contracted by TrPs. Your foot can't clear the ground during stride; your toes may catch and drag and ankles may be "weak" and their motion painful. These TrPs also send pain and tenderness to the front of the ankle. This pain can spill over to the top of the great (or big) toe, and be misdiagnosed as gout; the big toe can hurt so much you can't wear shoes. There may be severe burning pain from the knee down the leg to the foot that may be called "anterior shin splints." These TrP symptoms can worsen when climbing stairs or steep hills, or otherwise stressing the muscle.

Tibialis anterior weakness is a key factor of foot instability (Gefen 2001). Instability of gait and the ankle can have major repercussions, especially in the elderly, leading to debilitating or even fatal falls. Reduced ankle dorsiflexion may lead to increased risk of ankle sprain (de Noronha et al. 2006). These TrPs can cause painful motion of the ankle without evidence of joint injury, leading to accusations of hypochondria. You may have a medical history of ankle injury that "never quite healed" and frequent buckling of the ankle. Tibialis anterior TrPs are common causes of "growing pains" in children and adolescents. The referral pattern may be confusing, as many TrPs in other areas have smaller referral patterns inside or close to this pattern. Check for excessive wear of the rear lateral shoe heel—that's a sign of TrPs lurking in the tibialis anterior.

Notable Perpetuating Factors: Walking over uneven or slanted ground or up steep hills, prolonged standing, trauma, tightness in the calf muscle, Morton's foot, immobility, and use of repetitive quadriceps or knee-extension exercise machines. Catching your toe on something during walking can instantly activate these TrPs. Janet Travell's notes (in the Gelman Library University Archives, Washington DC) mention that these TrPs can develop secondary to peripheral artery disease. One of the authors (Starlanyl) has seen these TrPs in soccer players, dancers, and in a receiver in American football who danced on the football field, twisting and turning, gaining yardage and tibialis TrPs. Tibialis anterior muscle fibers show decreased exercise tolerance and capillary interface in patients with COPD (Eliason et al. 2010). There's a strong correlation between the severity of COPD and the decrease in the muscle-to-capillary interface.

Hints for Control (Patients): If you sleep on your back, brace your feet against a pillow or rolled blanket under the covers at the bottom of the bed. This will avoid having your feet in prolonged dorsiflexion. Slow, deep, stripping massage can inactivate these TrPs (Travell and Simons

1992, p. 365), but be careful not to exceed pain tolerance, especially in cases of coexisting FM. Self-massage can be useful. Release calf tightness so that the front of the leg can also relax—yes, you may need to work on TrPs in the *back* of the leg to ease TrPs in the *front* of the leg. Use a tennis ball against the floor, or a roller or knobber tool. Use your fingers to *gently* ease away fascia that's stuck to the bone and other tissues. Some people are convinced it can only be separated by tearing away the tissue. This makes as much sense as using a chain saw to cut a loaf of bread. Unless you want to risk (further) central sensitization, don't allow this—not to *any* part of your body. A home stretch program tailored to your needs is important. Proceed carefully, as stretching this muscle can result in a reactive cramping of the instep/arch of the foot. Massage and stretch the foot first, and keep hydrated.

Hints for Control (Care Providers): Check for possible L5 nerve compression, anterior compartment syndrome (ACS), or tendon rupture. Diffuse tightness and tenderness over the tibialis anterior belly may be fibrosis, which can mask ACS. Athletes with unbalanced musculature who over train have a tendency to develop ACS, and that condition itself can cause or perpetuate TrPs. It isn't uncommon for patients with CMP, FM, and multiple coexisting conditions (especially insulin resistance) to have painfully tight, swollen limbs. Be attentive to possibilities and interactions. Foot drop and foot slap may have myofascial rather than neurological origins. Palpate both tendons as potential TrP sites. Problems at the proximal tendon–bone junction and the tendon may set up a delayed muscle soreness that expands the pain referral areas and increases pain frequency, leading to central sensitization (Gibson, Arendt-Nielsen, and Graven-Nielsen 2005, 2006). Check both inferior and superior retinacula for TrPs. Don't just add orthotics. Correct the *causes* of gait irregularities and excessive pronation.

Stretch: This is a difficult muscle to stretch. A standing quadriceps stretch where you hold the front of your foot will stretch the tibialis anterior, but will be too far for many people. Sitting down on the shinbones stretches this muscle, but can place undue stress on the knee joints. The best way to keep the tibialis anterior supple is good hydration and regular massage. Self-massage on this muscle is great, but be gentle to your thumbs. From a seated position, use a water-based lubricant and apply long, gliding strokes, stopping for a moment on any painful points for a few seconds while asserting pressure without increasing the pain beyond 8 out of 10 on the pain scale. Try easing the tissue gently off the bone: this will stretch and lengthen the muscle and also soften tight muscle fibers. Find a good massage therapist and visit regularly.

Tibialis Posterior
Latin *tibialis* means "relating to the shin"; *posterior*, "behind."

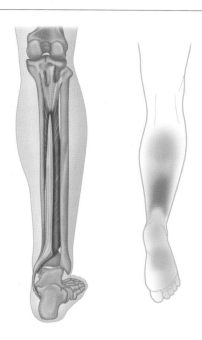

What It Does: This is the prime foot inverter, rotating the forefoot and pulling it upward and inward. It prevents excessive pronation of the foot.

Kinetics Comments: The tibialis posterior lies deep beneath the soleus. Its top tendon attaches to the top of the leg bones, and its long lower tendon passes behind the inner ankle and then branches out, attaching to many bones that form the arch of the foot. This muscle and its tendons help to keep body weight evenly distributed over the foot. The more unbalanced the musculature and the more excess weight we carry, the harder these tissues have to work to maintain balance. TrPs here are a clue that foot muscles already have TrPs. Fallen arches are often the result of a process that begins with stress from weakened and fatigued foot muscles (Emmerich, Wulkner, and Hurschler 2003). The tibialis posterior attempts to compensate, further stressing tendons and muscles. The entire kinetic chain then compensates, causing increased tension on more tissues.

TrP Comments: These TrPs are a common source of pain in the Achilles tendon and/or on the sole of the foot, especially while using the muscle. Orthotics may cause intense pain when they press on one of the referral areas. Weakness in this muscle causes extensive pronation. Tibialis posterior muscles laden with TrPs are likely to develop cramp-like pain when kept in the shortened position. Immobility is your enemy, as are contraptions designed to artificially induce contracture of the muscles. Yes, such devices are actually manufactured. They are called high heels. Existence of tibialis posterior TrPs over a prolonged period can create flat feet. When these TrPs exist, other TrPs are lurking in the surrounding muscles. These TrPs are often mistaken for (or called) plantar fasciitis, Achilles tendinitis, or posterior shin splints.

Notable Perpetuating Factors: Running or jogging (especially on a slanted, uneven, crowned, or irregular surface), TrPs in the foot and muscles in other areas, wearing badly worn or inappropriate shoes (including high heels), Morton's foot and other foot irregularities, chronic postural overload, hypermobile or hypomobile joints, and the use of calf-raise exercise machines.

Hints for Control (Patients): Wear sensible shoes. Confine walking and running to smooth, level surfaces as much as possible. Stretch well and often, not forgetting the Achilles tendon. You can often work the tibialis posterior using the opposite knee if you cross the lower leg to be worked over the other knee and press. This muscle is deep. Adjust pressure of the upper leg according to pain tolerance. Check for TrPs in surrounding muscles. Stretch and exercise foot muscles using a golf ball between the foot and the floor. A roller tool may be helpful for both the leg and the foot. Early tibialis posterior TrPs may be successfully inactivated by stretch alone (Patla and Abbott 2000), but don't be fooled into thinking that if the pain goes away, the TrPs go away. Keep working latent TrPs as well as TrPs in other areas, and identify and control perpetuating factors.

Hints for Control (Care Providers): Rule out deep posterior compartment syndrome and posterior tendon conditions. The size and shape of the tibialis posterior lower tendon can vary, and variations could contribute to "tibial stress syndrome" (yes, another description); this is *not* an indication for surgery (Saxena, O'Brien, and Bunce 1990). Parts of the tendon attachments are palpable, but, because this muscle belly is so deep, find indications of TrPs by history and ROM. Look for consequences of prolonged tibialis posterior TrPs, such as varus deformities of the foot. If the patient's toes curl to provide stability as they walk, the long toe flexors may be trying to compensate for a tibialis posterior weakened by TrPs. Check the entire kinetic chain for functional impairments. When tissues covering the tibialis posterior are extremely tight, manual treatment may be insufficient. FSM, ultrasound, galvanic stimulation, and other forms of electrical therapy may be useful for softening the tissues. This must be carried out in conjunction with the identification and control of perpetuating factors and a home self-treatment plan.

Stretch: Movement is the key. This is a deep muscle in the posterior compartment of the leg. Massaging the plantar tissues of the foot can help keep this muscle supple. Squatting to 90 degrees with the ball of the foot slightly elevated is a nice dynamic way to lengthen this muscle.

Popliteus and Surrounding Attachments

Latin *poples* means "ham (hollow of the knee)."

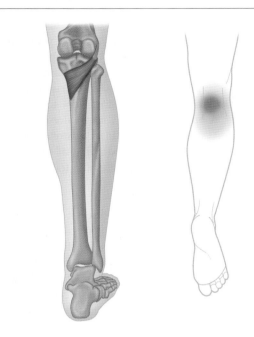

Popliteus muscle and referral pattern.

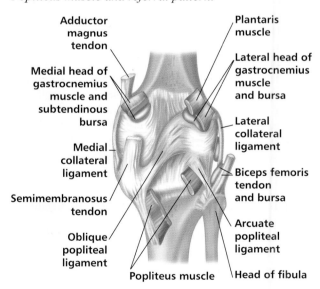

Popliteus muscle (cut) and surrounding attachments.

What It Does: Works with attachments to help control the knee joint. It helps rotate the thigh outward when the foot is on the ground, and releases the knee from a standing locked position, initiating knee flexion. Working with the medial hamstring, it assists in rotating the leg inward when the leg is not bearing weight.

Kinetics Comments: Knee anatomy is complex, and the popliteus is at the center of the action. It's a team player: in the medical literature it may be referred to as the "popliteus muscle-tendon unit" or something similar. The popliteus may contain a variety of receptors that allow it to function as a "dynamic guidance system" or a "kinesthetic knee joint monitor" (Nyland et al. 2005). A healthy popliteus and its associated connective tissues may play critical roles in preventing knee injury and facilitating rehabilitation after injury. The popliteal tendon pulls the lateral meniscus backward, and may prevent it from being damaged as frequently as the medial meniscus. When tendon and muscle are tight from TrPs, this protection is diminished.

TrP Comments: These TrPs make it painful to straighten the knee fully. They refer pain to the back of the knee, especially when you crouch, run, walk downhill, or go down steps. The TrPs tend not to hurt as much during sleep, when the muscle is relaxed, but reintroduce themselves as leg stiffness when you get out of bed and try to walk. TrPs in the popliteus muscle or tendon may be misdiagnosed as popliteal tendinitis or Baker's cyst. You can see how TrPs can cause tendinitis as the muscles contractured by TrPs put tension on surrounding tissues. Restrictions of the popliteal artery have been documented (Chernoff et al. 1995), as has popliteal vein entrapment (Misselbeck et al. 2008), but patients involved were not checked for TrPs although vein entrapment occurred shortly after a patient started an exercise program. Popliteal vascular compression due to myofascial compression in asymptomatic patients often occurs during leg position changes (Erdoes et al. 1994). Surrounding tissues should be checked for TrPs.

Notable Perpetuating Factors: Dysfunctional movement patterns, OA of knee or hip, using leg-curl machines or repetitive squat exercises, and unaccustomed running or walking downhill. One of the authors (Starlanyl) has seen patients develop popliteus TrPs after a mountain hike; the hikers had been transported to the top of the mountain and then walked down. High heels simulate a never-ending downhill walk and are major perpetuators. TrPs in the muscle or tendon can also be initiated from trauma due to abrupt starts and stops with a bent knee, called an active pivotal shift; this action may occur in sports such as tennis, hockey, and football. Dancers and gymnasts are also exposed to active pivotal shift, as are people with cognitive deficits, who may frequently stop abruptly in mid stride to turn and retrieve what they've forgotten.

Hints for Control (Patients): Sweeps with an ice cube in a face cloth from mid calf to the knee towards the outside may release tension from the upper gastrocnemius as well as the popliteus.

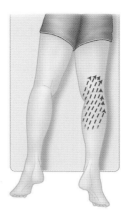

After ice, rewarm the area and then move the knee though its ROM. An elastic bandage around the knee may help control pain, but avoid prolonged restriction of circulation or immobilization. Avoid use of tools on this area, as it contains many delicate structures such as blood vessels.

Hints for Control (Care Providers): TrPs in this muscle may limit extension to less than 7 degrees (Kostopoulos and Rizopoulous 2001, p. 208). If treatment does not result in immediate release, suspect TrPs in other muscles or other causes of restriction such as spinal pathology. Stretch and spray or ultrasound may be useful for releasing the popliteus, as may any non-pressure method. Consider the blood vessels and nerves here, and be cautious when doing manual work—no elbows, please! Check the tendon as well as the muscle. Popliteus TrPs can contribute to hyperpronation and also be caused by it. Identify and treat the initiator, such as weak thigh muscles. If the posterior cruciate ligament has been injured, these TrPs may be the major pain generator. When popliteus muscle TrPs are chronic, look for a TrP at the lower attachment point. Check the heads of the gastrocnemius too. One of the authors (Starlanyl) suspects that TrPs in the popliteus and in the lower tendon of the sartorius, gracilis, and semitendinosus muscles are associated with some cases of pes anserine bursitis and/or retinacular TrPs. The association has been observed in several patients, but each had multiple conditions with no definitive initiators.

Stretch: Sit on the floor with your knees double hip-distance apart. You can point your toes away from or towards your face, as long as it feels good. Try reaching forward and back, gently rocking and mobilizing not just the popliteus, but all the muscles and fascia along the posterior kinetic chain. Philip Beach, a friend of one of the authors (Sharkey), calls this the "long sitting posture." Philip advises to bend the knees gently if you feel this position places too much pressure on your lower back.

Peroneus (Fibularis) Longus, Brevis, and Tertius

Greek *perone* means "a buckle."
Latin *fibula* means "a buckle"; *longus*, "long"; *brevis*, "short"; *tertius*, "third."

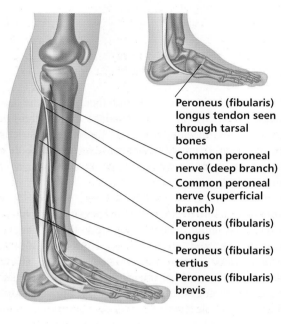

- Peroneus (fibularis) longus tendon seen through tarsal bones
- Common peroneal nerve (deep branch)
- Common peroneal nerve (superficial branch)
- Peroneus (fibularis) longus
- Peroneus (fibularis) tertius
- Peroneus (fibularis) brevis

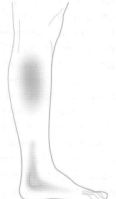

Peroneus (fibularis) longus.

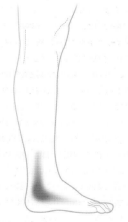

Peroneus (fibularis) brevis.

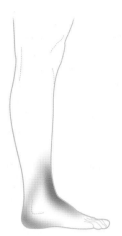

Peroneus (fibularis) tertius.

What They Do: When the foot is bearing body weight, all three peroneus muscles help raise the outside edge of the foot off the floor (eversion). The longus and brevis work with the tibialis posterior to plantar flex the ankle joint and enable pronation. The longus also helps maintain the transverse arch of the foot. The longus and brevis assist in keeping the body in an upright position over the foot during the stance phase of the gait cycle, helping control sideways sway; this becomes more obvious during a one-legged stance. They also help us keep our balance when we run, especially over rough, uneven ground. Although the brevis seems to be more effective than the longus in everting the foot (Otis et al. 2004), it can have a tendency to over-invert the foot, which puts stress on the tendons and ankle joint, leading to frequent inversion sprains. The tertius does its best to prevent over-inversion, and may serve to check the brevis. Unlike the other peroneals, the tertius is involved with foot dorsiflexion rather than plantar flexion.

Kinetics Comments: Many anatomical variations exist in the peroneal muscles. In about 13% of people there is even a peroneus quartus muscle. The peroneus longus is, as its name suggests, long. Its lower tendon is long as well, and changes direction three times before it attaches to the inner side of the sole of the foot! Together with the brevis tendon, it travels around the back of the outside ankle bump (lateral malleolus) to attach underneath the foot. The common peroneal nerve (before it splits into the deep and superficial peroneal nerves) passes through the area between the fibula and the peroneus longus attachments. Nerve entrapment in that region has been documented by Ihunwo and Dimitrov (1999), and between the longus and the soleus by Jayaseelan (1989). We suspect peroneal nerves can be entrapped along their entire length. Each peroneal tendon can spontaneously rupture, and they can be affected, along with their muscles, by trauma in many ways. Any tightness of these muscles and/or tendons will have repercussions up and down kinetic lines. If the horizontal connecters such as the sacrotuberous ligament become involved, as they often do, kinetic lines on both sides of the body can be affected.

TrP Comments: Common symptoms of these TrPs are ankle pain/soreness and weak ankles; the ankle turns out and "sprains" easily. A true significant sprain causes ankle swelling—TrPs don't, but they can feel like a sprain. To complicate matters, anything that causes a sprain or fracture can also activate TrPs. Ankles weakened by TrPs can increase the likelihood of ankle fracture, yet the immobility of a cast is a TrP perpetuating factor. During a one-legged stance, peroneus TrPs can have you wobbling like a batted cat toy; when walking, we have our weight on one foot for some of the time, so this concerns everyone. The unsteadiness becomes more noticeable during prolonged one-legged stances, such as in martial arts. A wobbly leg is not a sign of a lack of practice, and practicing more will make it worse. Peroneus tertius TrPs can cause pain at the base of the Achilles tendon. This can be masked by tibialis posterior and/or soleus TrPs. These TrPs can entrap the deep and/or superficial peroneal nerve, resulting in a sharp, shooting pain down the side of the leg or the top of the foot and ankle that can stop you in your tracks. If the deep peroneal nerve is entrapped by the longus, you could have difficulty balancing. You may trip over your own feet, or develop a condition called foot drop. The TrPs' connection with foot drop is often missed, leading to incorrect assumptions and difficulties. You may also develop parathesias—unusual sensations and sensitivities on the ankle, top of the foot, and toes.

Notable Perpetuating Factors: Trauma, Morton's foot, high heels, sock compression, flat feet, prolonged immobilization, ill-fitting or worn shoes, shoes with pointed toes and/or narrow toe box, gait irregularities, hyperpronation, crossing the leg at the knee, resting the calves on a hassock, prolonged plantar flexion, unequal leg length, and twisting or spraining the ankle towards the outside. Any condition that contributes to lateral loss of balance, such as vestibular dysfunction, can stress leg muscles as they attempt to keep the head and trunk aligned over the foot, encouraging TrP formation. Peroneal nerve entrapment can be perpetuated by compression stockings or socks (Travell and Simons 1992, p. 385).

Hints for Control (Patients): Rotate your ankle using your hand to help in circling the ankle; if the circle is more like a square, these TrPs are probably part of your life. Massage and tennis-ball work may help, but avoid nerve compression. Intermittent stretch and cold may give relief, with ice sweeps and positioning of the foot as indicated in the figure.

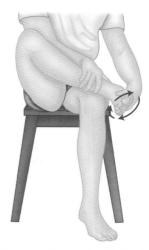

Rewarm the tissues afterwards. Moist heat alone may ease the tightness. Bring perpetuating factors under control.

Hints for Control (Care Providers): Many forms of neuromuscular manual work are effective for peroneal TrPs. Be attentive to the position of the peroneal nerves when using manual compression techniques. Ultrasound and other forms of electrotherapy may be helpful. Inspect the foot and the gait for abnormalities. Check for TrPs in the gluteus minimus and/or tibialis muscles. Especially after any trauma, be alert to the possibility of a rupture or tear of the tendons, remembering that they can rupture spontaneously. Injection of local anesthetic in TrPs in the proximity of the peroneal nerve can result in temporary paralysis of the muscle and the patient's inability to walk or bear weight on that leg until the anesthetic wears off.

Stretch: To bring these muscles though their ROM, sit on a chair or on the floor, and rest the ankle of one leg on the front of the other, above the knee (i.e. across the quadriceps). Hold your foot in your hands and gently plantar flex it. With your hands, turn or rotate your foot up towards the ceiling (inversion). While you do this, you can add the extra dimension of massage by pressing your thumbs into the plantar tissues of the sole, encouraging a gentle softening within the foot. You are in control of the speed of the stretch and the amount of thumb pressure.

Long Flexors of the Toes
(flexor digitorum longus,
flexor hallucis longus)
Latin *flectere* means "to flex."

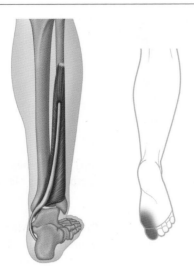

Flexor hallucis longus.

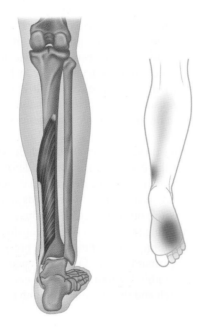

Flexor digitorum longus.

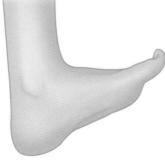

Dorsiflexion.

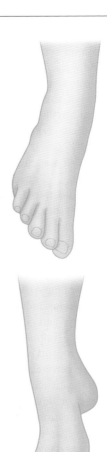

Eversion.

Inversion.

What They Do: Work together to point (plantar flex) the toes. The flexor digitorum longus flexes all the toe joints except for the great toe, and helps to plantar flex the ankle joint and invert the foot. The flexor hallucis longus (*hallucis* is Latin for "of the great toe") flexes the great toe and helps boost the foot, propelling the body forward while walking. It also helps plantar flex the ankle joint, and assists in inverting the foot. If you ever leap for joy and manage to get straight up and down successfully, you have these muscles to thank. They are involved in both take-off and landing during a two-legged vertical jump.

Kinetics Comments: These muscles prevent foot slap after heel strike as you walk; helping the foot clear the ground during the phase of the gait cycle when the leg swings free. In essence, they prevent you from stumbling over your own feet, but, if you have TrPs, they may fail in this task.

TrP Comments: Although these TrPs can cause the foot and/or toes to feel weak, the chief symptom is pain on the top of the foot, especially when you stand or walk. This can be most noticeable after you've been off your feet for a while. As you walk, the foot may not clear the ground and "slaps" the ground instead, as may the rest of you shortly thereafter. TrPs in the flexor hallucis longus affect the great toe and the pad behind it, and are often mistaken for gout. These conditions can coexist.

If the big toe can't raise itself sufficiently, it can catch when you try to climb stairs—you want to avoid this. A wake-up stretch may prompt a rush to get up as the toes cramp. TrPs can cause toe cramps when the involved toes are extended, which may occur when you take that first step when you arise. Ouch!—that gets your day off on the wrong foot. These TrPs can be part of growing pains in children and adolescents. One of the authors (Starlanyl) has noticed that in patients with FM, the spillover pain can extend much higher than shown on the diagram. TrPs in the flexor digitorum longus muscle, if not treated promptly, may contribute to the development of hammer toe or claw toe.

Notable Perpetuating Factors: Prolonged plantar -flexion, stumbling and falling, local trauma immobilization, inappropriate footwear, Morton's foot, anything that encourages the foot towards hyperpronation or instability, running or walking on uneven ground or soft sand, using calf-raise machines, peroneus and/or tibialis TrPs, and/or hypo- or hypermobility of the ankle and foot.

Hints for Control (Patients): Try ice sweeps down the muscle (not just along the referral pattern), followed by rewarming. Maintain a neutral position of the foot during sleep. Keep the legs and feet warm, but avoid garments with constricting elastic. Stretch frequently during the day. Discard shoes after they are worn down. The cost of good shoes is an investment in good health.

Hints for Control (Care Providers): Ask about painful feet, and get specifics. Many patients don't remember a time when their feet didn't hurt, and they may not be aware that leg muscles can cause foot pain. Note whether passively flexing the toes to full range hurts. Check for radiculopathy of the lower lumbar vertebrae. Look for signs of entrapment of the deep branch of the peroneal nerve, caused by impingement of the extensor digitorum longus TrP taut band against the fibula. Tightness in the flexor digitorum longus in early childhood can cause bone deformity, and must be promptly diagnosed and treated as soon as possible.

Stretch: If you have access to a swimming pool and the water is sufficiently warm for patients with TrPs, it may help to walk around in the pool. Take exaggerated, long strides in slow motion, with the body immersed to waist level. On dry land, exercise the muscles by trying to pick up objects with your toes; it's best to do this standing, but sitting is just fine.

Soleus

Latin *solea* means "a leather sole" or "a sandal."

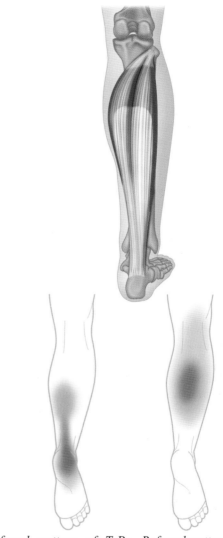

Referral pattern of TrPs in the area of the muscle slightly above a hand's width higher than the ankle crease.

Referral pattern of TrPs in the gastrocnemius muscle bellies above the tendons.

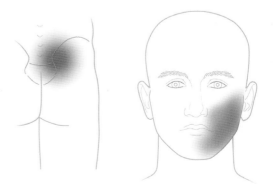

These are referral patterns of TrPs in the base of the calf muscle belly (gastor) area.

What It Does: Keeps us from falling forward while we stand, and stabilizes the knee and ankle. It helps point the toes of the foot, and allows us to stand on the ball of the foot. Because of large-diameter vein pockets, a tough fascial covering, and large open veins above, the soleus muscle provides major pumping action to return blood to the heart as its motion helps pump blood from the legs back to the center of the body for reoxygenation. The soleus and gastrocnemius are the primary plantar flexors of the ankle.

Kinetics Comments: The soleus is a deep muscle, lying underneath the gastrocnemius. These two muscles work together, and join to form the Achilles tendon. Unlike the gastrocnemius, the soleus doesn't directly affect the knee. The soleus can refer pain to, and interact with, the sacroiliac joint and TMJ. Anything that interferes with this process interferes with reoxygenation of the blood, and can cause a global energy crisis affecting the whole body. This sets the stage for the formation of TrPs everywhere.

TrP Comments: Upper soleus TrPs tend to refer to the sacroiliac and pelvic areas, and are more likely to interfere with the venous pump, causing ankle and foot swelling. In conjunction with the musculovenous pump, they can cause symptoms of calf and foot pain with edema of the foot and ankle. Because of large-diameter vein pockets, a tough fascial covering, and large open veins above, the soleus muscle provides major pumping action to Because of large-diameter vein pockets, a tough fascial covering, and large open veins above, the soleus muscle provides major pumping action to return blood from the legs to the upper body for reoxygenation. In combination with the plantaris tendon, upper soleus TrPs can be involved in posterior tibial nerve, vein, and/or artery entrapment. They can contribute to craniosacral dysfunction and/or dental malocclusion. We have found that the jaw referral pattern from TrPs at the base of the calf muscle is not unusual, as has been reported elsewhere. It seems to be fairly common in people with CMP and FM. TrPs in the outer edge of the soleus tend to refer pain to the mid calf; TrPs in the lower part of the muscle may be more likely to cause heel pain.

Soleus TrPs often cause growing pains in the calf. They can cause or contribute to ankle stiffness. Ankle ROM can increase immediately and significantly after even one soleus TrP release (Grieve et al. 2011). TrPs in the soleus can cause unbearable heel pain, contributing to or causing what is often described as plantar fasciitis. These TrPs can also be mistaken for Achilles tendinitis. Walking uphill or up and down stairs may be difficult or impossible. Patients with gastrocnemius and soleus TrPs may have a flat-footed, stiff-legged gait, making it difficult to walk on uneven ground, or walk fast. Soleus TrPs don't cause nocturnal calf cramps, but heel pain

from soleus TrPs may feel worse at night. Carol Shifflett (2001) has noticed that the TrP referral pattern may appear in the sacroiliac joint and then reappear in the face and jaw to cause jaw pain and TMJD symptoms, including toothache. She mentions several patients who had never had headaches until they caught shrapnel in the calf or ripped an Achilles tendon (pp. 42, 101).

Notable Perpetuating Factors: Immobility, cold drafts, wearing skates and ski boots with inadequate supports, using calf-raise exercise machines, unequal leg length, trauma, high heels, tissue compression by chair edges and leg rests, prolonged kneeling, or frequent stooping over. Overworking muscles is the most common cause of soleus TrPs. When a foot with smooth-soled shoes on hard slippery surface slips out at toe-off during the gait cycle, the soleus must check the slide. Rigid-soled shoes that allow only ankle and no toe movement can cause TrPs, as the stiff sole increases the lever arm that the soleus must work against. A near-fall can sometimes be as damaging as a fall, especially if you have muscle imbalance that causes a lot of "near misses." The soleus can grow thick as it tries to constantly prevent its owner from falling. At one time, it was easy to tell a train conductor by their thick soleus muscles. A trained eye can still pick out someone with forward-sway imbalance, as the soleus muscles are relatively overdeveloped.

Hints for Control (Patients): The soleus responds to self-treatment better after a warm bath or shower, followed by stretching. Ice sweeps or stretch and spray may help the tightness, but be attentive to controlling perpetuating factors, especially muscle imbalances. Keep massaging, and work the muscle with a tennis ball, and attend to muscles and attachments around the soleus.

Hints for Control (Care Providers): Many techniques such as strain/counterstrain and contract/relax can be helpful for releasing this muscle. Manual TrP therapy plus self-stretching can significantly ease plantar heel pain (Renan-Ordine et al. 2011). A bulging, tight soleus may be a sign of TrPs and forward-sway balance problems. Look for contributory proprioceptive, optical, and vestibular dysfunctions. Check the SI joint and ligaments in the lower spine. Soleus TrPs may often be the cause of "heel spur pain"; there may be bilateral spurs but only one heel hurts.

Stretch: Stand with one foot directly behind the other, heel to toe. Holding a wall or other support, "sit down" slowly, going only as far down as feels comfortable. Keep your feet flat on the floor. Return to the upright position, change feet, and repeat.

Plantaris
Latin *planta* means "sole of the foot."

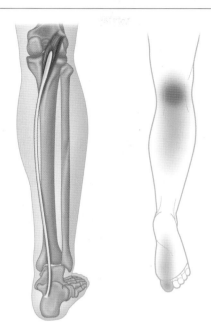

What It Does: A weak flexor of the knee and plantar flexor of the ankle. Its long tendon, the Achilles, helps propel the body in running, walking, and jumping.

Kinetics Comments: The plantaris can vary anatomically—it can have one muscle belly or two, separated by a tendon. This muscle can become entrapped between the tibial nerve and its branches (Nayak et al. 2009), or join with the soleus to entrap the popliteal artery (Turnipseed and Pozniak 1992). The plantaris has the longest and strongest tendon in the body—the tendocalcaneus, also known as the Achilles tendon. Achilles fibers are unusual, spiraling by as much as 90 degrees, allowing the tendon to withstand extraordinary strain. The plantaris is mostly covered by the gastrocnemius, and is sometimes considered to be its accessory muscle.

TrP Comments: Superficial diffuse calf pain from plantaris TrPs may be accompanied by swelling of the muscle. The popliteal artery can be entrapped by the soleus and plantaris muscles, or by Achilles tendon fascia. Symptoms of popliteal artery entrapment include rapid fatigue of the calf, and muscle cramp. When the plantaris is tight and swollen from TrPs and entrapment, a pillow or support under the knees can cause pain. These TrPs may cause parathesias such as numbness or tingling on the surface of the foot. They can activate while the plantaris is being heavily used, such as when running on an incline or jumping, and occur more often in athletes. Plantaris TrPs are often misdiagnosed as Achilles tendinitis. Prompt and effective treatment of the TrPs, if they are the sole cause of the pain, will result in prompt and effective pain relief.

Notable Perpetuating Factors: Sports injuries, inappropriate shoes, and anything that stresses the soleus. Prolonged cooling of tired, immobile legs is also a factor and can occur when using air conditioning on a long drive, or lingering outdoors in a breeze after long periods of unaccustomed activity.

Hints for Control (Patients): Maintain feet in a neutral position while sleeping on your back. A cold compress may be more helpful than heat for entrapment pain, although moist heat can ease tightness and fluid flow. Use what works for you. Massage before and after exercise and work. Warm up before and cool down after.

Hints for Control (Care Providers): Look for a plantaris TrP commonly lurking between the two heads of the gastrocnemius. Swelling behind the knee and patient intolerance to pressure in that area, such as from a support or even a pillow, is an important clue to the possible presence of plantaris TrPs. The plantaris and gastrocnemius can often be treated together when using manual therapies, including stretch and spray, as these muscles have similar attachment areas.

Stretch: This muscle requires the knee to flex and extend in order to bring it through its full ROM; since it attaches to the heel bone, plantar flexion and dorsiflexion also need to be included. The plantaris originates just above the knee joint posteriorly, and attaches to the heel by its long lower tendon, so movements such as kicking and jumping will stretch this little muscle that is so well hidden at the back of the knee. The single-leg, forward-bending, standing stretch with the toes pointed away should suffice for most people.

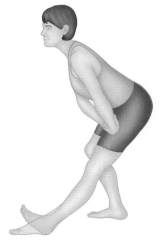

Lean into the stretch slowly, until you feel a mild, comfortable stretch. Return to standing upright. Then stretch the other leg. Dorsiflexing the foot in this stretch position may result in a burning sensation in tendons behind the knee, so please proceed with caution. Discover what works best for you.

Long Extensors of the Toes and the Ankle Retinaculum
(extensor digitorum longus, extensor hallucis longus)
Latin *extendere* means "to extend"; *retinacula*, "rope."

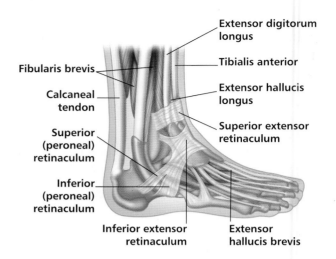

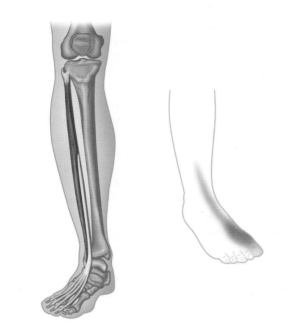

Extensor digitorum longus.

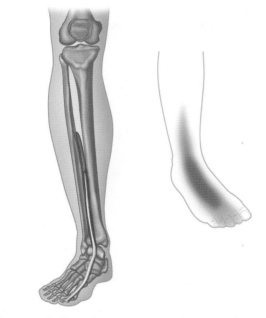

Extensor hallucis longus.

What They Do: The long extensors maintain the plantar arch and help draw the toes upward to allow the foot to clear the ground during walking, running, and climbing stairs. The extensor hallucis longus extends the joints of the great toe and helps to dorsiflex the foot at the ankle. The extensor digitorum longus extends the four smaller toes, helped in part by the lumbrical muscles. The retinaculum is a network of fascial tissue that helps keep the tendons in place; it contains a receptor network that we're just beginning to understand.

Kinetics Comments: These muscles lie between the tibia and the fibula, help prevent foot slap following the heel strike of the gait cycle, and help control posture sway. The great toe doesn't have lumbrical or interossei muscles and depends on the extensor hallucis longus to extend it. The retinaculum holds the tendons, and contains a vast number of proprioceptors that may provide important feedback to the brain concerning foot location in relation to surrounding objects (Stecco et al. 2010). Retinaculum TrPs may be why you stub your toe so often.

TrP Comments: These TrPs cause pain primarily over the top of the foot. Patients may complain that their foot feels weak; they may fall over their feet when the foot doesn't clear the ground during stride. Long extensor TrPs can cause toe cramps that seem more common at night or early morning. TrPs in the extensor digitorum longus can initiate extensor substitution in which the toes are excessively contracted. At first, this occurs during the swing phase of stride to compensate for weak muscles. Without intervention, the condition will progress until the toes remain contracted. This can lead to claw or hammer toes. Foot drop may result if taut TrP bands in the extensor digitorum longus entrap the deep branch of the peroneal nerve against the fibula.

Toe extensor TrPs can be part of "growing pains" in childhood and adolescence. Vittore et al. (2009) indicated that weakness in these muscles has been implicated as a cause of flexible flat feet in childhood, with no mention of TrPs. We suspect that many researchers are studying the result of TrPs unawares, and that numerous problems could be treated successfully by manual therapy at a young age, thus preventing a great deal of pain, dysfunction, and associated costs later. The ankle retinaculum can be a cause of chronic pain after injury (Demondion, Canella, and Moraux 2010). Retinaculum TrPs feel like small, hard nodules, just under the skin; they refer pain locally and inward. As far as we are aware, this is the first text to mention retinacular TrPs.

Notable Perpetuating Factors: Muscle overuse, trauma, unaccustomed prolonged walking, walking on uneven ground, immobility, hypermobility of the joints in the foot, repetitive kicking, catching the toes on the ground when kicking a ball, dancing en Pointe or demi Pointe in ballet, crossing the legs at the ankles, or wearing high heels. Extensor TrPs can interact with lower lumbar spinal dysfunction and/or a tight Achilles tendon.

Hints for Control (Patients): Keep lower legs and feet warm and free from drafts. Control perpetuating factors. Soak feet in warm water, and then mobilize the foot areas that are stiff and tight using hand massage, helping feet and toes stretch in all directions. Work your feet with a golf ball and your legs with a tennis ball. Get circulation and energy flowing. TrPs in the retinaculum respond to barrier release and finger pressure release. The retinaculum is not separate from the fascia, but is a specialized fascia that allows tendons to run or glide smoothly beneath. The best intervention is massage, mobilizing this tissue in every direction.

Hints for Control (Care Providers): In ballet dancers and athletes such as taekwando players, check for possible injury to the extensor hallucis longus tendon, as well as for TrPs. Trigger toe due to "a constricting lesion" in the tendon of a ballet dancer has been reported (Ozkan et al. 2006), and this may have been a TrP. If these TrPs do not respond to the usual therapies, check for metabolic conditions and nutritional insufficiencies. Foot drop caused by TrP nerve entrapment can respond immediately to treatment. Retinaculum TrPs don't feel the same as TrPs in the underlying tissues—they move differently, as they are confined to the retinacular tissue.

Stretch: Sit comfortably. Raise one leg slightly and use a pedal motion up and down for a while. Repeat with the other foot. Vary the exercise by tilting each foot slightly inward or outward.

Superficial Intrinsic Foot Muscles
(extensor digitorum brevis, extensor hallucis brevis, abductor hallucis, flexor digitorum brevis, abductor digiti minimi)
Latin *superficialis* means "relating to the surface"; *intrinsecus*, "situated within."

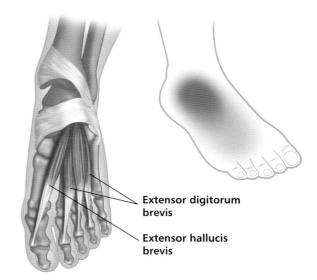

Extensor digitorum brevis

Extensor hallucis brevis

Extensor digitorum brevis and extensor hallucis brevis. This referral pattern is common to both muscles.

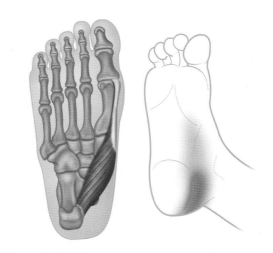

Abductor hallucis.

215

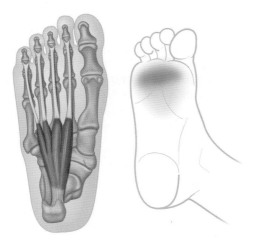

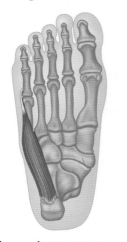

Flexor digitorum brevis.

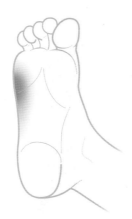

Abductor digiti minimi.

What They Do: Stabilize the foot when the body is in a one-legged stance. This position is not reserved for martial artists and those who enjoy hopping about: it is part of walking. These muscles join with others to set the body in motion when we walk or run.

Kinetics Comments: These TrPs cause unbalanced and uncoordinated gait. If only one foot is affected, you may limp; when both feet have these TrPs, you're fortunate if you shuffle along. Unbalanced gait affects multiple kinetic chains as you struggle to walk without causing pressure on these TrPs. It hurts, so you walk less and sit more, and the whole body pays. When patients have flat feet, the abductor hallucis and flexor digitorum brevis compensate for the lack of an arch—they work harder. Those muscles are also recruited to compensate for hypermobile ligaments and other foot irregularities. As they weaken with the extra burden, other muscles are recruited to help them, and a TrP cascade is born.

TrP Comments: You may have expensive orthotics, yet they're too painful to use. You may own too many pairs of shoes, but none are comfortable. When the complaint is sore feet, these TrPs are often the reason: they cause pain and tenderness to the foot, but not to the ankle or above, although they can be mistaken for a sprained ankle. It hurts to stretch these muscles because they're tight and inflexible, and walking endurance is profoundly limited. These TrPs frequently cause intolerance to orthotics, and can cause severe aching even when the foot is not holding weight. Unfortunately, some patients may turn to surgery for relief if their care providers don't know TrPs. Superficial intrinsic foot muscle TrPs can cause fallen arches. If you have fallen arches and bend your toes upward, you may feel taut bands of TrPs stretching across where the arch would be. If it's TrP-caused, there are no other pathologies, and you can control all perpetuating factors, this condition may be reversible.

Notable Perpetuating Factors: Inappropriate or ill-fitting shoes, trauma, Morton's foot, hyperpronation, muscle imbalances, joint dysfunction, walking or running over uneven ground, or anything that causes a limp or other gait irregularity. These TrPs are often first activated in childhood by shoes that don't fit. We traumatize our feet all the time and think nothing of it: stub the toe, bang the side of the foot on the hearth, trip on a curb. You rub the foot and forget it—but muscles remember. If you sit on a wheeled chair at a desk or workstation and the floor is hard and slippery, your feet may periodically move the chair back to the workstation. This causes cumulative trauma and can form these TrPs. Insurance companies would save money in the long term if TrP therapists evaluated workstations—and assessed the workers, too.

Hints for Control (Patients): Abductor hallucis TrPs respond to massage. The abductor digiti minimi and flexor digitorum brevis need stretching, because they tighten the sole of the foot. Wear appropriate, well-fitting shoes. Pamper your feet. They carry you all day, so give them the comfort they deserve. After a hot day on your feet, soak them in cool water: it's amazing what relief this provides. On cold days, soak them in warm water. Any day, any weather, give them a gentle massage. Move muscles in as many ways as you can.

Hints for Control (Care Providers): TrPs in the extensor digitorum brevis or extensor hallucis brevis may cramp the foot and refer pain to the instep in children and in adults. When children complain of heel pain, check the abductor hallucis. Entrapment of the posterior tibial nerve and its branches by the abductor hallucis muscle and/or by TrP taut bands (or anatomical variations) can cause tarsal tunnel syndrome (Travell and Simons 1992, p. 512). Stretch and spray and other cold therapies should be avoided in patients with impaired circulation or metabolic conditions such as diabetes. The abductor hallucis and flexor digitorum brevis may contribute to static arch support in flat-footed persons. These patients need TrP relief, not hard orthotics. After TrP inactivation, appropriate arch supports may be useful.

Stretch: Use a rolling tool (a narrow rolling pin works) or golf ball to exercise your feet. Practice picking up marbles with your toes for about five minutes. See how your feet respond, and increase or decrease the workout the next day accordingly.

Deep Intrinsic Foot Muscles
(quadratus plantae, flexor hallucis brevis, adductor hallucis, flexor digiti minimi brevis)
Latin *intrinsecus* means "situated within."

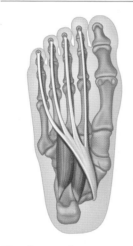

Quadratus plantae.

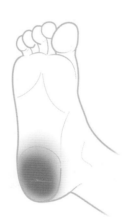

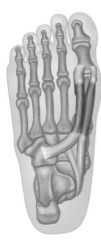

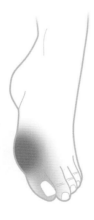

Flexor hallucis brevis.

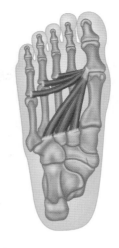
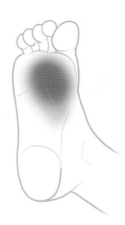

Adductor hallucis.

What They Do: Prepare the foot to move the body.

Kinetics Comments: When the foot hurts, the hip, knee, and ankle are stressed from trying to avoid pressure on the painful areas. Muscle imbalances and articular dysfunctions in the foot may lead to pain and dysfunction in any part of the body.

TrP Comments: Quadratus plantae TrPs refer pain and tenderness to the bottom surface of the heel, and are often misdiagnosed as plantar fasciitis. Taut bands crossing the arch area of the foot may originate in this muscle. Muscle imbalance from TrPs in the adductor hallucis and abductor hallucis can contribute to bunion formation. Referred pain from the flexor hallucis brevis covers the bunion pad area of the first toe, and may spill over to include all of the first toe and much of the second toe. There are often TrPs where the flexor hallucis brevis tendon attaches to the heel bone. This area is tension sensitive, and TrPs here are a frequent cause of heel pain, often called plantar fasciitis. The adductor hallucis TrPs send pain to the ball of the foot, as well as locally. TrPs in the transverse head of this muscle can cause a strange fluffy feeling of numbness under the metatarsal heads, and a sensation that the skin over the ball of the foot is swollen. It can feel as if the area is tightly stuffed with dry cotton balls. The pain from deep intrinsic foot TrPs is most noticeable when you get up in the morning. Until the plantar fascia and muscles stretch out, the first steps you take can be severely painful, and may feel as if you are walking over broken glass. You might also have numbness of the foot, or feel as if your foot is swollen. The use of orthotics with any of these TrPs can produce intolerable agony.

Notable Perpetuating Factors: Any cause of immobility (such as shoes that restrict toe movement), trauma to the toes and feet, Morton's foot, calluses, hyperpronation, hyper- or hypomobility, inflexible soles, walking or running on uneven terrain, soft soles that are too flexible with inadequate metatarsal support, walking on soft sand, wearing wet socks in cold weather (especially if muscles are fatigued), gout, Achilles tendinitis, plantar fasciitis, flat feet, diabetic neuropathy, and tarsal tunnel syndrome.

Hints for Control (Patients): Stretching and deep, slow massage of these muscles is helpful in conjunction with warm soaking. Discard ill-fitting or worn shoes. Unless you have a structural deformity, orthotics are usually unnecessary. You need soft cushioning, not hard orthotics, but not cushioning that makes your shoe too tight. We do not advise people with impaired circulation to use intermittent cold therapy.

Hints for Control (Care Providers): Distinguish between a fixed flat foot due to tarsal coalition and a relaxed pronated flat foot; the latter responds more quickly to conservative therapy. Include gait and posture analysis in posture evaluation. These TrPs interact with low lumbar and upper sacral dysfunction.

Stretch: See Superficial Intrinsic Foot Muscles.

Lumbrical and Interosseous Muscles of the Foot

Latin *lumbricus* means "earthworm"; *inter*, "between" or "among"; *osseus*, "bony."

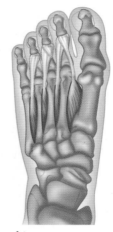
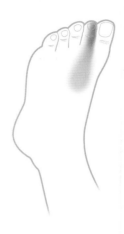

Dorsal interosseous.

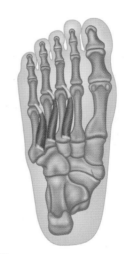
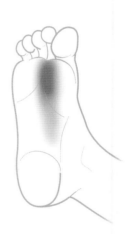

Plantar interosseous.

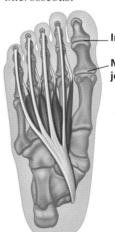

Interphalangeal joint

Metatarsophalangeal joint

The lumbrical and interosseous muscles are also part of the deep intrinsic foot muscles, and they have similar referral patterns.

What They Do: The lumbricals help flex all but the great toe at the metatarsophalangeal (MP) joint, and extend the lesser toes' interphalangeal (IP) joints. The dorsal (top) interosseous muscles work with the plantar (underneath) interosseous muscles to flex the MP joints. The plantar interossei are always underfoot. The dorsal interossei are very powerful: when we engage in vigorous twisting and turning of the foot, they control the direction of the toes to allow the long and short toe flexors to perform their own jobs. The interossei are involved in flexing many joints in the foot, helping the forefoot stabilize, as well as helping to maintain the foot arches.

Kinetics Comments: The lumbricals work with the flexor digitorum longus to prevent the toes from clawing inward when they push off during the gait cycle. They also help us dig into soft sand when we walk across it in bare feet. The lumbricals contain many sensory fibers, and research is needed concerning their importance.

TrP Comments: Lumbrical TrPs cause local pain, weaken the muscles, and restrict joint play, and so may contribute to any foot deformity or pain; one of the authors (Starlanyl) suspects they cause proprioceptive dysfunction. Interossei TrPs cause pain and tenderness locally along the side of the toe, and send pain to the ball of the foot behind each toe; they're often misdiagnosed as arthritis. TrPs in the first dorsal interosseous muscle can cause tingling in the great toe, and may be mistaken for gout. Inactivating dorsal interosseous TrPs may result in the disappearance of hammer toes, especially in patients who have not had them for long.

Notable Perpetuating Factors: Shoes that are too tight, coexisting area conditions (such as gout or arthritis), Morton's foot, trauma to the toes, and calluses.

Hints for Control (Patients): Ensure that all your shoes provide your toes with sufficient support and room. The shoe that seems to fit while you are sitting may not fit when you stand. If you wear shoe inserts, wear them when you try on shoes, and make sure that your shoes are wide enough for your feet. Tend your feet at least as well as you tend your face: keep the skin supple with lotion, and soak and clean them carefully.

Hints for Control (Care Providers): Ligaments around the interossei may have TrPs, especially those proximal to the tarsometatarsal joints. TrP injections of the feet are particularly painful, and should be avoided if at all possible. Use manual therapy and gentle ultrasound. Invest some time in creating handouts for teaching your patients how to care for their feet, and give them individual instruction when required.

Stretch: Curl the toes of one foot. Using your hand, uncoil the toes one at a time, finishing by extending all the toes together in one big stretch. Repeat with the other foot. Exercise bare toes by picking up marbles with them. Wiggle your toes around periodically during the day—if your shoes are not roomy enough to wiggle your toes, they don't fit!

13 Beyond the Myofascia

Introduction

When Travell and Simons wrote their definitive medical texts on trigger points, they laid the foundation; it is up to the rest of us to continue the work. For decades, clinicians and scientists such as David G. Simons, Robert D. Gerwin, John CZ Hong, and others kept TrP medicine alive, adding new pieces of the puzzle. Many continue to do so, and TrP research is rapidly expanding, thanks to a new generation of investigators such as Cesar Fernandez-de-las-Penas, Hong-You Ge, and Jay Shah. Little has been done intentionally on non-myofascial TrPs. As we were preparing this book, the most surprising thing to us was the amount of TrP research done inadvertently by investigators who are unaware of TrPs. It was obvious to us that these papers concern TrPs, even though TrPs are not mentioned.

We know that skin TrPs are common, and that active skin TrPs typically cause sharp pain and moderate to severe stinging or numbness. Tendon TrPs are common and have specific referral patterns. Some of the attachment TrPs in Travell and Simons' trigger point manuals are tendon TrPs. Subcutaneous TrPs may cause severe postsurgical pain that refers in an unanticipated way (Hendi, Dorsher, and Rizzo 2009). Postsurgical pain can be prevented or greatly minimized by the injection of local anesthesia along the surgical site before the incision is made. Some sprains initiate TrPs in the joint capsules: for example, one ankle sprain caused four joint capsule TrPs (Travell 1951). Each of these TrPs referred pain to the ankle and foot. Skin TrPs in the lower abdomen may cause urinary frequency and urgency as well as pain that seems to originate from the kidney (Simons, Travell, and Simons 1999, p. 956). Periosteal TrPs were also reported, with associated autonomic symptoms (pp. 43–44). We offer the following insights and possibilities in our exploration of TrPs in realms transcending the myofascia.

Scar TrPs: The Tip of the Iceberg

Laparotomy may leave behind unexpected deep scarring that can be activated by a simple abdominal massage. Scars that cause pain and other symptoms are called active scars. They not only cause pain, but also cause dysfunction. Such scars have formed without healthy independent layering of the tissues (Kobesova et al. 2007), and can affect posture, gait, and spinal flexibility. Scars may activate years after the original trauma. Even if a forty-year-old patient understands the concept of myofascial TrPs, she or he may not associate a paralyzing pain shooting from the knee to the hip with a knee scar from falling off a bike as an eight-year-old. Due to their nature, scars are considered to be deep tissue, even if parts of them are on the surface. The visible part of the scar, if there is one, is only the tip of the iceberg. Until a thorough history is taken and a manual examination of tissue mobility is done, there is no way to know the extent of stuck tissue beneath the surface. During the history taking and examination, one should document any scars and note their origin. When standard myofascial therapies don't work, frequently the reason is untreated active scar TrPs, as discovered by Lewit and Olanska (2004). These authors found that in a series of 51 postsurgical pain patients, the scar TrPs were the primary pain generators. Incidental appendectomy or ovary removal may have been done through the hysterectomy incision, leaving unnoticed internal scarring that can be far-reaching with no external scar.

Even a vaginal hysterectomy may cause massive vaginal cuff scarring with TrPs, and there may even be TrPs in a surgical drain site (Cummings 2003b). Scar tissue may form around spinal joints, causing restricted vertebrae, with spinal muscles compensating by moving too much and too hard. Irritation and sympathetic nervous system hypersensitivity (sensory overload) may result. Active TrPs in abdominal scars frequently refer to the back (Valouchova and Lewit 2009), but they could cause pain in the same abdominal region as the scar (Kobesova et al. 2007). The good news is that, even if a scar has caused significant pain for decades, manual treatment can often relieve the pain. When there is a wound, that area must be guarded from movement and covered to promote healing. In general, the process of scarring takes two to three weeks. Once the scar has finished its formation, protecting and sealing the wound, the scar by its nature tends to put tension on surrounding tissues. This can have a ripple effect. The scar is a barrier: it is a barrier to movement, and the body was designed to move. That movement restriction can, over time, cause other tissues to stick together. Releasing the scar and related adhesions may release tight tissues elsewhere along the kinetic chain. Scar release hurts. The tissue being separated is literally being torn apart. It must be done as gently as possible, working from as many areas as possible (see Chapter 14).

Ligaments: The Ties That Bind

Healthy ligaments are shock absorbers. When ligaments are tight and rigid with TrPs or calcification, bones may be pulled out of healthy alignment in relation to other structures, and the kinetic chain compensates. The effects of short, tight pelvic ligaments are obvious to experienced t'ai chi chuan players as they mindfully transfer weight from one foot to another. Many martial arts moves take advantage of the opponent's tight ligaments, just as they do of tight muscles, by targeting them as the weak links in the kinetic chain.

Ligament TrPs are described by Simons, Travell, and Simons (1999, p. 43); Hackett (1958, pp. 27–36) also described them thoroughly but, as was mentioned in the *Trigger Point Manual*, there were problems with the prolotherapy that Hackett recommended. Healthy ligaments are elastic. Prolotherapy is the injection of irritating substances into the tissues that further shortens those tissues. It is permanent scarring. One must be very

cautious with the use of prolotherapy, a name originated by Dr. Hackett. Prolotherapy was recommended by Dr. Hackett for weak ligaments. However, we believe that prolotherapy should be reserved for intrinsically hyperlax ligaments that have lost their elasticity, after any TrPs and facet joint problems have been treated. In cases of apparent long ligaments, when the ligament *seems* long due to compensational rotation of the attached bone, the cause is functional. Once the postural rotation is corrected (if the ligament hasn't lost its elasticity), the ligament returns to its normal length, but if it has been scarred by prolotherapy it cannot do so. One should treat the rotation and its perpetuating factors, including the myofascial TrPs.

Hackett referral pain patterns include hip joint ligament referral down the leg to the big toe, sacrotuberous and sacrospinous ligaments referring pain to the heel, and the iliolumbar ligament referring pain into the groin and vagina, with the acknowledgement that the iliolumbar ligament can cause any unexplained vaginal, testicular, or groin pain. The sacrotuberal, inguinal, sacrospinous, and other deep stabilizing ligaments can form TrPs that can entrap nerves and blood vessels. Sacroiliac joint stability is maintained by strong intrinsic and extrinsic ligaments. The sacrotuberous and sacrospinous ligaments are extrinsic (long) ligaments. As well as stabilizing the pelvis, they may have significant proprioceptor functions (Varga, Dudas, and Tile 2008), so it is of vital importance to preserve their integrity.

The sacrotuberous ligament has deep ties with the erector spinae and also the long dorsal sacroiliac ligament (Vleeming et al. 1996). It contains the coccygeal branch of the inferior gluteal artery, and is connected to the

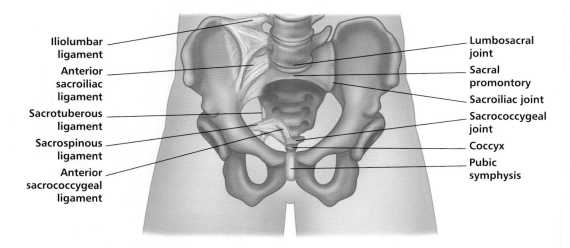

Pelvis with ligaments, anterior view.

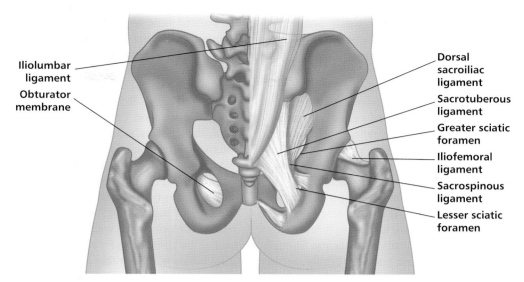

Pelvis with ligaments, posterior view.

sacrum, the coccyx, and the obturator fascia. The balance of the pelvic structures can be profoundly affected by TrPs in the sacrotuberous ligament, resulting in low back pain and postpartum pelvic pain. A tender point that can be found in the sacrotuberal ligament can be treated by massage and other mechanical therapies. This point can be connected to a reflex chain that contracts the lumbar erector spinae and affects the pelvic region as well, as noted by Lewit and Kolar (2000); it is also associated with backache, neck pain, and headache, as well as vocal dystonia. These authors mentioned the possibility that this tender point could be linked with a TrP in the coccygeus muscle underneath the ligament (p. 525).

The pudendal nerve can be entrapped between the sacrotuberous and sacrospinous ligaments (Robert et al. 1998). Presently, the common practice is to surgically sever the sacrotuberous ligament to relieve the resulting perineal pain. Perhaps manual TrP work or injections would be a better first option, allowing time to treat other TrPs that impact these structures. For example, in 50% of humans, the origin tendon of the long head of the biceps femoris is continuous with the sacrotuberous tendon (van Wingerden et al. 1993); therefore TrPs in the biceps femoris may create tension in the sacrotuberous ligament, which could then create tension in other structures.

The long posterior sacroiliac ligament is a critical link between the legs, spine, and arms, and its tension can have far-ranging effects on multiple kinetic chains. The tightness of these ligaments is affected by pelvic torsion. During pregnancy, the pelvic ligaments are relaxed, and the sacrotuberous and sacrospinous ligaments *must* relax for birth to proceed normally. The birthing process and recovery are much easier for baby and mother if the pelvic ligaments are free of TrPs. The time to check this is before conception if possible, or as soon after as practical.

The fibular collateral ligament has a referral pattern that may be masked by TrPs in the vastus lateralis muscle or tendon. Look at the anatomy of the knee or any other complex joint and think what havoc TrPs residing in ligaments there can cause. One must proceed cautiously, as TrPs could be the body's way of compensating for hyperlax ligaments. Tendons are relatively inflexible compared to ligaments. Keep the tendons free to minimize stress. TrP injections with local anesthetics in close proximity to the peroneal nerve may cause temporary paralysis or the peroneal muscle.

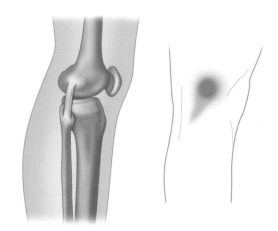

Fibular collateral ligament.

Taut bands running horizontally across the spinal column have been discovered. Each band begins on one side of the spinal column and crosses the spine to the other side. To our knowledge, these have not previously been described in the literature. One of the authors (Starlanyl) has them, and they have been palpated by myofascial TrP experts including TrP therapists and an MD, a DO, a chiropractor, and an acupuncturist. Some bands are in the cervical spine, while others are in the thoracic spine and low back. Similar taut bands across the spine have been found in five other patients, and I have corresponded with more patients and care providers who have palpated similar bands. Each patient had CMP with coexisting erector spinae TrPs, but these taut bands are not associated with those TrPs. Each patient had suffered previous whiplash trauma. Whiplash can occur at spinal levels other than the neck during falls, sports injuries, and other traumas. We know the TrPs exist, but don't yet know their origin. The leading speculation is that they may be anterior longitudinal ligament (ALL) TrPs. The ALL is often damaged during whiplash, especially during rear impacts. Injuries to the ALL may result in neck instability (Stemper et al. 2006), leading to further TrPs. Pain-generating nerves from irritated discs run through the ALL. They don't run fast enough to outpace the pain—they carry it—and substance P (a neurotransmitter) is found there as well (Coppes et al. 1997). Substance P is released when a TrP twitches, adding to the pain burden. The ALL has not yet been tested for the presence of other substances commonly found in the vicinity of TrPs. With aging, the ALL sometimes calcifies, which may be worsened or even caused by the presence of TrPs. TrPs may also occur in the supraspinal ligament. We look forward to more research on this subject.

The Geloid Mass

Justine Jeffrey, this author's (Starlanyl's) myotherapist, discovered masses of gelatinous tissue over resistant TrPs on some of her patients. These geloid, rubbery, clearly definable, discrete masses with palpable boundaries often had the same tactile sensation as that of a silicone implant. We referred to them as "myoblobs," until David Simons renamed them "geloid masses." My description matched one he remembered from an article by Essam Awad (1973). I read the article and agreed. Two studies followed (Starlanyl et al. 2001–2), building on the conclusion of Dr. Awad that these masses were largely glycosaminoglycans, especially hyaluronic acid. The geloid masses occurred in patients with both FM and CMP, and all the patients in the second Starlanyl study had both thyroid resistance and insulin resistance. This meshed with the finding of others that resistance to both of these hormones often occurred in the same patients (Garrison and Breeding 2003). Conversations followed with JB Eisinger, who had found that thyroid resistance was common in FM (Eisinger 1999).

Tissue overgrowth has been linked with excess glycosaminoglycans (Mariani et al. 1996). I had observed tissue overgrowth in the form of ingrown hairs, thick scars, adhesions, fibroids, and overgrown cuticles in patients with FM and CMP. John Hong wrote that he had observed tissue overgrowth in his patients with CMP,

but only in those who also had FM. After our first study (Starlanyl and Jeffrey 2001), I found that the geloid masses responded to the application of hyaluronidase, but one needed to avoid its application on joints. It was difficult and expensive to obtain, so we swam metabolically upstream. George Roentsch, a member of our research team, compounded T3 cream for the second study. His T3 formulation is available free on the website of the International Association of Compounding Pharmacists. We have since found that many of these patients do not test low in typical thyroid testing, but do respond to T3 cream. This is typical in cases of thyroid resistance. After reading our papers, Dr. Awad called. He was sure that what we described was what he had biopsied so long ago. One of his coworkers, Fritz Kottke, agreed that, yes, the geloid mass was what they had studied (Ibrahim, Awad, and Kottke 1974). A friend saw the study and emailed me to say that he thought he recognized the geloid masses in one of his patients (Ozgocmen 2001); his description sounded like an early-stage geloid mass. We discussed the possibility of T3 topical cream, but hyaluronidase is more efficient and significantly easier to obtain in Turkey than in the USA. The patient responded. Dr. Kottke had been mentor to Dr. Simons, as Dr. Simons had been to Dr. Hong and me. The research was reproducible, and spanned the boundaries of time and distance. Research published as this book was being written sheds new light on the importance of the hyaluronic acid and fascia connection (Stecco C et al. 2011). There is a substantial layer of deep connective tissue, rich in hyaluronic acid, between deep fascia and deeper skeletal muscle, and lesser layers contained within the deep fascia. Hyaluronic acid (also called hyaluronan), is a critical element that determines tissue stiffness. It affects the sliding motion between fascia and muscle, and between different layers of fascia. Hyaluronic acid is hydroscopic; it attracts water and holds it like a sponge. This attribute turns deep fascia into a reservoir of wastes, toxins and excess fluid that may be a key to interstitial swelling in chronic pain and dysfunction. This concept may hold a potential treatment of TrPs with hyaluronidase, and indicates that the use of cosmetics and medications containing hyaluronic acid must be reassessed for some patients with chronic pain.

The Dural Tube

The dural tube (also called dural or thecal sac) is modified fascia in an elongated membranous cylinder that extends from the brain to the end of the spine. It protects the spinal cord and nerve roots and keeps them bathed in cerebrospinal fluid. Dural rigidity is associated with headaches (Dean and Mitchell 2002). Injury to the coccyx can cause headaches due to dural tube restrictions (Upledger 1987, p. 119). When the dura is tighter than optimum, there is more chance that minor bony irregularities or disc bulging will become pain producing. Any flexion of the body can cause tension in the spinal cord (Harrison et al. 1999). The head-forward position puts the spine in a degree of tension, which is one reason it is a perpetuating factor and can lead to a propensity for greater damage during subsequent trauma. The dural tube can be released to ease compression in the CNS. This compression can happen from any stressor, especially trauma—even the trauma secondary to facet injections. Much of the work done in dural tube release is in the realms of osteopathic medicine, chiropractic, and manual release therapies such as neuromuscular therapy and cranio- and myofascial release. Manual techniques for release of a tight dural tube should include release at the crura (see Diaphragm). Exercises such as the pelvic tilt and touching chin to chest help to stretch the dural tube and keep it flexible (Manheim 1994, p. 146).

Cardiac TrPs: The Heart of the Matter

TrPs discussed elsewhere in this book are located in striated skeletal muscle. The pericardium—the sac surrounding the heart—is a type of modified fascia, as are the dural tube and the perineum. Cysts may occur in the pericardium and can cause chest pain, shortness of breath, cough, and/or abnormal heartbeat—symptoms that are also caused by TrPs elsewhere. Occasionally they occur after trauma, but usually we are not sure why they form. We generally don't become aware of their presence unless they are the types that grow and cause problems. Might some of these cysts be TrPs? One of us (Sharkey) believes so (and the other author agrees)—the thought came to him while contemplating a heart that he held in his hand. Although the muscle of the heart is smooth muscle it is striated, just like skeletal muscle, and is somewhat similar to skeletal muscle in its constitution. The myocardium is intercalated, which means that if only one fiber receives an electrical stimulus, that stimulus will spread across all heart fibers. The possibility of myocardial TrPs has not been mentioned elsewhere, to our knowledge. We believe it's worth considering whether cardiac TrPs can exist. If they can, what symptoms are they producing? Which treatment protocols are best? With the numerous imaging diagnostic tools now available, we call upon researchers to go where no one has gone before.

A Gut Reaction

The iliocaecal valve lives between the end of the small intestine and the beginning of the large intestine; this valve prevents contents from moving backward. It may refer pain, although the patterns have not been confirmed. It can be aggravated by constipation and other gut irritations, and can activate psoas TrPs and perhaps TrPs in other areas as well. Trigger areas that referred pain to the abdomen and multiple sites outside the abdomen have also been discovered in the esophagus, small intestine, and colon (Moriarty and Dawson 1982). Could TrPs occur throughout the gastrointestinal system? Layers of the inner abdominal wall lining that suspend the organs and hold them in place are called mesenteries. David G. Simons raised the possibility of TrPs in the intestinal mucosa (Simons, Travell, and Simons 1999, p. 959), and I (Starlanyl) had several discussions with him about the possibility of TrPs there and in the mesentery tissues. We suspected that they were common. (We also believed that ducts throughout the body could be entrapped by TrPs as well.) The mesentery is a type of fascia, and entrapment of blood vessels by TrPs in the mesentery could contribute to mesenteric ischemia and inflammation. This is currently only speculation, but manual TrP work done on the abdominal area can have profound results. On patients with CMP and central sensitization, even exceedingly gentle work aimed at the deep interior must proceed with care, as it could inadvertently set off massive TrP cascades if multiple TrPs exist in many tissue layers, with consequential release of substances in amounts too large to be processed and eliminated readily.

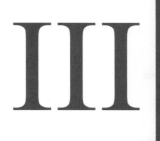

WHERE DO WE GO FROM HERE?

Now that we've looked at individual TrPs, it's time to learn how to deal with multiple TrPs, expanding on the material in Chapter 4. Like the rest of this book, this part is for both patients and care providers; after having read through it, you can then use this book as a working reference. TrP medicine is complex. It is appropriate for care providers to refer to the book during the history taking, exam, and treatment—especially at first. Patients and care providers need to understand this. The process will become easier and faster as you gain more experience. Chapter 14 covers the mysteries of history taking, physical exams, and treatments; in each of these areas, the patient is a valuable, contributing member of the health care team. We conclude in Chapter 15 with a discussion of FM and TrPs in the twenty-first century.

14 Solving the Puzzle: History, Exam, and Treatment

Preparation for an Appointment

Care providers, this chapter will cover mysteries, and they aren't the kind you read on a rainy weekend. They shouldn't actually be mysteries, but modern medicine has evolved into something that doesn't always work well for FM, TrPs and CMP. It tends to rely on tests and other things that aren't applicable, and dismiss things that don't show up. If your patient has both FM and extensive CMP, don't be dismayed if the early pattern charts are almost entirely marked in, with overlapping types of symptoms and colors every which way. Your patient may need multiple charts for each color. This complexity of pain and dysfunction may actually understate the truth, because there may be layers of TrPs yet to manifest. You will be working with your patient to bring about healing through TrP therapy and teamwork. Your patient, with your help, will evolve into a vital resource for you both. Right now, you both have a lot to work on. It is a start, because you *are* working on it. This chapter will help you use the history, symptoms, ROM and palpation to locate TrPs to identify the most troublesome TrPs and perpetuating factors. As the TrPs are treated and the perpetuating factors come under control, individual TrP patterns will be revealed on the charts. Give it time.

Patients, optimize appointments by bringing a current symptom pattern chart for each visit. A blank sample chart can be found at the end of this chapter—make copies of it to use. Start working on your chart long before the appointment, whenever you remember important things you want to say. This is especially important if you have FM as well. You can keep adding to the chart until you hand it over, but keep it brief and clear. You may want to make a color copy for yourself. If you don't have access to color copies and have different types of pain, you may want to make several charts; one for each type of pain or symptom. The reason may become evident once you look at the chart. If you have a lot of overlapping pain and other symptom coverage, you may also need several charts. Referral patterns are identified by areas that *aren't* covered as well as those that are, so be precise, and note other symptoms that may hold clues to the location of the peripheral symptoms. If you have peripheral pain generators other than TrPs, such as arthritis, other joint problem or diabetic neuropathy, include those. Include even temporary pain generators such as sprains, as they may add to symptoms of central sensitization.

If you keep a notebook of dated symptom charts it will help detect patterns and potential perpetuating factors. Gee, every time Aunt Nellie visits I get this pain in my neck … Is it your Aunt Nellie? Or does she sit in a corner chair and you have to crane your neck to hear what she says? You get the picture? Now you need to draw it. Include notes on non-pain sensations, such as loss of balance or bloating. For pain areas, note the nature of the pain (stabbing, burning, etc.), as that may be an important clue. Note areas of swelling or other localized symptoms. A notebook of the charts will also help keep a record of your progress. If you work with your medical team on control of perpetuating factors and peripheral symptom causes, you will have progress, but it may be hard to realize it otherwise. As one TrP is resolved, another may awaken. Don't be dismayed. This is progress. You are dealing with unwinding fascia. Some of us have tissues so tight that we can't see the muscles move under the skin when we use them. What a triumph when this changes.

Make copies of the sample blank chart at the end of this chapter; use it to record what you feel. This will help keep your medical appointments efficient, and also provide a record for you and your care providers. In the sample chart, there's a space for notes on symptom quality. Note the approximate dates each symptom appeared. If you don't remember the dates the first time, give the approximate month and year. Don't let that inability frustrate you. Frustration won't help you remember, and it can hurt. You don't need any more hurt. You'll develop a habit of noting when a new symptom appears. Mention what you've tried to control symptoms—what helps and what doesn't. Write down the three or four main questions you want answered on the next medical visit, and list any prescription or other needs. Make your notes clear and brief, and limit them to what's significant, including any changes. If you need a more expanded version for yourself, put it on a separate paper. Your care provider must be able to read it. You have limited time together. Writing legibly isn't easy for some of us. Take your time. It will help you use every minute with your care provider wisely.

Leave space for your care provider's comments and instructions. Whenever you add a new medication or change dose, update your other care providers. Keep a list of medicinal teas, herbs, and other over-the-counter (OTC) medications you take regularly (e.g. eye drops, nasal sprays, antacids, herbal remedies, laxatives), as well as OTC topical preparations (e.g. antihistamine creams). Updated lists of medications, supplements, and a brief history, including surgeries (type, reasons for, date, outcome), should be part of your home medical records. Keep a list of all illnesses and allergies (including food). It's good to have a list of nonmedical therapies you use. Include all forms of bodywork and mindwork and self-therapies. Maintain records of any medications you have tried and how they affected you, the dose, who prescribed them, and when. Samples of many forms for this have been provided (Starlanyl 1998), and you can tailor them to meet your own needs. Retain copies of relevant test results as well. All this material should go with you when you see a new doctor, and some should be with you when you travel. You're a vital part of the treatment team, with your own responsibilities and duties. Empower yourself by learning all you can to avoid pain, dysfunction, and trips to the Emergency Department. Learn to manage what you have and control the symptoms as much as possible. Pay attention to what your body is trying to tell you. You can't complain that your medical team isn't listening to you if you won't listen to your own body.

Care providers, your new suspected or known CMP and FM patients may not trust you at first. They may have suffered through, and paid for, all manner of tests, treatments and procedures. Many may have been unnecessary. They may have been denied needed answers and understanding as well as treatments, medications, and support; thus even validation, and hope. The system may have been cruel and unfair to them, and they may be expecting more of the same. They may feel hopeless, helpless, or angry; they may be physically and emotionally drained and frustrated. It takes courage for them to take one more chance. They have done so—they have come to you. You may have to convince them that you can make a difference when so many others have promised but failed to deliver, and then placed the blame on their patient. Take the time to earn their trust, because they are worth it. These patients may come with hefty records: some of the material inside will be significant, but some important conclusions may be erroneous.

Scan the charts for relevant gems before the first appointment, because you will need every minute you have together—and more. These patients may have been labeled with psychological ills because previous care providers didn't recognize TrP symptoms. They might have been given physical therapy to "strengthen" muscles weakened by TrPs, and then blamed when the therapy didn't work. They may have problems remembering sequential events, and be labeled "tangential" because of their previous history deliveries. Or they could have been classified as hypochondriacs or malingerers. Notes from an astute bodyworker may reveal the presence of taut bands and contraction knots, indicating the presence of TrPs. You can't treat CMP without the patient's cooperation and commitment: you need to rely on your patient (and sometimes your patient's companions) to supply needed information. If central sensitization—which may or may not have been labeled FM—is present as well, and you attempt to treat the FM without treating the myofascial TrPs, the best that you can expect is that the TrPs will become latent. Those little land mines will wait until an activating factor creates a massive boom, with your patient at ground zero. TrP treatment and control of perpetuating factors is a critical part of FM management strategy (Ge et al. 2011). Current research suggests that "assessment and treatment of concurrent TrPs in FMS should be systematically performed before any specific fibromyalgia therapy is undertaken" (Giamberardino et al. 2011).

If your new patient has CMP, or you suspect it, you need to spend time with them—more than the current system provides. If you only suspect CMP, schedule a "meet and greet" session during which you can get an idea of possible TrPs and coexisting conditions. An intake assessment may require several hours, and may need to be broken up into segments. There is danger in palpating areas, and perhaps activating TrPs, without treating. There is a tremendous amount of work dealing with CMP, but, eventually, an educated patient does most of it. CMP is a high-maintenance condition, and that work is amplified by FM too. With this book, your lives will become easier. If you are fortunate, your patient will come in with this book. If they don't, see that they go out with it: it will save time, money, and effort. This book gives patients tools they need. Eventually, they will be more specific with regard to TrPs when making appointments: instead of "my shoulder hurts," the appointment may be made for "probable coracobrachialis TrP activation with possible levator scapulae involvement." You get more specific information from educated patients. Education is part of your job. Anticipate that, in future visits, your patient will bring their charts partly filled in; during the visit, more information may be added Ensure that your first instructions for completing the charts are clear. Check with your patient that. Ensure that your first instructions for completing the charts are clear and legible, and check that they've been understood. You may want to make a color copy of each symptom chart as part of your progress notes. Especially if your patient also has FM or other cognitive challenge, s/he needs written instructions, including any action notes specifying what each of you needs to do before the next appointment. For example, you may need to order tests for coexisting conditions or provide stretches, and your patient may need to get tests done, modify a diet, and/or add exercises.

If your new patient comes in totally unaware of TrPs, charts and other important data, part of the first visit may be spent helping her or him fill out that chart. This is especially true if s/he says that everything hurts. You may be able to find one area that isn't totally colored in. It's education time—with these conditions it's always education time—and it's a start. And education goes both ways. You may be surprised at what your patients can teach you if you listen and observe. Find TrPs by means of history, symptoms, ROM, and palpation. As TrPs are treated and perpetuating factors brought under control, individual TrP patterns will be revealed. Other patients may come in with localized TrP pain, but in time you may find that there are TrPs all over their bodies. An educated patient will understand that this isn't a sign that things are getting worse under your care: it is simply that latent TrPs are being revealed and treated. Unraveling CMP cannot be rushed. You needn't spend extra money on diagnostic equipment: you already have what you need to diagnose TrPs—your eyes, ears, fingers, and brain. Develop (in t'ai chi terms) your ability to focus your intention to use those parts of your body as information gatherers during the diagnostic process. Learn how to use them, and invest the time you need to gain experience in their diagnostic use. You need to learn to coordinate these investigative tools that you've been given, and hone your talent to find and heal TrPs. Investing time and effort in this process will teach you priceless diagnostic skills. You will become more attentive to life; to observe, and to make connections. Base your questions on patient history and symptoms, and word them carefully. For example, avoid phrases that can lead to misunderstandings, such as "working at a computer"; the patient may work for four hours a day at a computer, and then play computer games or correspond via email for an additional six hours. Become familiar with Chapter 6 and the concept of perpetuating factors, and modify questions accordingly. Remember, it doesn't take an active TrP to cause symptoms: muscle cramps, for example, can be imitated by latent TrPs (Ge et al. 2008b).

History

The body is an ecosystem, but it isn't a closed ecosystem—there are sensory impacts, environmental impacts, medicinal impacts, etc. Some care providers learn how to take a history as part of the process of differential diagnosis, but differential diagnosis tends, by its nature, to be exclusive. With chronic pain there are usually multiple causes contributing to that pain, only one of which is myofascial, and a list of perpetuating factors. More complex cases may involve multiple coexisting conditions and layers of perpetuating factors, only some of which may be evident at first meeting. The central sensitization and biochemical imbalances of fibromyalgia may add yet another dimension. Care providers, you need to reframe what you've learned into the dynamics of interactive diagnoses. Patients, you need to acquire skills to take your own history, because your history holds clues to your symptoms, TrP locations, and perpetuating factors. You are the authority on your own history. Do you remember when the pain or other predominant symptom first started? If so, what was happening in your life around that time? Can you remember times when your symptoms changed or new symptoms appeared? What changed in your life just before or at that time? Learn to look for patterns—not just symptom patterns, but life patterns as well. The clues are all there, waiting to be discovered. When you take a medical history, think outside the box: this is most easily done by not putting yourself inside the box in the first place. Look for connections. The history should indicate if the pain pattern is stable, or if it has evolved over months or years. Neither FM nor CMP is progressive. Any worsening or addition of symptoms is an indication of uncontrolled perpetuating factors.

During ideal history taking sessions, patients and care providers work together as a team to hunt for clues. This is not standard medical practice. Patients may not mention important symptoms or occurrences during the history-taking process for several reasons: they may be in denial, or they may think they'll be considered irrational if they mention how they fling objects into the air when they try to pick them up, or that they become nauseated watching an airport carousel for luggage. Patients new to you may be considerably apprehensive about how you will treat them, adding to their stress level. Patients may not remember a specific physical or psychological trauma, and/or they may have PTSD. If they are in chronic pain and/or have FM, they may not be able to remember all important events, and the significance of some events may become apparent only as new symptoms appear. Patients may be unaware of a repetitive strain, especially postural strain. (Casually taken photos—not staged, professional ones—can offer great clues to postural problems.) Family members, especially spouses, educated in this discovery process may be great resources. Encourage the patient to seek constructive feedback from family and friends, taking extra care that it isn't turned into an adversarial process. For those patients who live alone, an overnight guest might help uncover clues to sleep abnormalities or other perpetuating factors. During history taking, note faulty and potentially destructive movement patterns, including breathing patterns. For example, sitting with legs crossed is often done to compensate for weak QLs. The first history is a time for ideas to emerge, and is only the beginning to a process that never ends. What happens today is tomorrow's history.

When I (Starlanyl) lectured about these conditions in Brittany, we had a morning session for care providers and an afternoon session for patients. During lunch, a doctor with new awareness in his eyes came up and spoke of his regret for not being able to also attend the afternoon session due to office hours. He gestured to the TrP diagrams and gently admitted, "I must go and apologize to my patients." Such a compassionate and honest revelation is uncommon. Yet the process of learning in medicine is just that; a process that never ends. You can learn nothing if you think you already know everything. Patients who have become educated about FM and CMP may have had previous experiences with defensive, suspicious, or even hostile care providers. They may have been labeled as exaggerators or considered obsessed with their health because of their knowledge of medical terms and their conditions. Everyone needs to accept that patients are an integral and valuable part of the health care team, and fluid communication among team members is essential. Patients and care providers need to learn that it's safe to be specific, and to ask questions, and to admit that there is something they don't know. Both need to learn to trust each other, and to communicate freely. This means dialogue: "It hurts when I move my arm."—"When you move your arm how? Can you show me?" The patient may not know what triggers the symptom pattern until he or she repeats the exact motion, and that motion can indicate to the educated care provider where some of the TrPs are. The extent and nature of ROM restriction may give some indication of their severity, and to possible coexisting conditions. In cases of active CMP, the arm may always hurt, but a particular movement may cause it to hurt more. Taking histories for CMP patients may take much longer than for other patients, especially if FM co-exists, but many resources including time may be saved in the long run. However, insurance, legal and other systems need to become educated to this reality: for example, it is necessary to educate hospitals with policies censuring doctors who have an "inadequate" number of surgical referrals. Many surgeries may be preventable with early TrP identification and treatment.

Exam

Although much of this section is written for care providers, our readers who are patients need to read it too. Patients need to know what to expect in an exam. There are ways in which patients can help to make the exam more efficient, and that often means preparation is required. Patients may already be aware of significant factors, such as restriction of movements or gait irregularities. Patients can learn to be specific—for example, rather than saying "I trip a lot," say that "I trip often when I am going up the stairs" or "Sometimes I trip going across a flat floor." Patients may be able to save time by making a separate chart showing any scars, lumps, or asymmetries. Before the first appointment, or if CMP and FM are just now being considered, it's a good time for patients to examine their lives. Make a list of what affects your health the most, and how. This is valuable information; keep it brief and clear.

If you as a patient are aware of many symptoms in many areas, you and your care provider must decide together, before the exam, which are the four most important and life-altering symptoms that must be addressed today. These might include symptoms that could affect the ability to sleep, eat, breathe, maintain balance, or move. The clues to the locations of the perpetrators and/or TrP contributors are in the history and your charts. Care providers, plan to examine thoroughly only areas that can be treated in some way. Both parties must know the current level of pain before the exam, and then agree on a level that will not be exceeded during the exam. This can be very difficult if, using a scale of 1 to 10 with 10 being the worst possible pain, the patient is normally at an 8 or above. These numerical scales can only compare one patient's pain from one time to another. They are relatively worthless for comparing one patient's pain to another's. Patients need to specify what some numerical value means to them. For example, one patient might say that at a level 9 pain, they are bedridden and cannot prepare food for themselves, but can make it to the bathroom when necessary and they can take care of their personal hygiene. Another patient might have an entirely different numerical scale. Patients, it doesn't help anyone when you attempt to compare your pain to that of another person with these conditions. It can generate a lot of negativity. If one person can do a task at their pain level 7, it doesn't mean you can do that task at your level 7, or that you should try. Life is a compilation of variables, not an equation of absolutes. When you begin to compare, nobody wins. Avoid situations where nobody wins. Do the best you can with what you've got, and never feel guilty.

Some patients may need to take a little extra medication well before the exam to minimize the possibility of the exam aggravating FM. Palpation may activate TrPs, so the examiner should palpate deeply only those muscles that s/he or another care provider on the team will treat that day, remembering that effects of the exam may be delayed. Patients can become quite ill after an exam because of materials released through movement and palpation (see Chapters 3 and 13). The exam has truly already begun during history taking, with observation as the patient gestures, speaks, and moves around. Likewise, during the exam proper, the history taking and dialogue continues. ROM testing with goniometer measurements helps to find TrPs, can help track treatment success or failure, and will provide insurance documentation. Superb range-of-motion charts are available from Round Earth Publishing (Finn and Shifflett 2003). Depending on symptoms, check for gait irregularities, and sitting and standing postures; just as in t'ai chi chuan, it's often the transitions between postures that are the most difficult to execute and that relay the most important information.

The keys to manual examination are palpation, positioning, and patience. Palpation is the art of intentionally touching tissues to examine and discover what those tissues have to tell you about the body's condition. Examiners need to develop a fine sense of touch. Palpation for TrPs, especially in CMP patients with FM, is a *gentle* art. Keep in mind that other texts and resource materials are generally concerned with single muscle TrPs, and the pain those single TrPs cause has been described as "intolerable" and "torture." These patients are dealing with a multitude of interactive TrP symptoms that may also be amplified by FM. Respect that interaction, and respect your patient for persevering in spite of all that may have occurred before.

Examiners, remember that pressing on a TrP causes the symptom pattern. With multiple interactive TrPs you may activate multiple TrPs. Please don't deliberately provoke the TrP local twitch response if you can avoid it, because every time a TrP twitches, it releases toxic substances and the area becomes more acidic. If the patient has many TrPs—and they can have hundreds—those noxious biochemicals add up during and after an exam. Your patient may feel achy and miserable for days, and perhaps weeks, especially if FM amplifies the experience. Minimize TrP activation during exams. Please don't intentionally try to create a twitch response. *Avoid strumming palpation on taut bands*: it causes needless pain. Educate your fingers to minimize the production of unnecessary pain. Encourage a stream of feedback from your patient as you examine. Modify your technique to meet your patient's sensitivity.

There are resources to help learn the art of palpation (Chaitow 2010; Earls and Myers 2010); training is also available and desirable. You must still put in the time with your fingers palpating tissues. Practice how to use the direction of the muscle fibers to identify the muscles, and how to move your fingers gently across the fibers to encounter the taut bands. Bodyworkers have the definite advantage here. Doctors often are disadvantaged, in this modern world where touch between doctor and patient is often discouraged. So how do you get experience? Not on your patients, although every patient you touch can teach you something. Start by paying attention to *everything* you touch, focusing mindfulness and intention. Practice feeling the lines on the head of a coin. Pay attention to the muscles under the surface when you stroke your pets. Become more familiar with touching your own skin, and develop a feel, literally, for the layers of tissues underneath.

While you are sitting watching television or listening to music, palpate. For those who have their own TrPs, search out those lumps and ropy bands under your own skin. It's often easier to palpate taut bands and contraction knots on a limb that is stretched three-quarters of the way out. Move the limb around, noting how certain TrPs are more amenable to palpation from some positions than from others. Find out if the addition of a light lotion or oil or even water helps or interferes with your sense of

the tissues. Start with flat palpation, using the tips of the fingers, with your hand held parallel to the body surface being examined. This form of palpation is often the most useful for light exploration of superficial areas.

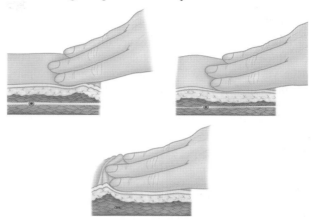

Flat palpation.

You'll develop "the touch" for changes in tissue texture, and any irregularities: the skin may move fluidly in one area, and in others may seem stuck. What do you feel in the tissues over bone or near scars? This type of palpation can be modified into a versatile treatment technique for patients and care providers.

Pincer palpation is also an excellent technique to master, but please start with light, gentle pressure.

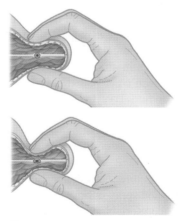

Pincer palpation.

This technique is handy when you're working close to the edges of muscles; especially when you can "get around" each side of them, such as parts of the SCM. You may be able to run the edge of the properly positioned muscle between your thumb and fingers until you encounter contraction knots. If the history and the referral pattern indicate a possible TrP in the vicinity and you cannot palpate it, see if you can find the taut band and follow it to the TrP. Positioning is critical in the art of palpation for TrPs: try different alignments of the muscle. Palpation is a science as well as an art, and much of the muscle positioning has been mapped out; for example, Travell and Simons (1992) devote many pages and diagrams to positioning the quadratus lumborum muscle. Careful positioning is necessary in palpating for location of deep TrPs, as well as for many therapies, including stretch and spray, and TrP injections.

At times, TrP locations may be resistant to palpation due to fibrosis, obesity, swollen tissue, or other coexisting conditions. The patient's pain tolerance must guide how deep you can go and how much area you can palpate. Meaningful feedback is critical to a successful exam. Patients, tell your examiner what you feel and how you are feeling; this isn't the time to chat about your goldfish. Let your examiner know if you think s/he may be close to a TrP, or when the target has been acquired. Both patients and care providers might want to ask relatives and friends to allow you to practice your palpation technique on them, but be gentle—they may have latent and unsuspected TrPs. A patient may wish to teach friends and family how to do a light palpation by demonstrating on an accessible TrP, but be sure they know to be very gentle. Just let them run their fingers gently over the surface of the skin to feel the contraction nodule. It's a chance to educate them about the reality of the TrPs causing many of your symptoms. At one time, "X" spots were used as *guidelines* to the most common locations of motor endplate zones, because that's where we thought most common TrPs were located. We've learned that motor endplates are found more extensively throughout muscles than just in the endplate zone (Gerwin 2010, p. 333), which means you can't find all the TrPs simply by looking at diagrams and checking the "X" spots. You need an understanding of anatomy, and you need to palpate all of the muscle and its attachments. We're gaining a new appreciation of the importance of TrPs in attachments such as tendons and ligaments. You can't get palpation experience looking at diagrams, or find TrPs by looking at pictures—you must *do*.

The patient must be as comfortable as possible during the exam and for TrP assessment. Patients with FM and CMP may require extra medication and/or therapy such as stretch and spray during and after the exam. The room must be comfortable to the patient in temperature, without drafts. The more relaxed the muscle, the easier it is to palpate, so it is important that patients avoid tensing in anticipation of pain. It often helps to put a muscle being palpated into a partial stretch. While it is important that latent TrPs must be treated (Ge and Arendt-Nielsen 2011), *the* exam is not the time. For now you are finding (and eventually treating) active TrPs causing the previously agreed-upon four most significant symptoms. Attachment TrPs may be harder to palpate, as this area is frequently tighter and more likely to be scarred, fibrotic, or calcified. You palpate with the fingertips. Palpation *requires* short, smooth fingertips and fingernails. You can't palpate successfully if you have fingernails like hawk talons or calluses like steel guitar players. Keep nails short, with no ragged edges. Take care of your hands. Practice touching lightly, so that the eyes of your fingers see all that they are able.

Examiners may need to figure out a way to take notes during the exam, including a sketch of—yes—another body chart. In CMP, TrP contraction nodules in thicker muscles may occur in clumps as large as a grapefruit. The tissues around such a clump may be so tight and swollen with infiltrates that it feels like one huge nodule until some of the interstitial swelling is reduced, and such a clump may be covered with a geloid mass. TrPs are not homogeneous: the feel of each contraction nodule depends on many variables, including the amount and variety of biochemical infiltrates and excess fluid the area contains. Some contraction nodules resemble ball bearings, marbles, or even tiny hard seeds; the last can often be found around nerve endings. Sketch in any stuck tissue, but unless positively necessary, such as for reactive cramping, don't treat *during* the exam. Passively move the muscle to check if there is a crackling or popping sound when the joint is moved. Write down the presence of dermographia and location of geloid masses. Sketch atypical patterns of hair loss on the body and head, which can occur along TrP referral patterns and may be mistaken for stress reactions or other conditions.

Treatment

Patient education is a major part of treatment. For example, patients must understand that pain caused by such-and-such a motion is an important clue to where the TrPs are located, and that continually avoiding that motion will only lead to further loss of function. Each patient is unique: a specific therapy may be more successful on some patients at different times, may not work at all on others, and may even make some worse. Finding out why may be an important part of identifying subgroups of FM, but the presence, location and number of TrPs must be taken into consideration. One thing is always certain—you need to identify and control as many perpetuating factors as soon as possible and as completely as possible. Also, any therapy program must start cautiously and slowly. A successful TrP treatment will release those toxic substances and stored wastes from the myofascia and surrounding tissues. This is true even for the gentlest therapy, and CMP patients may have a lot of TrPs to release. The body's detoxifying system can handle only so much waste and toxic matter at a time, and the rest continues to circulate in the body until it can be processed and eliminated.

Each new therapy must start cautiously until the patient's tolerance is found. For example, the positive experience of deep sleep from sodium oxybate therapy can restore the balance of some biochemicals (those that are rebalanced during deep sleep), causing release of some muscle tension, causing activation of some TrPs, thus causing a temporary increase in pain and other symptoms. This could lead to a mistaken belief that these symptoms are drug side effects rather than TrP activations that are part of the healing process. That could be why so much of the sodium oxybate side effects list reads like a list of possible TrP activation symptoms. The dose of sodium oxybate for CMP and FM patients who can't get deep sleep otherwise should be started much lower than that for narcolepsy patients or patients with only FM and a few TrPs. It must be titrated slowly upwards, with frequent patient feedback and careful monitoring, especially at first, to achieve deep sleep with the lowest possible dose. One needs to be familiar with the whys and wherefores of drug actions and interactions, as well as the mechanisms of FM and TrPs, when dealing with these conditions and medication therapy.

All actions have consequences. For instance, obese individuals on a healthy diet may already be dealing with the release of toxins, as these are often stored in the body fat (Tremblay et al. 2004). When such a patient is also treated for TrPs, the released materials are additive, and increased fatigue and aches might, again erroneously, lead one to believe that the treatments are doing harm. Ease up on therapy according to patient tolerance: treatments must be scheduled so that the patient is able to recover from one treatment before going to the next. When the health of the patient has improved to the extent that there are fewer toxins released and detoxification pathways are improved, more frequent therapies can be scheduled. The system is currently set up to expect more frequent treatment right after an injury or new diagnosis, and less frequent treatment as a patient improves. This is not what most patients with CMP and FM need.

For both patients and care providers beginning on the healing road together, there may be the temptation to take on too much at once, or to feel totally overwhelmed by the enormity of the task. Travel on any road one step at a time. After the first exam, prepare a plan together. It would be marvelous to immediately be able to identify and map all TrPs, but it's not always possible or even advisable to do so. It may have taken some doing and more than a bit of time to get the patient in the situation s/he is in now, and there's no quick fix. Of course, there are always people who will say that there is, and they'd be happy to sell it to you. If you've read this whole book, you have some idea of the complexity of TrPs, FM and how they interact. So unless you can get a contract in writing how that miracle diet or herb or whatever is going to identify and fix your ill-fitting furniture, erase that head-on collision, or vanquish those coexisting medical conditions, shoo that denial dragon away. You can't wave a magic wand. Well, you can, but it won't do any good. Don't be overwhelmed by what you *can't* do: focus on what you can. Target the four most significant symptoms. Identify all known and suspected perpetuating factors and decide what needs to be done to control the known

ones and investigate the suspected ones. That may mean tests (such as a sleep study), exercise regimens (including correct breathing technique), and dietary changes. The patient may need to start journals (sleep, diet, pain level, exercise) so that suspected problems can be documented. That includes keeping a record of treatments too. These are high-maintenance conditions, and there is no cure yet. But there can be significant improvement in quality of life, treating symptom management, and even remission. Breathing correctly doesn't take extra funds, but the results can be profound.

The process may be overwhelming, so it's best to break it into parts. Some things may seem unchangeable, but that perception too may change with time. Make a list of what can be changed. For the primary care provider (PCP), this is also the time for the first medication check, and the start of vitamin and mineral supplementation if needed. Schedule appointments for tests and treatments. Address sleep dysfunctions and other life-altering issues. During future visits, the PCP needs to include time to check brief journal summaries (the patient prepares these), compliance with scheduled therapies and, at first, test results.

Any chronic pain conditions may be accompanied by information-processing deficits, and fibromyalgia may bring its own cognitive deficits, so please write down any instructions for patients. If there are stretches prescribed, the patient needs to demonstrate an understanding of them by performing each one in front of the appropriate care provider. Supply a written direction sheet on every new exercise. Handouts are great time-savers in chronic pain treatment; they help prevent communication failures and may therefore save time, money, and even lives. Patients and care providers need to become comfortable using this book as a reference during treatment. CMP is too complicated to expect anyone to remember all of these patterns along with all of the information that goes with each one. Familiarity takes experience, and that takes time and effort.

Proprioception and autonomic function may be impaired in CMP in many ways: there may be coexisting conditions, and/or multiple nerve and blood vessel entrapments. FM central sensitization amplifies TrP symptoms and may amplify any treatment side effects. There may be layered TrPs, especially if the muscle is a complex one such as the levator ani. So where do you start? Well, that depends on the four symptoms your patient has picked and what kind of care provider you are, and will vary with the patient and the circumstances. For example, pelvic asymmetries must be corrected before leg length, but unequal leg length may be contributing to pelvic asymmetries. Pain is almost always a major perpetuating factor. If patients are on narcotics or other heavy medication and have substantial pain, check the spine. If history indicates abrupt or repetitive trauma, check the spine. If the TrPs don't respond to adequate treatment, check the spine. The spine is a major pain and dysfunction interaction site. TrPs are associated with disc pathology, at least in the cervical (Hsueh et al. 1998) and lumbar (Samuel, Peter, and Ramanathan 2007) areas; one of the authors (Starlanyl, unpublished work) has found this true of spinal facets as well. Typical forward and backward bending tests for disc vs. facet pain may not work if TrPs are part of the equation, because these motions may aggravate TrPs causing some of this pain. The TrP taut bands may also be "guarding" the spine. Appropriate imaging, which may include flexion/extension X-rays, may reveal perpetuating factors. There are non-surgical options for controlling spinal nerve pain; patients may require a combination of these, including spinal, nerve and facet blocks and FSM. TrP injections may prevent some degenerative disc pathology. We don't know. So much time has been wasted trying to deny the existence of TrPs and FM. It's much more cost-effective to prevent them.

Care providers should consider adding TrP therapists to their health care team. For example, dentists must be able to provide minimum TrP work to have success in equilibration when patients have head and neck TrPs. Stretch and spray could save much harm in the dental world. Handouts on TrPs are available for some dental, medical and mental health specialties (Starlanyl, website). TrP medicine opens up a new range of treatment options, no matter what your field. Which therapies have worked for the patient in the past?—build on them. What therapies are available in your area?—it is to every care provider's advantage to know who's out there and can help. When dealing with CMP and FM, patients need a health care team. They work together, first on those four targeted symptoms. What kind of therapy lends itself to those problems?—be open to alternatives. There is a whole world of treatments beyond the scope of this book to consider. Therapies often complement each other, but many aren't currently covered by insurance. One must proceed with caution with any new therapy, or any new area of therapy, for patients with CMP. Therapies that may be beneficial in the long term may cause extra symptoms in the short term due to TrP activation. Go into every new therapy with the knowledge that no matter how gentle, it may provoke TrP activation. Remember that perpetuating factors often have perpetuating factors.

Bodywork

No book can cover all types of bodywork, although some have been described by Starlanyl and Copeland (2001), and neuromuscular aspects have been covered by Sharkey (2008). In every type of bodywork, therapists vary greatly in their skill sets and experience. For example, some massage therapists do Swedish massage only, using five flowing strokes that calm the CNS and improve microcirculation. I (Starlanyl) have a massage therapist,

Lindsay Crossman, who is adept in that technique as well as in a variety of TrP skills, Vodder lymphatic drainage, and an abundance of other healing therapeutic options. She is constantly expanding her knowledge, as are the rest of my health care team. Patients and care providers, investigate. See who is available in your area. Patients, ask your support group. If you don't have one, start one. It soon gets around who is good and who isn't. You require an excellent PCP who understands your conditions. The letters after the name won't indicate what they know about FM and CMP. Many medical schools don't yet teach what is in this book. Ask what they know. Then vote with your feet, and demand options. Some craniosacral or myofascial release therapists have some of the education, but may lack "the touch." Patients with CMP and FM must be especially careful in choosing bodyworkers. Their bodyworkers must know and understand both of these conditions, or be willing to learn and listen. Even gentle Trager massage may cause such patients to be bedridden for a while if there is lack of understanding and dialogue before the massage begins. When CMP and FM coexist, any body work, therapy or exam can activate one TrP that develops satellites and can start a chain reaction of TrP activation, called a TrP cascade. Suddenly, all the TrPs in the whole body, or in one side, can be active, and everyone is wondering where all the pain came from. When toxic materials are released from the myofascia, cognitive function may be one of the first things affected, including communication skills. It is important to give the bodyworker feedback when necessary, and the bodyworker must be aware that the client may be profoundly affected by the treatment, either immediately, or as a delayed response.

General Bodywork Hints

Keep a list of anything that breaks the symptom cycle or can provide temporary relief. Here are some general bodywork tips:

- Care providers, with any type of treatment, address the less painful side first, if there is one, to diminish the chance of reactive cramping or rebound (Funt 2009).

- Adequate hydration is critical to healing. Patients should drink ample, healthy water before and after treatment, and keep it handy at all times.

- Healthy posture is a priority.

- Patients: move mindfully and efficiently, avoiding jerky motions. Use your body properly. Care providers: ensure that your work table doesn't place undue stress on you or your patients.

- Begin all posture exercises carefully, performing them without repetitions several times during the day, coordinated with proper breathing.

- A muscle with TrPs is already physiologically contractured and can't be strengthened until the TrPs are resolved. Be patient.

- Repetitive exercise is inappropriate for muscles with active TrPs.

- Find a healthy exercise that you enjoy and do it regularly.

Any bodywork can provoke an emotional response, including reliving of traumatic experiences. These emotions can include rage as well as terror or sorrow. Some forms of bodywork are more apt to provoke a response than others. Shedding tears as part of a somato-emotional release can be helpful, but be aware that other reactions are possible too. When treating patients with CMP and multiple coexisting conditions, including FM, preparation can be a life saver. There are four common stress responses: fight, flight, freeze, and startle. FM can amplify any stress reaction, and pain can provoke it. Remember, in FM, touch, smells, and sounds can be perceived and experienced as pain. Neurotransmitters can be unbalanced in FM, and they control the expansion and contraction of blood vessels, among other things. Care providers: monitor your patient's status during therapy and have an emergency plan in place for cases of sudden sensory overload. Your patient may be in a freeze or numb state and not able to clearly communicate to you the level of pain they are experiencing. This may rapidly advance to a startle or even shock state; appropriate care protocols may vary from decreasing as many stimuli as possible (dimmer lights, music shut-off, etc) and careful monitoring, or to shock protocol. Patients: keep a list of activating factors for your TrPs, a list of signs that indicate your symptoms are getting out of control, and a written plan to follow if and when that occurs (Starlanyl and Copeland 2001). Have necessities on hand if you must spend a prolonged time at home, and a list of contacts you can call on for help if needed.

Therapeutic Methods

A TrP is physiologically contractured tissue that requires physical techniques. Manual thrust chiropractic isn't appropriate for TrPs: if there's nerve entrapment, especially spinal, it could be both painful and harmful. Chiropractic Activator adjustments are often effective for bone realignment and may relieve pressure on other tissues. TrPs must also be treated and perpetuating factors brought under control, or the adjustment and the relief will be temporary, because the TrPs are still causing muscle contracture, and the bones may be pulled out of alignment by the tight muscles. Even if there is spinal or other pathology, it's often possible to significantly improve the symptom level and quality of life by treating the TrPs. TrP patients come in all varieties, from star athletes to cancer and HIV patients … from children to geriatric patients in nursing homes. Symptom relief is

a valuable gift to provide to anyone. Treat the patient, not the imaging or the lab test. It's better to under treat than over treat—small, gradual steps are best. Any changes must be facilitated through all the systems of the body. This requires energy, and TrP areas are already in an energy crisis. We need to identify a direction and destination for our treatments. That said, the care provider and the patient are dealing with a situation that is constantly changing and shifting like sand beneath the feet. Be prepared to change the plan on the basis of the response to the previous treatment.

Areas of very sensitive TrPs can be worked by stretching tight tissues *around* the TrP, gradually working your way to the TrP itself. Skin rolling, a technique whereby the upper area of skin is picked up and rolled along the tissues, is often impossibly painful and unproductive in TrP areas, especially for FM patients. The skin surface may be cemented to the subcutaneous tissues, which adheres to the tissues beneath, and so forth down to bone. Attempting to abruptly tear those tissues apart is akin to flaying your patient, causing mind-numbing pain. The patient may also experience delayed disorientation and other sensory overload effects for days, so seek gentler options. Check muscle attachments for TrPs. Many insurance companies are unaware that some muscles have more than one attachment, and a reimbursement may reflect this: educate them.

Barrier Release
In all therapy methods, the patient must be as comfortable as possible, and the muscle(s) to be treated must be well supported. Barrier release is a form of flat palpation that is extremely useful. If working on a limb, the muscle is slowly and gently lengthened until it begins to resist; there should be minimal if any additional pain—just resistance. The palpating fingers gently approach the area of the TrP, sliding across tissues in a flat plane until the tissues resist the progress of the fingers. At this point a palpable barrier has been encountered. Hold gentle finger pressure against this barrier until it releases, as if it is melting. This may process takes time. Take what it requires. It doesn't take a lot of pressure, but you may need to try an approach to the barrier from several different directions before you get a release. The fingers progress until they find a new barrier; work continues until all the barriers are gone or there has been as much treatment as can be tolerated. The same process may be needed with every taut band. The TrPs may, however, be too irritable to tolerate the pressure, and if the patient tenses in response, the process won't work. Moreover, excessive speed or pressure can increase pain and rupture the contraction knots. Work the fascia in a three-way stretch, restoring the elastic component and healing ground-substance deformation and tissue thickening. You are gently separating microadhesions. There can be blood vessel and nerve entrapments, so be mindful of those fragile structures. When there is a release, the

tissues beneath your fingers will shift—sometimes subtly, at times massively. This method is similar to scar TrP release. Be patient. Like the song says, breaking up is hard to do.

Scar Release

When the body fails to knit traumatized tissues neatly in corresponding independent layers, it can form adhesive scar tissue that alters the proprioceptive input of the whole region (Lewit and Kolar 2000). This, in turn, results in a variety of protective compensations that can disrupt entire kinetic chains. Scars can be trouble, even if they seem innocuous. Active scars may be clinically relevant to the current symptoms, even though they are some distance away. Especially if central sensitization (FM) is involved, there may be layer after layer of irregularly formed stuck tissue down to the bone, spreading out in all directions. The surface scar may be indicative of only a small portion of the tissue damage. TrPs in scars can cause sharp, lightning-like or electric pain. Tendons, ligaments, and bones may shift to accommodate scars and adhesions. Scars can introduce an unpredictable kinetic chain branch. Look for "increased skin drag in the area of the scar, increased resistance of the skin and the subcutaneous tissues to stretch and folding, and tenderness when exerting pressure on the tissue fold" (Lewit and Kolar 2000, p. 527). Only part of the scar may be active, although this may change as treatment progresses. Utilize the barrier release method—this doesn't involve pressing *on* the scar, but rather stretching surrounding tissue away from it. Gently mobilize large scars, especially when adhered to underlying bone. Respect FM pain amplification. Never attempt to tear the scar away from its surrounding tissue!

Approach a scar from some distance, granting it respect, as if cornering a wild and unpredictable creature (which in fact you are!) Use flat palpation, very lightly, until you feel the first barrier. By palpating the scar and the immediate surrounding tissue, you can feel where tissues are stuck, how deep they're stuck, and in what directions they are stuck. Next, start to work on the scar, keeping lines of communication open and encouraging feedback from the patient. Scar release hurts—the object is to get the maximum release with the minimum amount of pain.

Material from a lovely paper by Kobesova et al. (2007) about the treatment of an active scar is presented here with the permission of those authors. The article offers hope that, even after decades, TrPs in scar tissue may be effectively treated with tissue mobilization. Deep abdominal scars are common, can be extensive, and may be hidden and unsuspected. An appendix or ovaries removed during another surgery may leave no visible scar, yet cause severe pain when palpated. Such internal scars may be causing major kinetic chain disruptions. The active scar doesn't move freely against underlying structures: there is resistance to the skin stretching around it. Check to see if such a scar is involved in the patient's

chief complaint. If not, note it for future work and move on. If the scar is clinically relevant, barrier palpation and similar techniques are the least traumatic ways to release the scar. The goal is to increase tissue mobility. Start by stretching the superficial area around the scar, mobilizing the skin and the immediate area beneath the visible part of the scar. Please be as gentle as possible.

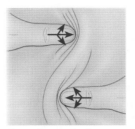

Stretching a soft tissue fold.

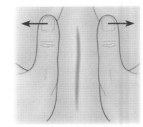

Skin stretch.

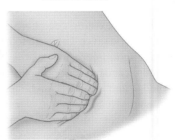

Deep palpation and barrier release of restrictions in the abdominal cavity.

Drawings reproduced with kind permission of Anna Kobesova.

Mobilize the tissue in as many ways as possible, always keeping within patient pain tolerance limits; work it using barrier release.

> Whether the clinician stretches or shifts the scar, there is always a free range in which little resistance is encountered. By our definition, the barrier is reached (engaged) at the first point of resistance. This definition implies that the physiologic barrier is soft; it easily gives and can be "sprung." Very gentle digital movement must therefore be used, which allows the first barrier of resistance to be palpated, and then the resistance gradually increases under the physiologic circumstances … Treatment involves engaging the pathological barrier and waiting; after a short delay, a release gradually occurs until the normal barrier is restored. (Kobesova et al. 2007)

Some patients can learn to self-treat scars within their reach. Any successful TrP treatment may produce multiple twitch responses. Some TrP twitches may go unnoticed: some may be very obvious. Remember, when a TrP twitches, over 30 irritating biochemicals are released into the body (Shah and Gilliams 2008). It's much better if those substances are on their way out, rather than being stored within the tissues. As these chemicals circulate, and until they have been released from the body, patients may feel toxic. They need to drink large amounts of water before and after therapy to dilute and help flush out these materials. Tolerance to treatments can vary considerably from patient to patient, and tolerance may vary depending on the treatment type for any given patient. One scar may take multiple sessions.

Indirect Therapy

Chronic pain almost always involves a myofascial component (Simons, Travell, and Simons 1999, p. 267). The interactive aspect between TrPs and many other conditions can be useful, as successful treatment of such a condition can help TrPs. For example, histamine is a big player in pain, and can be controlled by medications and some therapies. It is involved in immune reactions and allergies, and influences the action of some cytokines (Igaz et al. 2001), which play a part in FM. Histamine is one of the chemicals released during TrP twitches. Don't neglect the TrP component of other major illnesses. For example, TrP release may significantly improve the quality of life of cerebral palsy patients. One study (van Wilgen et al. 2004) found that 46% of post surgery cancer patients have myofascial pain adding to their symptoms. For example, TrP therapy for terminally ill patients may allow them to eat, giving them a higher-quality life.

Patients with multiple illnesses may find that what helps one condition may worsen another. For example, people with arthritis are often given those little marble-like balls to exercise their fingers, but such repetitious work can rapidly worsen coexisting TrPs. Arthritis pool therapies may include repeatedly lifting jugs filled with water overhead. The TrPs are going to complain, loudly—perhaps not immediately, but patients may not be able to lift a teacup the next day. Pool temperature must be higher for CMP therapy than for arthritis; pools that are adequately heated for arthritis may lead to dangerous cramping in some TrP patients. A temperature of 90°F (about 32°C) is good, but may be difficult to find.

Stretching

The concept that stretching can magically solve many pain problems is a myth. Most muscles will begin to rip and tear when they're elongated by more than 5–7% of their resting length. If muscle receptors are functioning correctly, the fibers and associated fascia are desperately trying to resist lengthening by contracting or stiffening. If tissues are tight from TrPs, movement is the key. Any involved (TrP-laden) muscle needs to be completely relaxed in order to be fully stretched, and that can be problematic. Stretching may ease central muscle TrPs but aggravating attachment TrPs. If hyperlax (often called hypermobile) tissues are involved, care must be taken not to overstretch: both the patient and the bodyworker may be unaware that hypermobility is a factor until the TrPs are resolved. We believe that some TrP formation is the body's attempt to compensate for hyperlax ligaments; these TrPs return quickly after treatment, as they exist because associated ligaments have lost the ability to stiffen—their first line of defense. Stretch only within a healthy ROM, not the maximum possible, and stretch in a dynamic manner. Holding static stretches can

result in the lengthening of more "plastic" tissues (such as ligaments). A combination of muscle inhibition and overstretched or "lax" ligaments is a recipe for formation and perpetuation of TrPs.

> Standard stretches can leave shortened areas unaffected while further separating overstretched sarcomeres and firing off protective anti-stretch reflexes. This is why (static) stretching as "warmups" in exercise class can decrease flexibility. It is also why "strengthening" exercises can leave muscles weaker: more shortening of the already over-shortened fibers, further stretching of over-stretched ones. In contrast, stretching against resistance dramatically increases ROM because it restores both types of abnormal fibers to normal resting lengths. Stretching under load pulls the over-stretched sarcomeres back together while pulling the shortened ones apart. (Shifflett 2011, p. 84)

Dynamic ROM stretching involves taking a muscle through its full, healthy ROM by actively contracting its antagonist muscle—the muscle that works to balance it—so that the muscle stretch slows down towards the end of its range. This stretching is a functional elongation of all muscles involved in any specific action. We don't encourage the holding of a stretch end-point; the muscle should keep moving (dynamic), without bouncing or any other types of coercion. Dynamic ROM stretching is moving as nature intended, and should include rotations where possible, ensuring lengthening of the tissues in their order along the kinetic chain. We aren't forcing a stretch, only maintaining the available healthy ROM.

Tennis-ball Stretch

There are many ways to use a tennis ball to stretch muscles and treat TrPs. Rest your back, buttocks, or thigh on the tennis ball against the seat while in an automobile or during a long meeting. Press gently and hold it for a few minutes or less—avoid impairing microcirculation. Move your body on the ball from one side of the taut band to the other, as feels comfortable. Keep the pain level in check: if this hurts too much, start with a softer surface such as a sofa. Don't use too much pressure, as it can cause rebound tightening. When you can work the TrPs without excessive post-exercise soreness the next day, use a harder work surface. Practice using the ball against a wall. It takes a while to learn to keep the ball in place while you work the TrPs, so don't get frustrated if the ball escapes to the floor and you need to retrieve it—persevere. Remember to work on the sides of your body with the ball. Working on the floor with a tennis ball is very beneficial, but can be more painful because it's harder to control the amount of pressure. The first time you try ball work, go over each area once or twice lightly, then see how you feel the next day and modify treatment accordingly. FM patients especially have a tendency to lose track of how much bodywork they are doing. Use a timer. Don't use the ball across the spine or tailbone. Use deep belly breathing while you work with the ball, and keep hydrated.

A tennis ball in a knee sock can be useful for accessing hard-to-reach back areas, and you won't have to keep retrieving it. Knot two tennis balls together in a knee sock to use as a roller along the sides of your spine. Work those paraspinal muscles against the wall or on the floor. When you find TrPs, see which movements aggravate them, and which ones help. What do they tell you about your posture? If the aches and pains move from side to side, that's actually good: you're working out some TrPs, and other ones are clamoring for attention.

Stretch and Spray

This is not recommended for the cold intolerant. Many who are familiar with TrPs are used to the phrase "spray and stretch." However, we start the *stretch* first, to stimulate the muscle spindles; this is then followed by the vapocoolant *spray*, to deactivate the muscle spindles via cooling (Sharkey 2008). The spray direction follows muscle fiber arrangement and can be applied during stretch, *from muscle origin to insertion*. Each sweep should be close to and along side, but not directly over, the previous one, with no breaks between the sweeps. The spray pattern is specific to each muscle or part of a muscle and the muscle must be rewarmed after the spray. The muscle is then put through a *passive healthy ROM stretch three times*. Muscle positioning during spray is crucial. Many of the specific muscle spray patterns are shown in Simons' and Travell's texts (Simons et al. 1999; Travell and Simons 1992), and some can be found on the Internet. Patients need diagrams. Care providers need to remember, *spray from muscle origin to insertion*. This method is also useful in combination with TrP injections.

Patients, if you have clinically significant accessible TrPs, sufficient mobility, and the ability to learn safe technique, your care providers may teach you basic stretch and spray and help you get a spray prescription. It is even better if you have a willing, trainable partner who can assist, but they need training by the professional, and also need written directions to follow. The way you stretch and spray is important, and there are safety considerations, but your care provider will give you training and written instructions. It is important that time is invested by your care providers in preparing handouts and education—this may prevent emergency calls to your PCP during the night or on weekends. Self-treatment may provide sufficient pain relief to enable you to sleep, or to get yourself to your PCP's office.

For some muscles, the handout must include balancing safety, because some areas are difficult to reach. When beginning this therapy, start slowly, with one bottle—some people are sensitive to the spray, and others cannot master the method. *Asthmatics should not attempt to use vapocoolant, and everyone must learn to cover sensitive areas, as well as the mouth and nose to avoid breathing in expelled fumes or mist.* Check in advance that you will not have an allergic response to the spray. During the treatment you may need someone else present for health and safety reasons. Rewarming is a significant component of the therapy (Bahadir et al. 2010), and logic dictates that's true for ice stroking as well.

Ice Stroking

Ice stroking uses ice instead of vapocoolant spray. Ice is less expensive, safe for the environment, and (unless we continue to destroy said environment) more accessible. To avoid chilling the muscle directly, water can be frozen in a paper cup, or as an ice cube placed in a washcloth. The object is to cool the surface in swift strokes; not freeze the muscle. Ice stroking works best when used in the same pattern as stretch and spray. Care providers: if you suggest ice stroking, train your patients and supply written handouts for each muscle technique. Ensure that the patient does not become chilled during the procedure, or the skin harmed. The ice must flow gently and swiftly over the surface in the proper direction, and the surface rewarmed immediately before the patient stretches again. Muscles stretch better when they are warm and supple. This therapy takes a fine hand and experience—and experience takes time.

As you try any therapy, think about what it's doing. Cold shrinks blood vessels, and therefore decreases circulation. Cold reaches the brain faster than pain signals—so does touch. You can try overloading pain receptors with touch: experiment with light skin brushing or even a feather's touch, but both of these have been known to provoke a TrP twitch response. Heat expands blood vessels to help bring circulation into an area. Find out what works for you.

Needling

TrP injection therapy has been around for a long time, but acupuncture has been around a lot longer. Dry needling of TrPs without anesthetic is becoming more popular, because more people can do it than can do TrP injections with local anesthetic. Research indicates that it is the needling that relieves the tension caused by the TrP rather than the substance injected (Lewit 1979). Studies have been done on the merits of dry needling versus injection, but it is one of the authors' (Starlanyl's) opinion that much of the variation in success is due to the skill of the practitioners. TrP injections can be quite painful, and local anesthetic can minimize the pain. This can be an important consideration when there are multiple TrPs to be injected and central sensitization is an issue. Some local anesthetics are significantly toxic to muscles, and the one that is least toxic should always be chosen. *Steroids are not part of accepted typical TrP injection therapy.* It's vitally important that pain levels be monitored and under control, since the body can only endure so much before it reacts. (See Bodywork section in this chapter.) Some of the best care providers have had experience with TrP injections or needling causing sufficient pain to send a patient into shock. Logic would indicate that this is more likely to occur if the patient also has FM, has insufficient pain control, or both.

It's beyond the scope of this book to teach TrP injection techniques, but good training is available. Forms of needling, in our opinion, need to be professionally taught, along with many other TrP techniques, as part of professional medical and dental training. Even with experience and observation, many practitioners do not perform TrP injections properly. When a TrP is marked with a guideline "X," the temptation is to look at the picture, take aim at the location of the "X" spot on the patient, and then inject. That's not how a TrP injection is done. *TrP injections require careful positioning of the patient, careful palpation of the TrP, careful injection of all TrP areas in the contraction nodule, and full ROM stretching after the area is injected. It is inappropriate for the care provider to say, "I've injected. Now you go home and stretch."* Stretching *must* be integrated as part of the injection process.

TrP injections, including those into ligaments and tendons, can quickly release quantities of entrapped material that must be processed by the same detoxification pathway used to detoxify alcohol, caffeine, and acetaminophen. Patients, be kind to your body and don't stress it with extra toxins. Drink a lot of good water. You may be in a brain fog for a while, and/or particularly achy, as the released materials circulate in your bloodstream until they can be processed. Some of us prefer that the TrPs are injected with a small amount of local anesthetic, and then:

> … the dry needle is used to eliminate the remaining tender spots. Stretching after the trigger point injection is the most integral part of the treatment. Not stretching after injection or needling is the same as receiving no treatment at all. (Doggweiler-Wiygul 2004)

Psychological Support

It is logical to have difficulty keeping positive in a negative environment, but pain may have positive aspects. It's a learning experience. One of the first things you learn is that you don't want to experience it. There are books and chapters (Starlanyl and Copeland 2001) devoted solely to mindwork and psychological support. Stress is caused by chronic pain, and many symptoms may be compounded by the nearly universal lack of awareness or misconceptions concerning FM, TrPs and CMP. Patients must cope with the invalidation that comes from having a condition that is poorly understood by family, friends,

coworkers, classmates, and (too often) members of their medical team. This book is part of an effort to change the way chronic pain is being treated. That's way too big a job for two authors, or even for all those now involved in FM, TrPs, and CMP. So, kind readers, we ask that you use this book to help us teach the whole world.

Patients with these conditions have often expressed to me (Starlanyl) their sense of being marginalized, misunderstood, isolated, and alone. They feel overwhelmed as they struggle to explain their symptoms to an unenlightened world. They wonder if anyone believes them, or if anyone cares. I invite them they look at this book's reference section. Then go to my website (www.fmcmpd.org) and look on the care provider side for References for Research Purposes. There they will find many hundreds of medical research journal articles titles, some which have annotated notes on why that particular research is important to them. In these pages, you have already come across some of those talented authors. These dedicated researchers work to reveal the secrets behind these and related conditions. They are our hope. Whenever you feel alone, be comforted that these people and others are searching for the answers to your questions, and they are succeeding.

Healthy, function-oriented, information-oriented support groups can provide great support. If you don't have a group, start one. Avoid moan and groan groups, since negativity is a perpetuating factor. Remember these rules:

- There are always options.
- If you make a mess, clean it up and keep going.
- Find ways to navigate obstacles.
- Delegate, delete, or modify frustrating or annoying tasks.
- If you fall down, control your fall as best you can; then get up and keep going.
- If you make a mistake, accept that we all do, and learn from it; don't act as if it's the end of the world, or it will be.

Patients with FM must understand that hypersensitivity has its benefits. You may be able to grow the best plants. When you talk to your plants, they talk back. Animals may come to you. You may have empathic connection with all beings. This may get you in a world of trouble as you respond to what others are feeling rather than what they are saying, but you also have a unique ability to understand that can be very useful to help others. A long time ago, I (Starlanyl) created a word, FMily, that signifies our connection. Each of us may share more with each other than we do with blood relatives. There is an instant bond when we meet. We can use that to help each other and comfort each other. It's a priceless connection that means a great deal. We are FMily. We understand.

Don't allow yourself to believe that you lack choices. Catch yourself if you start a negative inner dialogue. Chronic pain patients must have a zero tolerance for toxic relationships. That includes your relationship with yourself. Take a good look at your lifestyle. Learn to pace yourself. This goes for you too, care providers. My (Starlanyl) spiritual, t'ai chi, and FM and CMP communities are great support. Others with these conditions often provide instant understanding. Friends are the family you choose, but choose wisely. A stroll through the woods, a good book or film, losing yourself in music, or a "walk" through a picture can provide the distraction you need to get through a tough time.

Medications

You might not have considered some of the medications that can be of value for your symptom control toolkit. For example, remember histamine and the connections it has to chronic pain? An antihistamine may relieve some of the symptom burden, but be aware that diphenhydramine (one of the first known antihistamines) stimulates about a quarter of the population. Some people can't take it because a pill in the morning keeps them awake that night, yet others can use it as a sleeping aid when taken in the evening. Diphenhydramine should not, however, be used by the elderly. Any substance that helps in controlling a perpetuating factor can be of help in controlling the symptoms. This includes ice and moist heat.

Consider options for controlling coexisting conditions, especially anything that may help two or three conditions at once. For example, Xyrem (sodium oxybate) has been proven to provide deep-level sleep (Russell et al. 2011), and the lack of this type of sleep is a major perpetuating factor for both TrPs and FM. Deep-level sleep is when many neurotransmitters and hormones are balanced, and allowing the body to perform this natural balancing act can promote healing in a number of ways, along with the other benefits that deep sleep can bring. Right now, use of sodium oxybate is very limited in the United States because of concerns that it could be abused as a "date rape" drug. If you undergo a sleep study showing that you can't get deep-level sleep even with a CPAP, your insurance will probably cover this medication. You may be able to use a much lower dose than is common. The goal with any medication is to use the smallest amount that achieves the optimum effect. If you do have problems getting sufficient restorative sleep, use good sleep hygiene. Keep environmental stimuli low: try high-performance ear plugs (look in a gun shop) and a good, soft sleep mask with straps that won't cause TrPs. Make use of all sorts of tools in your symptom control toolbox. Atrovent Nasal Spray 0.06% (ipratropium bromide) is a prescription anticholinergic drug used to treat congestion and runny nose, which may be caused by some TrPs. TrPs are associated with excess acetylcholine at the motor endplate, so it may provide multiple benefits. It may also allow better breathing, sleep, and allergy control. Anything that provides, or allows the body to provide, more oxygen to the tissues can be a big plus. Congestion and postnasal drip may be side effects of the body's attempt to protect its tissues from acid reflux, so work on controlling GERD as much as possible with diet and other options.

The experimental use of hyaluronidase may be a way to get at the cause of the swelling and tightness of deep fascia (Stecco C et al 2011.) One must be very careful to avoid touching joints with this biochemical, use minimum amounts, and use only on those TrPs that are resistant to other treatments. It is experimental, and must be compounded in the USA (and is very expensive there.) In the United States, the few medications approved for FM have a very low success rate and often intolerable cause side-effects. Many patients suffer when their doctors prescribe higher and higher dosages in a futile effort to reduce opioid usage.

Patients with mouth, nose, genital, or rectal TrPs might find that the use of topical lidocaine ointment can relieve the pain temporarily. This may make internal TrP work (and even pelvic and rectal exams) bearable in spite of painful TrPs. It won't prevent TrP cascades. Topical oral anesthetics are available OTC in many countries, and may make work on oral and nasal TrPs endurable. Even if only 5% of some symptoms are relieved, it's a help. If you have spinal illness or other significant point-source generators, a 5% lidocaine patch can take another slice out of your pain burden. Percentages add up. Don't leave anything out of the toolbox, except your brain. You need to be able to think outside of the box.

Drawing blood may be extremely difficult and painful if TrPs lurk in the area of the draw. Pain tends to cause the blood vessels to constrict anyway, and TrPs can further restrict blood flow. Add to that vasoconstrictive medications such as antihistamines, and veins can become absolutely unsociable. After the additional pain of a few unproductive needle sticks, the veins may go into a witness protection program. This scenario may be minimized if the patient is well hydrated, relaxed, and warm. Before the blood draw, the most accessible vein area (and an alternative) can be prepared a few minutes in advance with a compounded topical muscle relaxant, such as diazepam or carisoprodol. This relaxes the tissues surrounding the vein, and can make all the difference. The use of a butterfly needle will greatly minimize the chance of a TrP cascade developing, during which TrPs could activate from the venipuncture site all along the kinetic chain. This activation could take a week or more of extra therapy and medication to quiet down.

Muscle relaxants can be of tremendous help during long trips and other periods of prolonged immobility: they may prevent TrP activation, and speed recovery from prolonged sitting, unanticipated hauling of luggage, and other perpetuators. Many patients with CMP and FM have found that regular use of a muscle relaxant can minimize the need for pain medication. Tight muscles hurt! Do be aware that benzodiazepines can lessen the pain-relieving ability of narcotics.

In the USA, the "war on drugs" has become a war on chronic pain patients and their care providers. The Drug Enforcement Agency focuses on drug abuse rather than drug use. Fear of prosecution results in frequent undertreatment of acute pain, with the consequence that more patients are developing chronic pain, requiring expensive pain medications that are hard on their bodies and minds. TrPs go unrecognized and patients are put through needless procedures, surgical and otherwise, in an attempt to control the symptoms. Pain generated by multiple TrPs and then amplified by FM central sensitization goes unrecognized, with consequences that, at best, constitute patient abuse, and, at worse, are orchestrated torture. Further potential aggravation of TrPs may go unrecognized, so CNS is further sensitized by inadequate pain control. Care providers may attempt to perform testing and other procedures on patients with FM central sensitization without extra medicinal support, even though these same procedures commonly require pain medications for healthy people. It is often erroneously assumed that the patients with pain are on sufficient medication already, forgetting that this medication is required just to control their existing pain. If the test must be aborted because of extreme pain, it's then blamed on the patient, rather than on the lack of adequate pain management. Hospital administrations tend to deny capability to institute adequate pain management of TrPs and FM. FM patients are regularly "weaned" off the very pain medications that work—the ones they need to prevent their central sensitization from becoming worse. The system needs to change.

Electrotherapies

In CMP, a muscle may fail to release because TrPs in another muscle are preventing its release. There may be scarring, shortened fascial wrappers, adhesions, fluid accumulation by excess hyaluronic acid, fibrosis, etc. This tightness may hurt, especially if FM coexists. Hypersensitivity works in many ways. Look for therapy options. Ultrasound, galvanic stimulation, microstimulation, and other electrotherapies including FSM can help soften tissues, with less trauma and fewer side effects, although all the concerns mentioned earlier regarding the release of noxious substances are relevant. FM may amplify this sensation, but FM patients may also be more sensitive and receptive to these therapies. Hypersensitivity has some good effects. The more effective the treatment, often the worse the patient may feel afterward. FSM can be especially helpful because it is effective for treating TrPs, FM, and many coexisting conditions, as well as perpetuating factors such as scars (McMakin 2011). It is extremely patient-friendly, but, as with all techniques, is only as effective as the person controlling the equipment. Investigate options.

After any treatment, soaking in a bath with Epsom salts and ground ginger may prevent some post-therapy soreness. Many herbs and supplements, such as omega-3 oils, are anti-inflammatory. Avoid strenuous activity after treatment; this includes stopping at the grocery store on the way home. The body is learning to realign itself, and that's hard work. Patient tolerance of any treatment depends on many variables, including what is happening in that patient's life and how much central sensitization is present. Reread Chapter 6; identify all the perpetuating factors you can and bring them under as much control as possible. This really is the key to successfully reducing symptoms. If TrPs persist, there are unidentified perpetuating factors. Find them.

How many treatments will it take? That's a question care providers are often asked by insurance companies. Chronic means chronic. It takes what it takes—there can be no set time limits or number of visits or treatments. Patients and conditions vary tremendously, and chronic pain medicine often seems to be a field wherein all constants are variables. Right now, the medical care system is broken. Right now, the patient pays for the shortcomings of the current system. There are things that can be done, such as treating all acute injuries and illnesses aggressively. That doesn't necessarily mean more medication; it does mean preventing as many new perpetuating factors as possible, and controlling the ones that exist. If TrPs continue, in spite of adequate treatment, something is perpetuating them. It may be impossible to control all of the perpetuating factors. Many other chronic illnesses aren't curable either, but they're controllable to some extent. FM and CMP are no different. They are just less understood by insurance companies and other third-party payers. It may take some time to educate your insurance company that treating TrPs will be cheaper for them than dealing with expensive surgeries, rehabilitation, and other long-term consequences of not treating the TrPs. The systems are broken, and that's resulted in a lot of broken people. We need to work together to put those people back together, and help them put their lives back together too. Together, maybe we can even fix the system. To successfully accomplish that task, we must change the way that chronic pain, and chronic pain patients, are treated.

The Referral Pattern Chart 1

Patient: _____   Care provider: _____   Date: _____

blue = pain; yellow = numbness; orange = tingling; green = cramp; purple = tightness

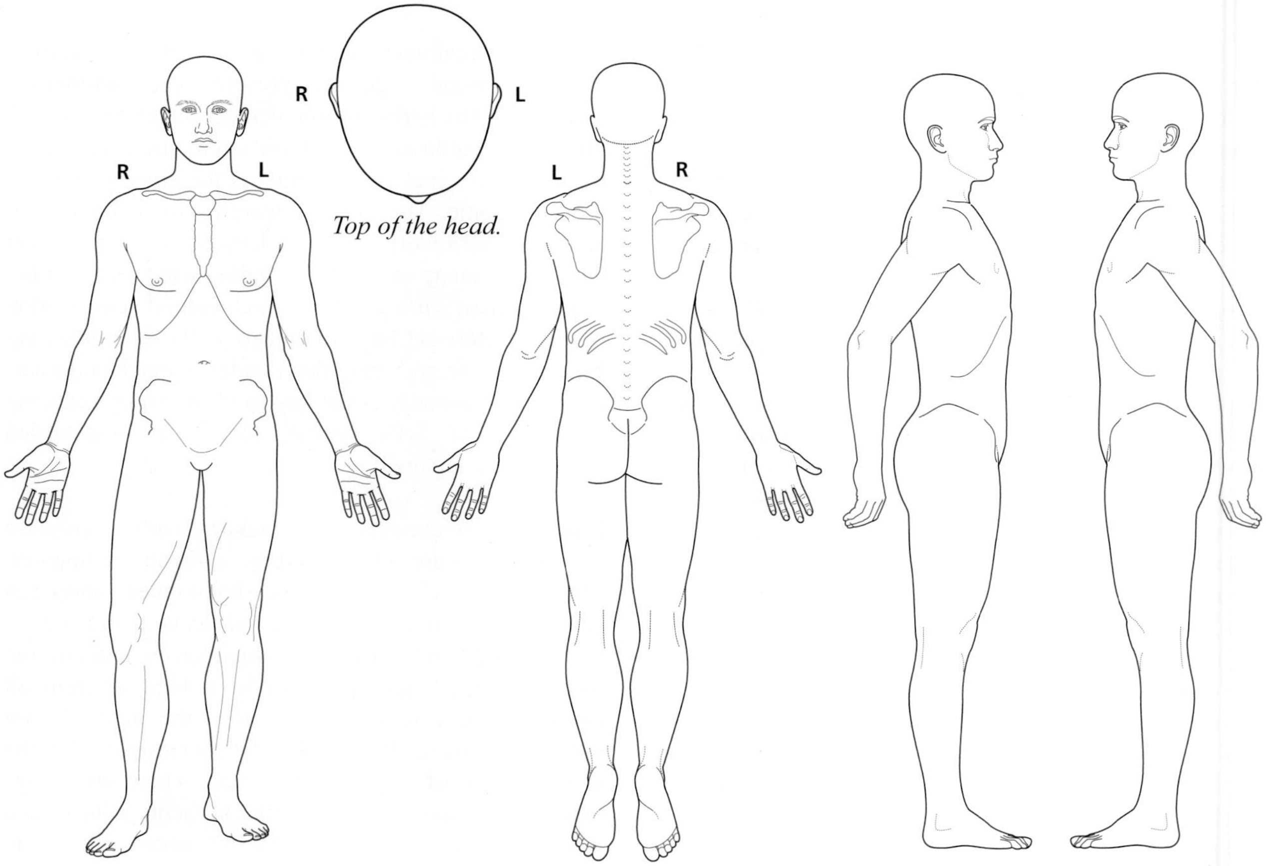

R   L

Top of the head.

R   L   L   R

L   R

Right side.   *Left side.*

Reason for visit: _____

Most distressing symptoms: _____

_____

Additional patient comments (quality and nature of pain, aggravating factors, what has been tried and results): _____

_____

_____

Changes: _____

Needs (including prescriptions, therapies or tests): _____

_____

_____

Action items (patient and care provider): _____

_____

The Referral Pattern Chart 2

Patient: _____ Care provider: _____ Date: _____

blue = pain; yellow = numbness; orange = tingling; green = cramp; purple = tightness

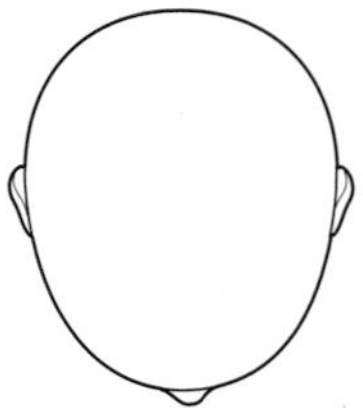

Top of the head.

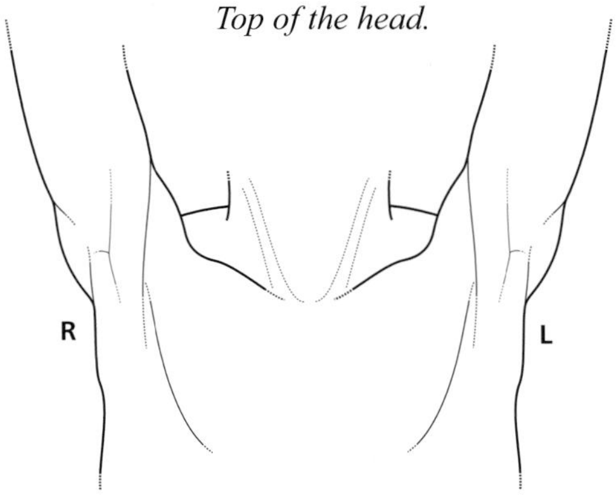

Underarm areas.

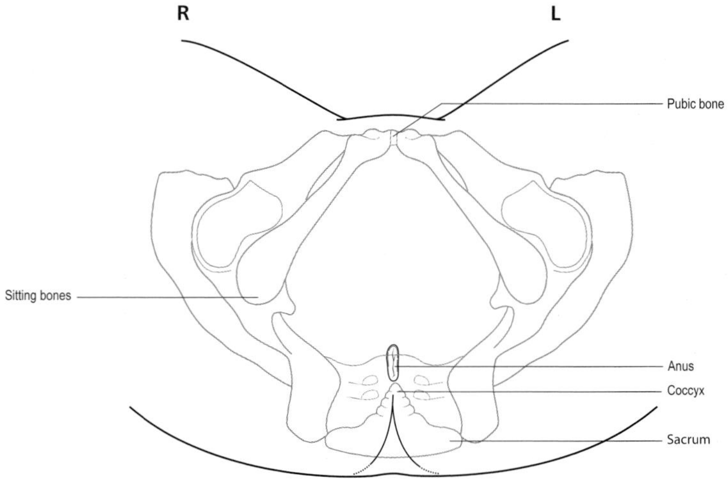

Pelvic area.

Additional patient input: _____

_____

_____

_____

Care provider comments: _____

_____

_____

_____

Action items patient: _____

Next visit: _____

Action items care provider: _____

_____

15 Trigger Points in the Twenty-First Century

Where We Are

If we immediately identify and treat individual TrPs and control their perpetuating factors, we can minimize the number of new cases of CMP that develop. At present, we have a large cadre of CMP patients, and they require appropriate care. We can improve their function and quality of life and prevent their conditions from worsening, although their numbers will grow as more care providers recognize TrPs. We now settle for descriptions such as "atypical MS" and "chronic low back pain" being used as diagnoses because of a general lack of TrP training. Insurance companies may label *billing* codes as "diagnostic", but most are only descriptions. Expensive and extensive procedures, including surgery, are being performed, yet pain and dysfunction often remain or return. Patients suffer with treatable symptoms because health care providers often fail to recognize TrPs. We all share a health care crisis and can't afford to continue with a system that creates more chronic pain patients as it wastes resources.

Patient quality of life with nonmalignant chronic pain is among the lowest of any medical condition. Managed health care focuses on finding a cure as quickly as possible, but chronic illness doesn't fit into that game plan. When patients aren't cured, care providers and patients may feel a sense of failure. But chronic means just that: the condition continues or recurs. Yet there is hope. All chronic pain conditions have that treatable TrP component. No matter how long symptoms have continued, TrPs respond to treatment. It's not easy to unravel the combination of FM and CMP. Each patient is unique, with an array of possible biochemical imbalances, sensitivities, TrPs and perpetuating factors. Nevertheless, FM and TrPs are treatable, and often preventable—and we know how to do it. It won't take billions of dollars. We may be able to save that once changes are implemented. We need training and some tweaks to the system. For example, any trauma signals the need for a subsequent TrP assessment. Emergency staff may recognize that FM can worsen after trauma, but need to learn that this happens because TrPs are activated, causing more pain and possible TrP cascades, sensitizing the CNS. They need to understand this, and also know how to minimize TrP activation. Acute trauma and its immediate treatment may mask the formation of new TrP cascades, so patients may fail to notice symptoms of CMP until months later. After any trauma, a routine follow-up in the form of a questionnaire could reveal developing chronicity.

We must climb out of the ruts that now entrench the wheels of medical progress. The majority of chronic pain patients receive inappropriate medical care, it costs more than they can afford, and it is not as effective as it could be. We already have teaching facilities to train specialists in TrPs and the identification and control of perpetuating factors. We need support for existing TrP schools, and for organizations such as the National Association of Myofascial Trigger Point Therapists in the USA. We need TrP training to be a part of medical education at all levels, insurance coverage for efficient patient education and preventative care, and a greater level of awareness of the variety of manual techniques available.

Presently, the process of obtaining adequate medical care can be frustrating; at times, it can even seem futile. For example, let's say that you have chronic low back pain and seek medical help. After extensive (and expensive) testing, you're told, "We know what you have. You have chronic low back pain." Everyone over the age of 40, however, will demonstrate some level of low back pathology. Too often, when care providers see low back pathology in imaging tests, they believe that the visible pathology must be causing the symptoms. They're treating what they see in the image; they're not treating the patient. Nothing is done for the soft tissue. So they correct the MRI, but the patient still hurts. The pathology visible in the image may not be causing the patient's symptoms. You can take a picture of a telephone and see that it's a telephone, but the picture can't tell you if the phone is ringing. You must interact with that telephone.

Janet G. Travell began describing TrPs in the 1940s, and David G. Simons wrote down her findings and added to them as co-author of the definitive myofascial medicine texts (Travell and Simons 1992; Simons, Travell, and Simons 1999). The first edition of Volume 1 of the Travell and Simons texts was published in 1983. The authors of these texts hoped that the medical establishment would read the heavily referenced text, grasp the new concept, and then implement the needed change in medical training. That didn't happen. They gave educational seminars. It still didn't happen. We're way overdue for an evolutionary leap in chronic pain management. Most FM and CMP patients have experienced at least one failure of the medical care system. Medical and dental students of all types need comprehensive training in the field of myofascial pain, and there must be a focus on preventative medicine, including (but not limited to) investigation and control of perpetuating factors. First aid training must include the basics of TrPs and FM. Some patients have uncontrollable perpetuating factors due to hereditary influences, severe coexisting conditions, or other issues. There is a need for global realization that chronic means chronic. When you have hundreds of TrPs, as many of us do, and have been ground up and left to lie on the wayside by the current medical system, you do the best you can with what you have to get the optimum medical care available. We must ensure that these patients get the care they deserve and the pain management they require.

Myofascial TrPs have been imaged by the Mayo Clinic and the National Institute of Health: they are real. That is not up for debate. One author (Starlanyl) now refers to CMP as Chronic Myofascial Pain and Dysfunction (CMPD), hoping to promote recognition that the dysfunctions caused by TrPs can be as disabling as the pain, are often misdiagnosed, and must be addressed as part of the treatable condition that they are. We are beginning to understand what happens when TrPs become chronic, and what chronic myofascial pain is. This includes the onslaught of chronic pain on the CNS, and how the brain responds, including the development of FM central sensitization. We know what we need to do. Now we must do it.

Janet Travell (1976) explained to the First World Congress on Pain in 1975:

> When injured, most tissues heal, but skeletal muscles "learn"; they readily develop habits of guarding that limit movement and impair circulation. Chronic pain, stiffness, and dysfunction of muscles result.

It's said that the wheels of medicine grind incredibly slow. Janet Travell wrote about myofascial TrPs before I (Starlanyl) was born. I'm 67. Those wheels have rolled over far too many patients during that time. The medical establishment must cease doing harm due to their refusal or inability to recognize and treat TrPs.

What We Need to Do

One of the most interesting things I (Starlanyl) discovered in writing this book is the volume of research that never mentions TrPs, and yet that's what the research is obviously about. (One of my saddest realizations is that, with the exception of TrPs anatomically restricted to males, I've had every one of them.) Many medical papers supposedly about FM actually describe coexisting myofascial TrPs. Their biopsies of FM patients are probably of coexisting TrPs (Simons 2010). Many FM research papers come to faulty conclusions because the researchers have ignored coexisting TrPs that are actually causing or contributing to symptoms. These researchers have no incentive to change the status quo, because they'd need to admit that their previous research conclusions might not be accurate. That huge amount of ambiguous research is one of the reasons that FM can seem so confusing. It's in the interest of some corporations (who fund some of that research) to shove as many symptoms as possible under the FM umbrella, because there's a lot of money to be made from "FM" medications. This situation is (very) slowly changing, as more researchers and clinicians grow to understand the importance of TrPs and the interaction between these conditions. In this book, we've connected some of that research. Studies have shown that low back and pelvic pain patients exhibit "specific, consistent, and distinct motion patterns … assumed to be functional compensation strategies, following altered neuromuscular coordination" (van Wingerden, Vleeming, and Ronchetti 2006). Now look in this book and see how TrPs cause much of this dysfunction that leads to pain and more dysfunction. It's in our power to stop the cycle of pain and dysfunction. *We must do so.*

Some of the frustration that primary care physicians feel with patients who have multiple "unexplained" symptoms would be remedied if the physicians had training in diagnosing and treating TrPs. Understanding the importance of perpetuating factors *must* be coupled with allowing sufficient time to discover them and bring them under control. We must develop prompt medical team communications. Presently, all too often, communications go only one way. They go to the PCP involved—and then the flow stops. One of the authors (Starlanyl) has read many medical records in which the bodyworker has described TrPs, indicated by lumps and ropy bands, restricted ROM, and referred symptoms patterns. The doctors still diagnosed the patients with "somatoform illness" or, in some cases, FM. Many care providers, including bodyworkers, are not allowed to diagnose. They *are* permitted, however, to note that the patient fulfills Travell and Simons' criteria for myofascial TrPs. We hope that they will clearly do so, and that those permitted to diagnose TrPs will become adequately trained to do so with ease and confidence. This book can help that process.

How We Need to Do It

In some cases, the seeds of CMPD may be planted before birth or in early childhood by some event that affects the neuroprogramming of movement patterns. Once **core muscles** are affected, respiratory, circulatory, and other biosystems are altered. In other cases, the first sign that something is wrong may be the development of central sensitization that may or may not be diagnosed as FM. We have no standard program for assessing for the development of early childhood TrPs or FM. Children have no reference point. They don't know what they're supposed to feel. They may not know that other children don't wake up tired, or have achy bones. More likely, the child will be scolded—and labeled as being "too sensitive" (i.e. a complainer), or a malingerer. By adolescence, the young adult may have "hypochondriac" or some other dismissive designation chiseled in stone on her or his medical chart.

The longer the initial phase of TrP therapy is delayed, the greater the number of treatments required and the less likely it is that complete symptom relief can be achieved (Simons et al. 1999, p. 56). We need aggressive treatment of acute pain. "For over 20 years the medical literature has carefully documented the undertreatment of all types of pain by physicians" (Rich 1997). We need prompt identification and treatment of acute TrPs to prevent chronicity and the development of central sensitization states such as FM, IBS, and migraines. In many countries—certainly the USA—pain medications and their regulation are in the domain of drug enforcers who focus their attention on drug *abuse* rather than on needful drug *use*. These drug enforcers know little about chronic pain management and patients who need these medications to function as normally as possible; they live in the world of drug dealers and abusers who use drugs to avoid functioning. Chronic pain patients who may require these drugs in order to function, and the doctors who prescribe them, often get caught in the crossfire. They require protection. They must be allowed to choose treatment options without interference from those who understand neither chronic pain management nor the basic concepts of these common but invisible chronic conditions. If there must be a "war", let it be a war on drug *abuse*, and not a war on chronic pain patients and their medication prescribers and pharmacies. The enforcers must focus on drug cartels, diversion, and *inappropriate* use of opioids. Let us educate drug enforcers, as well as the medical professionals and the public, about the necessity for adequate pain control and *appropriate* use of opioids.

There must be comprehensive curriculum changes in medical, dental, and legal training, and insurance codes must be revised. These are the baseline requirements—the necessary conceptual foundation for professional updating of skills to meet today's challenges in this field. They must be accompanied by a raised consciousness among the general public. Preventative medicine is paramount, as is the need for controlling perpetuating factors so that we're not just treating the same TrPs again and again. We have a steadily growing number of patients and care providers who are aware of TrPs. This book, along with other resources by the same authors, can provide the information needed to launch educational reform. Patients with FM, IBS, headaches, incontinence, vulvodynia, and other conditions that are fed by TrPs need to know that they *must* treat the TrPs and control the perpetuating factors, and, to help them do so, they require care providers who are educated in TrP diagnosis and management. We have a significant lack of care providers trained in TrP medicine, and those who are so trained must struggle to get insurance reimbursement and respect. Someday, TrP specialists of all types are going to be in great demand; when that day occurs, it will be a sign that we're on our way to fixing the system.

References

Abu-Samra M, Gawad OA, and Agha M. 2011. The outcomes for nasal contact point surgeries in patients with unsatisfactory response to chronic daily headache medication. *Eur Arch Otorhinolaryngol* 268(9):1299–1304.

Aktan Ikiz ZA, Ucerler H, and Ozgur Z. 2009. Anatomic variations of popliteal artery that may be a reason for entrapment. *Surg Radiol Anat* 31(9):695–700.

Anaya-Terroba L et al. 2010. Effects of ice massage on pressure pain thresholds and electromyography activity postexercise: A randomized controlled crossover study. *J Manipulative Physiol Ther* 33(3):212–219.

Anderson R et al. 2011. Safety and effectiveness of an internal pelvic myofascial trigger point wand for urologic chronic pelvic pain syndrome. *Clin J Pain* 27(9):764–768.

Anderson RC and Anderson JH. 1998. Acute toxic effects of fragrance products. *Arch Environ Health* 53(2):138–146.

Anderson RU et al. 2006. Sexual dysfunction in men with chronic prostatitis/chronic pelvic pain syndrome: Improvement after trigger point release and paradoxical relaxation training. *J Urol* 176(4 Pt 1):1534–1539.

Annis RF. 2003. Pronator quadratus—a forgotten muscle: A case report. *JCCA* 47(1):17–20.

Aparicio EQ et al. 2009. Immediate effects of the suboccipital muscle inhibition technique in subjects with short hamstring syndrome. *J Manipulative Physiol Ther* 32(4):262–269.

Arnstein P et al. 1999. Self efficacy as a mediator of the relationship between pain intensity, disability and depression in chronic pain patients. *Pain* 80(3):483–491.

Awad E. 1973. Interstitial myofibrositis: Hypothesis of the mechanism. *Arch Phys Med Rehabil* 54(10):440–453.

Bahadir C et al. 2010. Efficacy of immediate rewarming with moist heat after conventional vapocoolant spray therapy in myofascial pain syndrome. *J Musculoskel Pain* 18(2):147–152.

Berth A et al. 2009. Central motor deficits of the deltoid muscle in patients with chronic rotator cuff tears. *Acta Chir Orthop Traumatol Cech* 76(6):456–461.

Bertoni M et al. 2008. Administration of type A botulinum toxin after total hip replacement. *Eur J Phys Rehabil Med* 44(4):461–465.

Bewyer DC and Bewyer KJ. 2003. Rationale for treatment of hip abductor pain syndrome. *Iowa Orthop J* 23:57–60.

Bezerra Rocha CAC, Ganz Sanchez T, and Tesseroli de Siqueira JT. 2008. Myofascial trigger point: A possible way to modulating tinnitus. *Audiol Neurotol* 13:153–160.

Bilecenoglu B, Uz A, and Karalezli N. 2005. Possible anatomic structures causing entrapment neuropathies of the median nerve: An anatomic study. *Acta Orthop Belg* 71(2):169–176.

Blouin JS, Inglis JT, and Siegmund GP. 2006. Startle responses elicited by whiplash perturbations. *J Physiol* 573(Pt 3): 857–867.

Bretischwerdt C et al. 2010. Immediate effects of hamstring muscle stretching on pressure pain sensitivity and active mouth opening in healthy subjects. *J Manipulative Physiol Ther* 33(1):42–47.

Brisby H. 2006. Pathology and possible mechanisms of nervous system response to disc degeneration. *J Bone Joint Surg Am* 88(Suppl 2):68–71.

Brumagne S et al. 2008. Persons with recurrent low back pain exhibit a rigid postural control strategy. *Eur Spine J* 17:1177–1184.

Calandre EP et al. 2006. Trigger point evaluation in migraine patients: An indication of peripheral sensitization linked to migraine predisposition? *Eur J Neurol* 13(3):244–249.

Carriere B. 2002. *Fitness for the Pelvic Floor.* Stuttgart NY: Thieme.

Carrillo-de-la-Pena MT et al. 2006. Intensity dependence of auditory-evoked cortical potentials in fibromyalgia patients: A test of the generalized hypervigilance hypothesis. *J Pain* 7(7):480–487.

Chaitow L. 2010. *Palpation and Assessment Skills: Assessment Through Touch, 3rd ed.* Edinburgh: Churchill Livingstone.

Chao JD et al. 2002. Reduction mammoplasty is a functional operation, improving quality of life in symptomatic women: A prospective, single-center breast reduction outcome study. *Plast Reconstr Surg* 110(7):1644–1654.

Chen Q, Basford J, and An KN. 2008. Ability of magnetic resonance elastography to assess taut bands. *Clin Biomech (Bristol, Avon)* 23(5):623–629.

Chernoff DM et al. 1995. Asymptomatic functional popliteal artery entrapment: Demonstration at MR imaging. *Radiology* 195(1):176–180.

Colak T et al. 2009. Nerve conduction studies of the axillary, musculocutaneous and radial nerves in elite ice hockey players. *J Sports Med Phys Fitness* 49(2):224–231.

Coppes MH et al. 1997. Innervation of "painful" lumbar discs. Spine 22(20):2342–2350.

Corbel V et al. 2009. Evidence for inhibition of cholinesterases in insect and mammalian nervous systems by the insect repellant DEET. *BMC Biol* (Aug 5) 7:47–57.

Cummings M. 2003a. Referred knee pain treated with electroacupuncture to iliopsoas. *Acupunct Med* 21(1–2):32–35.

Cummings M. 2003b. Myofascial pain from pectoralis major following trans-axillary surgery. *Acupunct Med* 21(3): 105–107.

Dalmau-Carola J. 2005. Myofascial pain syndrome affecting the piriformis and the obturator internus muscle. *Pain Pract* 5(4):361–363.

Darnis B et al. 2008. Perineal pain and inferior cluneal nerves: Anatomy and surgery. *Surg Radiol Anat* 30(3):177–183.

Davidheiser R. 1991. Liabilities of competence. *Adv Clin Care* 6(1):44–46.

de Noronha M et al. 2006. Do voluntary strength, proprioception, range of motion, or postural sway predict occurrence of lateral ankle sprain? *Br J Sports Med* 40(10):824–828.

Dean NA and Mitchell BS. 2002. Anatomic relation between the nuchal ligament (ligamentum nuchae) and the spinal dura mater in the craniocervical region. *Clin Anat* 15(3):182–185.

DeMeo DL et al. 2004. Ambient air pollution and oxygen saturation. *Am J Respir Crit Care Med* 170(4):383–387.

Demondiaon X, Canella C, and Moraux A. 2010. Retinacular disorders of the ankle and foot. *Semin Musculoskel Radiol* 14(3):281–291.

Dick BD et al. 2008. Disruption of cognitive function in fibromyalgia syndrome. *Pain* 139(3):610–616.

Dilani Mendis M et al. 2009. Effect of prolonged bed rest on the anterior hip muscles. *Gait Posture* 30(4):533–537.

Doggweiler R. 2010. *Personal communication*, September 13.

Doggweiler-Wiygul R. 2004. Urologic myofascial pain syndromes. *Curr Pain Headache Rep* 8(6):445–451.

Doggweiler-Wiygul R and Wiygul JP. 2002. Interstitial cystitis, pelvic pain, and the relationship to myofascial pain and dysfunction: A report on four patients. *World J Urol* 20(5):310–314.

Dorey G et al. 2004. Randomized controlled trial of pelvic floor muscle exercises and manometric biofeedback for erectile dysfunction. *Br J Gen Pract* 54(508):819–825.

Dubousset J. 2003. Spinal instrumentation: Source of progress but also revealing pitfalls. *Bull Acad Natl Med* 187(3):523–533.

Earls J and Myers T. 2010. *Fascial Release for Structural Balance*. Chichester, UK: Lotus Publishing.

Eisinger JB. 1999. Hypothyroidism treatment: One hormone or two? [in French] *Myalgies* 2(Suppl 2):1–3.

Eken C, Durmaz D, and Erol B. 2009. Successful treatment of a persistent renal colic with trigger point injection. *Am J Emerg Med* 27(2):252e3–4.

Eliason G et al. 2010. Alterations in the muscle-to-capillary interface in patients with different degrees of chronic obstructive pulmonary disease. *Respir Res* 11:97.

Emmerich J, Wulkner N, and Hurschler C. 2003. Influence of the posterior tibial tendon on the medial arch of the foot: An in vitro kinetic and kinematic study [in German]. *Biomed Tech (Berl)* 48(4):97–105.

Erdoes LS, Devine JJ, and Bernhard VM. 1994. Popliteal vascular compression in a normal population. *J Vasc Surg* 20(6):978–986.

Esenyel M et al. 2003. Kinetics of high-heeled gait. *J Am Podiatr Med Assoc* 93(1):27–32.

Fernandez-Carnero J et al. 2007. Prevalence of and referred pain from myofascial trigger points in the forearm muscles in patients with lateral epicondylalgia. *Clin J Pain* 23(4):353–360.

Fernandez-de-las-Penas C et al. 2005. Referred pain from the trochlear region in tension-type headache: A myofascial trigger point from the superior oblique muscle. *Headache* 45(6):731–737.

Fernandez-de-las-Penas C et al. 2011. Referred pain from myofascial trigger points in head, neck and shoulder muscles reproduces head pain features in children with chronic tension type headache. *J Headache Pain* 12(1):35–43.

Finn R and Shifflett CM. 2003. Range-of-Motion Charts. Sewickley PA: *Round Earth Publishing.* www.round-earth.com.

Finnegan EM et al. 2003. Synchrony of laryngeal muscle activity in persons with vocal tremor. *Arch Otolaryngol Head Neck Surg* 129(3):313–318.

Fitzgerald MP and Kotarinos R. 2003a. Rehabilitation of the short pelvic floor. I: Background and patient evaluation. Int Urogynecol *J Pelvic Floor Dysfunct* 14(4):261–268.

Fitzgerald MP and Kotarinos R. 2003b. Rehabilitation of the short pelvic floor. II: Treatment of the patient with the short pelvic floor. Int Urogynecol *J Pelvic Floor Dysfunct* 14(4):269–275.

Fitzgerald MP et al. 2009. Randomized multicenter feasibility trial of myofascial physical therapy for the treatment of urological chronic pelvic pain syndromes. *J Urol* 182(2):570–580.

Funt LA. 2009. Personal communication, July 19.

Funt LA and Kinnie BH. 1984. *Anatomy of a Headache: The Kinnie-Funt System of Referred Pain*. St. Paul: European Orthodontic Products, Inc.

Galvez R. 2009. Variable use of opioid pharmacotherapy for chronic noncancer pain in Europe: Causes and consequences. *J Pain Palliat Care Pharmacother* 23(4):346–356.

Garrison RL and Breeding PC. 2003. A metabolic basis for fibromyalgia and its related disorders: The possible role of resistance to thyroid hormone. *Med Hypothesis* 61(2):182–189.

Ge HY and Arendt-Nielsen L. 2011. Latent myofascial trigger points. *Curr Pain Headache Rep* 15(5):386–392.

Ge HY et al. 2008a. Topographical mapping and mechanical pain sensitivity of myofascial trigger points in the infraspinatus muscle. *Eur J Pain* 12(7):859–865.

Ge HY et al. 2008b. Induction of muscle cramps by nociceptive stimulation of latent myofascial trigger points. *Exp Brain Res* 187(4):623–629.

Ge HY et al. 2009. Contribution of the local and referred pain from active myofascial trigger points in fibromyalgia syndrome. *Pain* 147(1–3):233–240.

Ge HY et al. 2010. The predetermined sites of examination for tender points in fibromyalgia syndrome are frequently associated with myofascial trigger points. *J Pain* 11(7):644–651.

Ge HY et al. 2011. Reproduction of overall spontaneous pain pattern by manual stimulation of active myofascial trigger points in fibromyalgia patients. *Arthritis Res Ther* 13(2):R48.

Gefen A. 2001. Simulations of foot stability during gait characteristic of ankle dorsiflexor weakness in the elderly. *IEEE Trans Neural Syst Rehabil Eng* 9(4):333–337.

Geisser ME et al. 2008. A psychophysical study of auditory and pressure sensitivity in patients with fibromyalgia and healthy controls. *J Pain* 9(5):417–422.

Gerwin R. 2010. Myofascial pain syndrome: Here we are, where must we go? *J Musculoskel Pain* 18(4):329–347.

Gerwin RD. 2001. A standing complaint: Inability to sit; An unusual presentation of medial hamstring myofascial pain syndrome. *J Musculoskel Pain* 9(4):81–93.

Ghalamkarpour F, Aghazedeh Y, and Odaaei G. 2009. Safe botulism toxin type A injection in patients with history of eyelid ptosis. *J Cosmet Dermatol* 8(2):98–102.

Giacomozzi C et al. 2005. Does the thickening of Achilles tendon and plantar fascia contribute to the alteration of diabetic foot loading? *Clin Biomech (Bristol, Avon)* 20(5):532–539.

Giamberardino MA et al. 2011. Effects of treatment of myofascial trigger points on the pain of fibromyalgia. *Curr Pain Headache* 15(5):393–399.

Gibson W, Arendt-Nielsen L, and Graven-Nielsen T. 2005. Delayed onset muscle soreness at tendon-bone junction and muscle tissue is associated with facilitated referred pain. *Exp Brain Res* 174(2):351–360.

Gibson W, Arendt-Nielsen L, and Graven-Nielsen T. 2006. Referred pain and hyperalgesia in human tendon and muscle belly tissue. *Pain* 120(1–2):113–123.

Glass JM. 2008. Fibromyalgia and cognition. *J Clin Psychiatry* 69(Suppl 2):20–24.

Glass JM. 2010. Cognitive dysfunction in fibromyalgia syndrome. *J Musculoskel Pain* 18(4):367–372.

Glass JM et al. 2011. Executive function in chronic pain patients and healthy controls: Different cortical activation during response inhibition in fibromyalgia. *J Pain* 12(12):1219–1229.

Gosker HR et al. 2007. Reduced mitochondrial density in the vastus lateralis muscle of patients with COPD. *Eur Respir J* 30(1):73–79.

Greenman PE, 1996. *Principles of Manual Medicine, 2nd ed.* Baltimore: Williams and Wilkins.

Griesen J et al. 2001. Acute pain induces insulin resistance in humans. *Anesthesiology* 95(3):573–574.

Grieve R et al. 2011. The immediate effect of soleus trigger point pressure release on restricted ankle joint dorsiflexion: A pilot randomized controlled trial. *J Bodyw Mov Ther* 15(1):42–49.

Gruneberg C et al. 2004. The influence of artificially increased hip and trunk stiffness on balance control in man. *Exp Brain Res* 157(4):472–485.

Hackett GS. 1958. *Ligament and Tendon Relaxation Treated by Prolotherapy, 3rd ed.* Springfield IL: Charles C Thomas.

Hains G et al. 2010. A randomized controlled (intervention) trial of ischemic compression therapy for carpal tunnel syndrome. *J Can Chiropr Assoc* 53(3):155-163.]

Harrison DE et al. 1999. A review of biomechanics of the central nervous system. Part II: Spinal cord strains from postural loads. *J Manipulative Physiol Ther* 22(5):322–332.

Hart FX. 2009. Cytoskeletal forces produced by extremely low-frequency electric fields acting on extracellular glycoproteins. *Bioelectromagnetics* 31(1):77–84.

Harvey G and Bell S. 1999. Obturator neuropathy: An anatomic perspective. *Clin Orthop Relat Res* (363):203–211.

Hatch GF et al. 2007. Role of the peroneal tendons and superior peroneal retinaculum as static stabilizers of the ankle. *J Surg Orthop Adv* 16(4):187–191.

Hendi A, Dorsher PT, and Rizzo TD. 2009. Subcutaneous trigger point causing radiating postsurgical pain. *Arch Dermatol* 145(1):52–54.

Henry SL, Crawford JL, and Puckett CL. 2009. Risk factors and complications in reduction mammaplasty: Novel associations and preoperative assessment. *Plast Reconstr Surg* 124(4):1040–1046.

Hodges PW, Sapsford R, and Pengel LH. 2007. Postural and respiratory functions of the pelvic floor muscles. *Neurourol Urodyn* 26(3):362–371.

Hooper MM et al. 2006. Musculoskeletal findings in obese subjects before and after weight loss following bariatric surgery. *Int J Obes (Lond)* 31(1):114–120.

Hsin ST et al. 2002. Myofascial pain syndrome induced by malpositioning during surgery: A case report. *Acta Anaesthesiol Sin* 40(1):37–41.

Hsueh TC et al. 1998. Association of active myofascial trigger points and cervical disc lesions. *J Formos Med Assoc* 97(3):174–180.

Hughes KH. 1998. Painful rib syndrome: A variant of myofascial pain syndrome. *AAOHN J* 46(3):115–120.

Hung HC et al. 2010. An alternative intervention for urinary incontinence: Retraining diaphragmatic, deep abdominal and pelvic floor muscle coordinated function. *Man Ther* 15(3):273–279.

Hungerford B, Gilleard W, and Hodges P. 2003. Evidence of altered lumbopelvic muscle recruitment in the presence of sacroiliac joint pain. *Spine* (Phila PA 1976) 28(14):1593–1600.

Ibrahim GA, Awad EA, and Kottke FJ. 1974. Interstitial myofibrositis: Serum and muscle enzymes and lactate dehydrogenase-isoenzymes. *Arch Phys Med Rehabil* 55(1):23–28.

Igaz P et al. 2001. Bidirectional communication between histamine and cytokines. *Inflamm Res* 50(3):123–128.

Ihunwo AO and Dimitrov ND. 1999. Anatomical basis for pressure on the common peroneal nerve. *Cent Afr J Med* 45(3):77–79.

Ingber RS. 2000. Shoulder impingement in tennis/racquetball players treated with subscapularis myofascial treatments. *Arch Phys Med Rehabil* 81(5):679–682.

Itza F et al. 2010. Myofascial pain syndrome in the pelvic floor: A common urological condition [in Spanish]. *Actas Urol Esp* 34(4):318–326.

Jacobs JA, Henry SM, and Nagle KJ. 2009. People with chronic low back pain exhibit decreased variability in the timing of their anticipatory postural adjustments. *Behav Neurosci* 123(2):455–458.

Jarrell J. 2003a. *Focus on pain presentation: Myofascial disorders and visceral diseases of the pelvis.* The Janet G. Travell MD Seminar Series (March 6–9), Orlando FL.

Jarrell J. 2003b. *Personal communication,* March 25.

Jarrell J. 2004. Myofascial dysfunction in the pelvis. *Curr Pain Headache* Rep 8(6):452–456.

Jeyaseelan N. 1989. Anatomical basis of compression of common peroneal nerve. *Anat Anz* 169(1):49–51.

Jones DS and Quinn S, eds. 2005–6. *Textbook of Functional Medicine.* Gig Harbor WA: Institute of Functional Medicine.

Kandt RS and Daniel FL. 1986. Glossopharyngeal neuralgia in a child: A diagnostic and therapeutic dilemma. *Arch Neurol* 43(3):301–302.

Karim MR et al. 2005. Enthesitis of biceps brachii short head and coracobrachialis at the coracoid process: A generator of shoulder and neck pain. *Am J Phys Med Rehab* 84(5):377–380.

Karski R 2002. Etiology of the so-called "idiopathic scoliosis". Biomechanical explanation of spine deformity. Two groups of development of scoliosis. New rehabilitation treatment; possibility of prophylactics. *Stud Health Technol Inform* 91:37–46.

Kerrigan DC et al. 2005. Moderate-heeled shoes and knee joint torques relevant to the development and progression of knee osteoarthritis. *Arch Phys Med Rehabil* 86(5):871–875.

Khazzam M, Patillo D, and Gainor BJ. 2008. Extensor tendon triggering by impingement on the extensor retinaculum: A report of 5 cases. *J Hand Surg Am* 33(8):1397–1400.

Kim SH et al. 2011. Spatial versus verbal memory impairments in patients with fibromyalgia. *Rheumatol Int* 32(5): 1135–1142.

Kobesova A and Lewit K. 2000. A case of a pathogenic active scar. *Australas Chiropr Osteopathy* 9(1):17–19.

Kobesova A et al. 2007. Twenty-year-old pathogenic "active" postsurgical scar: A case study of a patient with persistent right lower quadrant pain. *J Manipulative Physiol Ther* 30(3):234–238.

Kolbel T et al. 2008. Carotid artery entrapment by the hyoid bone. *K Vasc Surg* 48(4):1022–1024.

Kong A, Van der Vliet A, and Zadow S. 2007. MRI and US of gluteal tendinopathy in greater trochanteric pain syndrome. *Eur Radiol* 17(7):1773–1783.

Konitzer LN et al. 2008. Association between back, neck, and upper extremity musculoskeletal pain and the individual body armor. *J Hand Ther* 21(2):143–148.

Kooijman PG et al. 2005. Muscular tension and body posture in relation to voice handicap and voice quality in teachers with persistent voice complaints. *Folia Phoniatr Logop* 57(3):137–147.

Koolstra JH and van Eijden TM. 2005. Combined finite-element and rigid-body analysis of human jaw joint dynamics. *J Biomech* 38(12):2431–2439.

Kostopoulos D and Rizopoulous K. 2001. *The Manual of Trigger Point and Myofascial Therapy.* Thorofare NJ: Slack Inc.

Kotarinos, R. 2010. Personal communication, May 7.

Kumaresan S, Yoganandan N, and Pintar FA. 1999. Finite element analysis of the cervical spine: A material property sensitivity study. *Clin Biomech (Bristol, Avon)* 14(1):41–53.

Kundermann et al. 2004. The effect of sleep deprivation on pain. *Pain Res Manag* 9(1):25–32.

Kwak SD et al. 2000. Hamstrings and iliotibial band forces affect knee kinematics and contact pattern. *J Orthop Res* 18(1):101–108.

Labat JJ et al. 2009. Buttocks sciatic pain [in French]. *Neurochirugie* 55(4–5):459–462.

Leavitt F and Katz RS. 2006. Distraction as a key determinant of impaired memory in patients with fibromyalgia. *J Rheumatol* 33(1):127–132.

Leavitt F and Katz RS. 2008. Speed of mental operations in fibromyalgia: a selective naming speed deficit. *J Clin Rheumatol* 61(6):740–744.

Leavitt F and Katz RS. 2009. Normalizing memory recall in fibromyalgia with rehearsal: a distraction-counteracting effect. *Arthritis Rheum* 61(6):740–744.

Leavitt F and Katz RS. 2011. Development of the Mental Clutter Scale. *Psychol Rep* 109(2):445-452.

Leung AK et al. 1999. Nocturnal leg cramps in children: Incidence and clinical characteristics. *J Natl Med Assoc* 91(6):329–332.

Lewit K. 1979. The needle effect in the relief of myofascial pain. *Pain* 6(1):83–90.

Lewit K. 2010. *Manipulative Therapy: Musculoskeletal Medicine.* Edinburgh: Churchill Livingstone Elsevier.

Lewit K and Kolar P. 2000. *Chain reactions related to the cervical spine. In Conservative Management of Cervical Spine Syndromes, ed.* Murphy DR, 515–530. New York: McGraw-Hill.

Lewit K and Olanska S. 2004. Clinical importance of active scars: Abnormal scars as a cause of myofascial pain. *J Manipulative Physiol Ther* 27(6):399–402.

Litchwark GA and Wilson AM. 2007. Is Achilles tendon compliance optimised for maximum muscle efficiency during locomotion? *J Biomech* 40(8):1768–1775.

Liu ZJ et al. 2000. Morphological and positional assessment of TMJ components and lateral pterygoid muscle in relation to symptoms and occlusion of patients with temporomandibular disorders. *J Oral Rehabil* 27(10):860–874.

Loch C and Fehrmann P. 1990. Studies on the compression of the external carotid artery in the region of the styloid process of the temporal bone [in German]. *Laryngorhinootologie* 69(5):260–266.

Loeser RF and Shakoor N. 2003. Aging or osteoarthritis: Which is the problem? Rheum Dis Clin North Am 29(4): 653–673.

Loth S et al. 1998. Improved nasal breathing in snorers increases nocturnal growth hormone secretion and serum concentrations of insulin-like growth factor-1 subsequently. *Rhinology* 36(4):179–183.

Loukas M et al. 2008. An anatomic investigation of the serratus posterior superior and serratus posterior inferior muscles. *Surg Radiol Anat* 30(2):119–123.

Lowe JC et al. 1997. Mutations in the c-erbA beta 1 gene: Do they underlie euthyroid? *Med Hypo* 48(2):125–135.

Madill SJ and McLean L. 2010. Intravaginal pressure generated during voluntary pelvic floor muscle contractions and during coughing: The effect of age and continence status. *Neurolog Urodyn* 29(3):437–442.

Manheim CJ. 1994. *The Myofascial Release Manual, 2nd ed.* Thorofare NJ: Slack Inc.

Mariani G et al. 1996. Ultrastructure and histochemical features of the ground substance in cyclosporin A-induced gingival overgrowth. *J Peridontol* 67(1):21–27.

McCauliff GW, Goodell H, and Wolff HG. 1943. Experimental studies on headache: Pain from the nasal and paranasal structures. *A Res Nerv and Ment Dis Proc* 23:185–208.

McGill S. 2004. *Ultimate Back Fitness and Performance.* Ontario, Canada: Wabuno.

McMakin CR. 2011. *Frequency Specific Microcurrent in Pain Management.* Edinburgh: Churchill Livingstone Elsevier.

Meknas K, Christensen A, and Johansen O. 2003. The internal obturator muscle may cause sciatic pain. *Pain* 104(1–2) 375–380.

Mellick GA and Mellick LB. 2003. Regional head and face pain relief following lower cervical intramuscular anesthetic injection. *Headache* 43(10):1109–1111.

Menachem A, Kaplan O, and Dekel S. 1993. Levator scapulae syndrome: An anatomic-clinical study. *Bull Hosp Jt Dis* 53(1):21–24.

Misselbeck T et al. 2008. Isolated popliteal vein entrapment by the popliteus muscle: A case report. *Vasc Med* 13(1): 37–39.

Miyawaki S et al. 2004. Relationships among nocturnal jaw muscle activities, decreased esophageal pH, and sleep positions. *Am J Orthod Dentofacial Orthop* 126(5):615–619.

Moriarty JK and Dawson AM. 1982. Functional abdominal pain: Further evidence that whole gut is affected. *Br Med J (Clin Res Ed)* 284:1670–1672.

Muraoka T et al. 2008. Effects of muscle cooling on the stiffness of the human gastrocnemius muscle in vivo. *Cells Tissues Organs* 187(2):152–160.

Murata Y et al. 2009. An unusual cause of sciatic pain as a result of the dynamic motion of the obturator internus muscle. *Spine J* 9(6):e16–18.

Myers TW. 2001. *Anatomy Trains: Myofascial Meridians for Manual and Movement Therapists.* Edinburgh: Churchill Livingstone.

Nayak SR et al. 2009. Additional tendinous origin and entrapment of the plantaris muscle. *Clinics (Sao Paulo)* 64(1): 67–68.

Nelson J, Fernandez-de-las-Penas C, and Simons DG. 2008. Cervical myofascial trigger points in headache disorders. *Prac Pain Manage* 8(7):59–60.

Nelson-Wong E and Gallaghan JP. 2010. Changes in muscle activation patterns and subjective low back pain ratings during prolonged standing in response to an exercise intervention. *J Electromyogr Kinesiol* 20(6):1125–1133.

Nelson-Wong E et al. 2008. Gluteus medius muscle activation patterns as a predictor of low back pain during standing. *Clin Biomech (Bristol, Avon)* 23(5):545–553.

Nykand J et al. 2005. Anatomy, function, and rehabilitation of the popliteus musculotendinous complex. *J Orthop Sports Phys Ther* 35(3):165–179.

Ormandy L. 1994. Scapulocostal syndrome. *Va Med Q* 121(2):105–108.

Ostensvik T, Veiersted KB, and Nilsen P. 2009. Association between numbers of long periods with sustained low-level trapezius muscle activity and neck pain. *Ergonomics* 52(12):1556–1567.

Otis JC et al. 2004. Peroneus brevis is a more effective everter than peroneus longus. *Foot Ankle Int* 25(4):242–246.

Otoshi K et al. 2008. Case report: Meralgia paresthetica in a baseball pitcher. *Clin Orthop Relat Res* 466(9): 2268–2270.

Ozgocmen S. 2001. *Personal communication*, July 4.

Ozkan K et al. 2006. A previously unreported etiology of trigger toe. *J Am Podiatr Med Assoc* 96(4):356–358.

Park KM et al. 2010. The change in vastus medialis oblique and vastus lateralis electromyographic activity related to shoe heel height during treadmill walking. *J Back Musculoskel Rehabil* 23(1):39–44.

Patla CE and Abbott JH. 2000. Tibialis posterior myofascial tightness as a source of heel pain: Diagnosis and treatment. *J Orthop Sports Phys Ther* 30(10):624–632.

Pickering M and Jones JFX. 2002. The diaphragm: Two physiological muscles in one. *J Anat* 201(4):305–312.

Pirouzi S et al. 2006. Low back pain patients demonstrate increased hip extensor muscle activity during standardized submaximal rotation efforts. *Spine* 31(26):E999–E1005.

Powers CM 2010. The influence of abnormal hip mechanics on knee injury: A biomechanical perspective. *J Orthop Sports Phys Ther* 40(2):42–51.

Prateepavanich P, Kupniratsaikul V, and Charoensak T. 1999. The relationship between myofascial trigger points of gastrocnemius muscle and nocturnal calf cramps. *J Med Assoc Thai* 82(5):451–459.

Qerama E, Kasch H, and Fuglsang-Frederiksen A. 2008. Occurrence of myofascial pain in patients with possible carpal tunnel syndrome: A single blinded study. *Eur J Pain* 13(6):588–591.

Rask MR. 1984. The omohyoideus myofascial pain syndrome: Report of four patients. *J Craniomandib Pract* 2(3): 256–262.

Renan-Ordine R et al. 2011. Effectiveness of myofascial trigger point manual therapy combined with a self-stretching protocol for the management of plantar heel pain: A randomized controlled trial. *J Orthop Sports Phys Ther* 41(2): 43–50.

Reynolds KK, Ramey-Hartung B, and Jortani SA. 2008. The value of CYP2D6 and OPRM1 pharmacological testing for opioid therapy. *Clin Lab Med* 28(4):581–598.

Rich BA. 1997. A legacy of silence: Bioethics and the culture of pain. *J Med Humanit* 18(4):233–259.

Riot FM et al. 2004. Levator ani syndrome, functional intestinal disorders and articular abnormlities of the pelvis, the place of osteopathic treatment [in French]. *Presse Med* 33(13):852–857.

Robert R et al. 1998. An anatomic basis of chronic perineal pain: Role of the pudendal nerve. *Surg Radiol Anat* 20(2):93–98.

Robertson BL, Jamadar DA, and Jacobson JA. 2007. Extensor retinaculum of the wrist: Sonographic characterization and pseudotenosynovitis appearance. *AJR Am J Roentgenol* 188(1):198–202.

Rochier AL and Sumpio BE. 2009. Variant of popliteal entrapment syndrome involving the lateral head of the gastrocnemius muscle: A case report. *Am Vasc Surg* 23(4):535e5–9.

Rodriguez MA et al. 2009. Evidence for overlap between urological and non urological unexplained clinical conditions. *J Urol* 182(5):2123–2131.

Roehrs T and Roth T. 2005. Sleep and pain: Interaction of two vital functions. *Semin Neurol* 25(1):106–116.

Rogalski MJ et al. 2010. Retrospective chart review of vaginal diazepam suppository in high-tone pelvic floor dysfunction. *Int Urogynecol J Pelvic Floor Dysfunct* 21(7):895–899.

Ropars M et al. 2009. Anatomical study of the lateral femoral cutaneous nerve with special reference to minimally invasive anterior approach for total hip replacement. *Surg Radiol Anat* 31(3):199–204.

Rosomoff HL and Rosomoff RS. 1999. Low back pain: Evaluation and management in the primary care setting. *Med Clin North Am* 83(3):643–662.

Rubin JS, Blake E, and Matheieson L. 2007. Musculoskeletal patterns in patients with voice disorders. *J Voice* 21(4):477–484.

Ruiz-Saez M et al. 2007. Changes in pressure pain sensitivity in latent myofascial trigger points in the upper trapezius muscle after a cervical spine manipulation in pain-free subjects. *J Manipulative Physiol Ther* 30(8):578–583.

Russell IJ and Larson AA. 2009. Neurophysiopathogenesis of fibromyalgia syndrome: A unified hypothesis. *Rheum Dis Clin N Am* 35:421–435.

Russell IJ et al. 2011. Sodium oxybate reduces pain, fatigue and sleep disturbance and improves functionality in fibromyalgia: Results from a 14-week, randomized, double-blind, placebo-controlled study. *Pain* 152(5):1007–1017.

Sahin N et al. 2008. Demographics features, clinical findings and functional status in a group of subjects with cervical myofascial pain syndrome. *Agri* 20(3):14–19.

Saikku K, Vasenius J, and Saar P. 2010. Entrapment of the proximal sciatic nerve by the hamstring tendons. *Acta Orthop Belg* 76(3):321–324.

Salgueiro M et al. 2011. Is psychological distress intrinsic to fibromyalgia syndrome? Cross-sectional analysis in two clinical presentations. *Rheumatol Int* 32(11):3463-3469.

Samuel AN, Peter AA, and Ramanathan K. 2007. The association of active trigger points with lumbar disc lesions. *J Musculoskel Pain* 15(2):11–18.

Sanoja R and Cervero F. 2010. Estrogen-dependent changes in visceral afferent sensitivity. *Auton Neurosci* 153(1–2):84–89.

Saratsiotis J and Myriokefalitakis E. 2010. Diagnosis and treatment of posterior interosseous nerve syndrome using soft tissue manipulation therapy: A case study. *J Bodyw Mov Ther* 14(4):397–402.

Sato K and Nakashima T. 2009. Sleep-related deglutition in patients with sleep apnea-hypopnea syndrome. *Ann Otol Rhinol Laryngol* 118(1):30–36.

Saxena A, O'Brien T, and Bunce D. 1990. Anatomic dissection of the tibialis posterior muscle and its correlation to medial tibialis stress syndrome. *J Foot Surg* 29(2):105–108.

Schleip R, Klingler W, and Lehmann-Horn R. 2005. Active fascial contractility: Fascia may be able to contract in a smooth muscle-like manner and thereby influence musculoskeletal dynamics. *Med Hypotheses* 65(2):273–277.

Schneider-Helmert D. 2003. Do we need polysomnography in insomnia? *Schweiz Rundsch Med Prax* 92(48): 2061–2066.

Schneider-Helmert D et al. 2001. Insomnia and alpha sleep in chronic non-organic pain as compared to primary insomnia. *Neuropsychobiology* 43(1):54–58.

Schnider P et al. 1995. Increased residual urine volume after local injection of botulinum A toxin. *Nervenarzt* 66(6): 465–467.

Schwartz MJ, Offenbaecher M, Neumeister A et al. 2003. Experimental evaluation of an altered tryptophan metabolism in fibromyalgia. *Adv Exp Med Biol* 527:265–275.

Sedy J. 2008. The entrapment of dorsal nerve of penis/clitoris under the pubis: An alternative source of pudendal neuralgia [comment]. *Pain Physician* 11(2):215–224.

Shah JP and Gilliams EA. 2008. Uncovering the biochemical milieu of myofascial trigger points using in vivo microdialysis: An application of muscle pain concepts to myofascial pain syndrome. *J Bodywork Mov Ther* 12(4): 371–384.

Shah JP et al. 2005. An in-vivo microanalytical technique for measuring the local biochemical milieu of human skeletal muscle. *J Appl Physiol* 99(5):1977–1984.

Shah JP et al. 2008. Biochemicals associated with pain and inflammation are elevated in sites near to and remote from active myofascial trigger points. *Arch Phys Med Rehabil* 89(1):16–23.

Shamley DR et al. 2007. Changes in shoulder muscle size and activity following treatment for breast cancer. *Breast Cancer Res Treat* 106(1):19–27.

Sharkey JS. 2008. *The Concise Book of Neuromuscular Therapy: A Trigger Point Manual.* Berkeley CA/Chichester, UK: North Atlantic Books/Lotus Publishing.

Shifflett CM. 2011. *Migraine Brains and Bodies: A Comprehensive Guide to Solving the Mystery of Your Migraines.* Sewickley PA: Round Earth Publishing.

Shirley D et al. 2003. Spinal stiffness changes throughout the respiratory cycle. *J Appl Physiol* 95(4):1467–1475.

Sikdar S et al. 2008. Assessment of myofascial trigger points (MTrPs): A new application of ultrasound imaging and vibration sonoelastography. *Arch Phys Med Rehab* 89(11):2041–2226.

Simons DG. 2010. *History of myofascial trigger points. In Myofasziale Schmerzsyndrome, 1st ed.,* eds. Reilich P, Dommerholt J, and Groebli C. Germany: Elsevier GmbH.

Simons DG, Travell JG, and Simons LS. 1999. *Travell and Simons' Myofascial Pain and Dysfunction: The Trigger Point Manual, 2nd ed.* Vol. 1, Upper Half of Body. Baltimore: Williams and Wilkins.

Sirvent P et al. 2005. Simvastatin triggers mitochondria-induced Ca2+ signalling alteration in skeletal muscle. *Biochem Biophys Res Commun* 329:1067–1075.

Smith JD et al. 2001. Relief of fibromyalgia symptoms following discontinuation of dietary excitotoxins. *Ann Pharmacother* 35(6):702–706.

Smith M, Coppieters MW, and Hodges PW. 2005. Effect of experimentally induced low back pain in postural sway with breathing. *Exp Brain Res* 166(1):109–117.

Smith MT et al. 2009. Sleep disorders and their association with laboratory pain sensitivity in temporomandibular joint disorder. *Sleep* 32(6):779–790.

Smith RP et al. 1998. Obstructive sleep apnoea and the autonomic nervous system. *Sleep Med Rev* 2(2):69–92.

Smuts JA, Schultz D, and Barnard A. 2004. Mechanism of action of botulinus toxin type A in migraine prevention: A pilot study. *Headache* 44(8):801–805.

Snidvongs S, Nagararatnam M, and Stephens R. 2008. Assessment and treatment of pain in children. *Br J Hosp Med (Lond)* 69(4):211–213.

Solomon L, Schnitzler CM, and Browett JP. 1982. Osteoarthritis of the hip: The patient behind the disease. *Ann Rheum Dis* 41(2):118–125.

Starlanyl DJ. 1999. *The Fibromyalgia Advocate.* Oakland CA: New Harbinger Publications.

Starlanyl DJ. 2012. *Website: www.sover.net/~devstar.*

Starlanyl DJ and Copeland ME. 2001. *Fibromyalgia and Chronic Myofascial Pain: A Survival Manual, 2nd ed.* Oakland CA: New Harbinger Publications.

Starlanyl DJ and Jeffrey JL. 2001. The presence of geloid masses in a patient with both fibromyalgia and chronic myofascial pain. *Phys Ther Case Rep* 4(1):22–31.

Starlanyl DJ et al. 2001–2. The effects of transdermal T3(3, 3',5-triiodothyronine) on geloid masses found in patients with both fibromyalgia and myofascial pain: Double blinded N of 1 clinical study. *Myalgies* 2(2):8–18.

Staud R. 2006. Biology and therapy of fibromyalgia: Pain in fibromyalgia syndrome. *Arthritis Res Ther* 8(3):208.

Staud R. 2010. Is it all central sensitization? Role of peripheral tissue nociception in chronic musculoskeletal pain. *Curr Rheumatol Rep* 12(6):448–454.

Staud R. 2011. Peripheral pain mechanisms in chronic widespread pain. *Best Pract Res Clin Rheumatol* 25(2):155–164.

Staud R et al. 2003. Temporal summation of pain from mechanical stimulation of muscle tissue in normal controls and subjects with fibromyalgia syndrome. *Pain* 102(1–2):87–95.

Staud R et al. 2004. Maintenance of windup of second pain requires less frequent stimulation in fibromyalgia patients compared to normal controls. *Pain* 110(3):689–696.

Stecco A et al. 2011. RMI study and clinical correlations of ankle retinacula damage and outcomes of ankle sprain. *Surg Radiol Anat* 33(10):881–890.

Stecco C et al. 2011. Hyauronan within fascia in the etiology of myofascial pain. *Surg Radiol Anat* 33(10):891-896

Stecco C et al. 2010. The ankle reticula: Morphological evidence of the proprioceptive role of the fascial system. *Cells Tissues Organs* 192(3):200–210.

Stemper BD et al. 2006. Anterior longitudinal ligament injuries in whiplash may lead to cervical instability. *Med Eng Phys* 28(6):515–524.

Sucher BM. 1993. Myofascial release of carpal tunnel syndrome. *J Am Osteopath Assoc* 93(1):92–99.

Suttor VP et al. 2010. Evidence for pelvic floor dyssynergia in patients with irritable bowel syndrome. *Dis Colon Rectum* 53(2):156–160.

Tal S, Gurevich A, and Guller V. 2009. The approach to chronic pain management in the elderly [in Hebrew]. *Harefuah* 148(6):386–391, 411.

Talebian S et al. 2012. Postural control in women with myofascial neck pain. *J Musculoskel Pain* 20(1):25–30.

Tatar I et al. 2004. Innervation of the coracobrachialis muscle by a branch from the lateral root of the median nerve. *Folia Morphol (Warsz)* 63(4):503–506.

Tawk M et al. 2006. The effect of 1 week of continuous positive airway pressure treatment in obstructive sleep apnea patients with concomitant gastroesophageal reflux. *Chest* 130(4):1003–1008.

Teachey WS. 2004. Otolaryngic myofascial pain syndromes. *Curr Pain Headache* Rep 8(6):457–462.

Thomas AC, McLean SG, and Palmieri-Smith RM. 2010. Quadriceps and hamstrings fatigue alters hip and knee mechanics. *J Appl Biomech* 26(2):159–170.

Tomlinson SS and Mangione KK. 2005. Potential adverse effects of statins on muscle. Phys Ther 85:459–465.

Travell J. 1951. *Pain mechanisms in connective tissue. In Connective Tissues: Transactions of the Second Conference,* ed. Ragan C, 12–22. New York: Josiah Macy, Jr. Foundation.

Travell JG. 1976. *Myofascial trigger points: Clinical view.* In Advances in Pain Research and Therapy, vol. 1, ed. Bonica JJ and Albe-Fessard D, 919–926. New York: Raven Press.

Travell JG. 1977. A trigger point for hiccup. *J Am Osteopath Assoc* 77(4):308–312.

Travell JG and Simons DG. 1992. *Myofascial Pain and Dysfunction: The Trigger Point Manual.* Vol. 2, The Lower Extremities. Baltimore: Williams and Wilkins.

Treaster D et al. 2006. Myofascial trigger point development from visual and postural stressors during computer work. *Electromyogr Kinesiol* 16(2):115–124.

Tremblay A et al. 2004. Thermogenesis and weight loss in obese individuals: A primary association with organocholine pollution. *Int J Obes Relat Metab Disord* 28(7):936–939.

Tsai CT et al. 2009. Injection in the cervical facet joint for shoulder pain with myofascial trigger points in the upper trapezius muscle. *Orthopedics* 32(8):557.

Tsen LC and Camann WR. 1997. Trigger point injections for myofascial pain during epidural analgesia for labor. *Reg Anesth* 22(5):466–468.

Tsigos C and Chrousos GP. 2002. Hypothalamic-pituitary-adrenal axis, neuroendocrine factors and stress. *J Psychosom Res* 53(4):865–871.

Turnipseed WD and Pozniak M. 1992. Popliteal entrapment as a result of neurovascular compression by the soleus and plantaris muscles. *J Vasc Surg* 15(2):285–293.

Upledger JE. 1987. *Craniosacral Therapy II: Beyond the Dura.* Seattle: Eastland Press.

Vallejo MC et al. 2004. Piriformis syndrome in a patient after Cesarian section under spinal anesthesia. *Reg Anesth Pain Med* 29(4):364–367.

Valouchova P and Lewit K. 2009. Surface electromyography of abdominal and back muscles in patients with active scars. *J Bodyw Mov Ther* 13(3):262–267.

van der Pallts A, Veldhuizen AG, and Verkerke GJ. 2007. Numerical simulation of asymmetrically altered growth as initiation mechanism of scoliosis. *Ann Biomed Eng* 35(7):1206–1215.

van Wilgen CP et al. 2004. Morbidity of the neck and head and neck cancer therapy. *Head Neck* 26(9):785–791.

van Wingerden JP et al. 1993. A functional-anatomical approach to the spine-pelvis mechanism: Interaction between the biceps femoris and the sacrotuberous ligament. *Eur Spine J* 2(3):140–144.

van Wingerden JP, Vleeming A, and Ronchetti I. 2006. Differences in standing and forward bending in women with chronic low back or pelvic girdle pain: Indications for physical compensation strategies. *Spine (Phila PA 1976)* 33(11):E334–341.

VanHeest AE et al. 2007. Extensor retinaculum impingement in the athlete: A new diagnosis. Am J Sports Med 35(12):2126–2130.

Varga E, Dudas B, and Tile M. 2008. Putative proprioceptive function of the pelvic ligaments: Biomechanical and histological studies. *Injury* 39(8):858–864.

Verne GN et al. 2003. Reversal of visceral and cutaneous hyperalgesia by local rectal anesthesia in irritable bowel syndrome (IBS) patients. *Pain* 105(1–2):223–230.

Vilensky JA et al. 2001. Serratus posterior muscles: Anatomy, clinical relevance and function. *Clin Anat* 14(4):237–241.

Vittore D et al. 2009. Extensor deficiency: First cause of childhood flexible flat foot. *Orthopedics* 32(1):28.

Vleeming A et al. 1996. The function of the long dorsal sacroiliac ligament: Its implication for understanding low back pain. *Spine (Phila PA 1976)* 21(5):556–562.

Vogt L, Pfeifer K, and Banzer W. 2003. Neuromuscular control of walking with chronic low-back pain. *Man Ther* 8(1):21–28.

Vullo VJ, Richardson JK, and Hurvitz EA. 1996. Hip, knee, and foot pain during pregnancy and the postpartum period. *J Fam Pract* 43(1):63–68.

Vuong C et al. 2009. The effects of opioids and opioid analogs on animal and human endocrine systems. *Endocr Rev* 31(1):98–132.

Wallwork TL et al. 2009. The effect of chronic low back pain on size and contraction of the lumbar multifidus muscle. *Man Ther* 14(5):496–500.

Watanabe K and Akima H. 2010. Neuromuscular activation of vastus intermedius muscle during fatiguing exercise. *J Electromyogr Kinesiol* 20(4):661–666.

Weiner DK and Schmader KE. 2006. Postherpetic pain: More than sensory neuralgia? *Pain Med* 7(3):243–249; discussion 350.

Weiner DK et al. 2006. Chronic low back pain in older adults: Prevalence, reliability, and validity of physical examination findings. *JAGS* 54(1):11–20.

Weiss JM 2001. Pelvic floor myofascial trigger points: Manual therapy for interstitial cystitis and the urgency-frequency syndrome. *J Urol* 166(6):2226–2231.

Wellen KE and Hotamisligil GS. 2003. Obesity-induced inflammatory changes in adipose tissue. *J Clin Invest* 112(12):1785–1788.

Westgaard RH et al. 1994. Occupational and individual risk factors of muscular pain [in Norwegian]. *Tidsskr Nor Laegeforen* 114(8):922–927.

Whorwood CB et al. 2002. Increased glucocorticoid receptor expression in human skeletal muscle cells may contribute to the pathogenesis of the metabolic syndrome. *Diabetes* 51(4):1066–1075.

Williams DA et al. 2011. Perceived cognitive dysfunction in fibromyalgia syndrome. *J Musculoskel Pain* 19(2):66–75.

Williams EH et al. 2010. Surgical decompression for notalgia paresthetica: A case report. Microsurgery 30(1):70–72.

Wise D and Anderson A. 2008. *A Headache in the Pelvis, 5th ed.* Occidental CA: National Center for Pelvic Research.

Wu G et al. 2004. Spatial, temporal and muscle action patterns of tai chi gait. *J Electromyogr Kinesiol* 14(3):343–354.

Yahia A et al. 2010. A study of isokinetic trunk and knee muscle strength in patients with chronic sciatica. *Ann Phys Rehabil Med* 53(4):239–244.

Yamawaki Y, Nishimura Y, and Suzuki Y. 1996. Velopharyngeal closure and the longus capitis muscle. *Acta Otolaryngologica (Stockholm)* 116(2):774–777.

Yates BJ et al. 2002. Role of the vestibular system in regulating respiratory muscle activity during movement. *Clin Exp Pharmacol Physiol* 29(1–2):112–117.

Yoon SZ et al. 2009. A case of facial myofascial pain syndrome presenting as trigeminal neuralgia. *Oral Surg Oral Med Oral Pathol Radiol Endod* 107(3):e29–31.

You JY, Lee HM, and Luo HJ. 2009. Gastrocnemius tightness on joint angle and work of lower extremity during gait. *Clin Biomech (Bristol, Avon)* 24(9):744–750.

Young N and Blitzer A. 2007. Management of supraglottic squeeze in adductor spasmodic dysphonia: A new technique. *Laryngoscope* 117(11):2082–2084.

Index